ATLAS OF
FACIAL IMPLANTS

to
MARILYNN
KAIT
and
CHARLES

ATLAS OF
FACIAL IMPLANTS

Michael J. Yaremchuk MD FACS
Clinical Professor of Surgery, Harvard Medical School,
Chief of Craniofacial Surgery, Massachusetts General Hospital, Boston, MA, USA

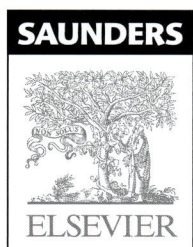

SAUNDERS

ELSEVIER

SAUNDERS
ELSEVIER

An affiliate of Elsevier Inc.

First published 2007

ISBN-13: 978-1-4160-0267-3
ISBN-10: 1-4160-0267-7

British Library Cataloguing in Publication Data
A catalogue record for this book is available from the British Library

Library of Congress Cataloging in Publication
A catalog record for this book is available from the Library of Congress

---

Notice

Medical knowledge is constantly changing. Standard safety precautions must be followed, but as new research and clinical experience broaden our knowledge, changes in treatment and drug therapy may become necessary or appropriate. Readers are advised to check the most current product information provided by the manufacturer of each drug to be administered to verify the recommended dose, the method and duration of administration, and contraindications. It is the responsibility of the practitioner, relying on experience and knowledge of the patient, to determine dosages and the best treatment for each individual patient. Neither the Publisher nor the author assume any liability for any injury and/or damage to persons or property arising from this publication.
The Publisher

Printed in China
Last digit is the print number: 9 8 7 6 5 4 3 2

ELSEVIER your source for books, journals and multimedia in the health sciences
www.elsevierhealth.com

Working together to grow
libraries in developing countries

www.elsevier.com | www.bookaid.org | www.sabre.org

ELSEVIER   BOOK AID International   Sabre Foundation

The publisher's policy is to use **paper manufactured from sustainable forests**

Commissioning Editor: **Sue Hodgson**
Development Editor: **Sharon Nash**
Project Manager: **Bryan Potter**
Design Manager: **Andy Chapman**
Illustrator: **Kip Carter**
Marketing Manager(s) (UK/USA): **Jeremy Bowes/Lisa Damico**

Contents

Preface

This atlas presents techniques I utilize for alloplastic implant reconstruction of the craniofacial skeleton. Both aesthetic and reconstructive applications are presented. In the cranium, alloplastic materials are used to protect the brain by replacing missing portions of the skull. In the internal orbit, they are used to support the eye by replacing lost portions of the orbital floor and walls. In other areas of the skeleton, alloplastic implants are used to restore or to augment craniofacial contours. Since many, if not most, clinical problems require more than just placing the implant, the book also includes adjunctive measures typically used to achieve the desired result.

The book is divided into four sections. The first section, *Background*, includes three chapters. Chapter 1 reviews indications for implant use, patient evaluation, and surgical planning. Chapter 2 presents the rationale for the use of alloplastic implants in the facial skeleton. It compares the host response to autogenous bone and the alloplastic materials frequently used today. This chapter also reviews implant related morbidity and complication rates presently documented. Chapter 3 overviews the technique of implant reconstruction whose goal is to produce an attractive face without post-surgical stigmata. In summary, this technique utilizes:

- Precise definition of the aesthetic goal based on the patient's skeletal morphology, its relation to normal value, and their desires for appearance.
- The use of inconspicuous incisions borrowed from aesthetic and craniofacial surgery to access the facial skeleton.
- Wide subperiosteal exposure of the area to be reconstructed.
- The use of strong, inert, biocompatible alloplastic materials for reconstruction.
- Screw fixation of the implant to the skeleton.

The remaining sections each describe implant applications for a horizontal third of the face. Section II addresses the upper third of the face. Its chapters describe reconstruction of the cranial vault and internal orbit. Section III addresses the midface. Its chapters describe augmentation of the infraorbital rim, the malar, and the piriform aperture, as well as the use of multiple midface implants. Section IV completes the book with chapters describing implant augmentation of the chin and posterior mandible. Each of these chapters includes a description of the relevant musculoskeletal anatomy, normal skeletal relations, a description of the surgical technique for implant placement and multiple clinical examples. All of the chapters in this book are expansions of scientific papers I have previously authored for the plastic surgery, craniofacial, ophthalmologic or neurosurgical literature.

This book builds on my ongoing surgical education. Special thanks go to those who taught me during my plastic surgery residency and early career at the Johns Hopkins Hospital. CT Su and Jack Hoopes demonstrated the importance of preoperative planning, meticulous technique, and attention to detail. Paul Manson introduced me to surgery of the facial skeleton and the utility of rigid fixation techniques to reconstruct it. Together with Joe Gruss, Paul revolutionized craniofacial fracture management in the United States by introducing and popularizing the concept and technique of extended open reduction and rigid internal fixation. Their influence is obvious in that the method of implant surgery presented here can be thought of as *Extended Open Augmentation with Rigid Implant Fixation*. Linton Whitaker was my preceptor during a craniofacial surgery fellowship at the Hospital of the University of Pennsylvania and the Children's Hospital of Philadelphia. Linton taught me how to examine both normal and disfigured faces. All of these master surgeons taught me that the aesthetic and reconstructive principles of plastic surgery are inseparable and intrinsic to all surgery of the face and facial skeleton. These concepts and techniques are the foundation of this atlas.

Acknowledgements

I am indebted to several individuals who were intrinsic to the production of this book. John Mesa, M.D., then a post-doctoral research fellow in our plastic surgery laboratory and now an intern in surgery at the Brigham and Women's Hospital, began the arduous task of assembling the clinical photographs used in this atlas. David Forristall (erf_consulting@comcast.net) skilfully completed it. Kip Carter, Chief of Medical Illustration Services at the College of Veterinary Medicine at the University of Georgia was willing to tackle one more project with me. His illustrations are obviously key to the presentation of this work. Finally, Sue Hodgson, Publishing Director for Elsevier, coordinated our efforts with great skill and professionalism.

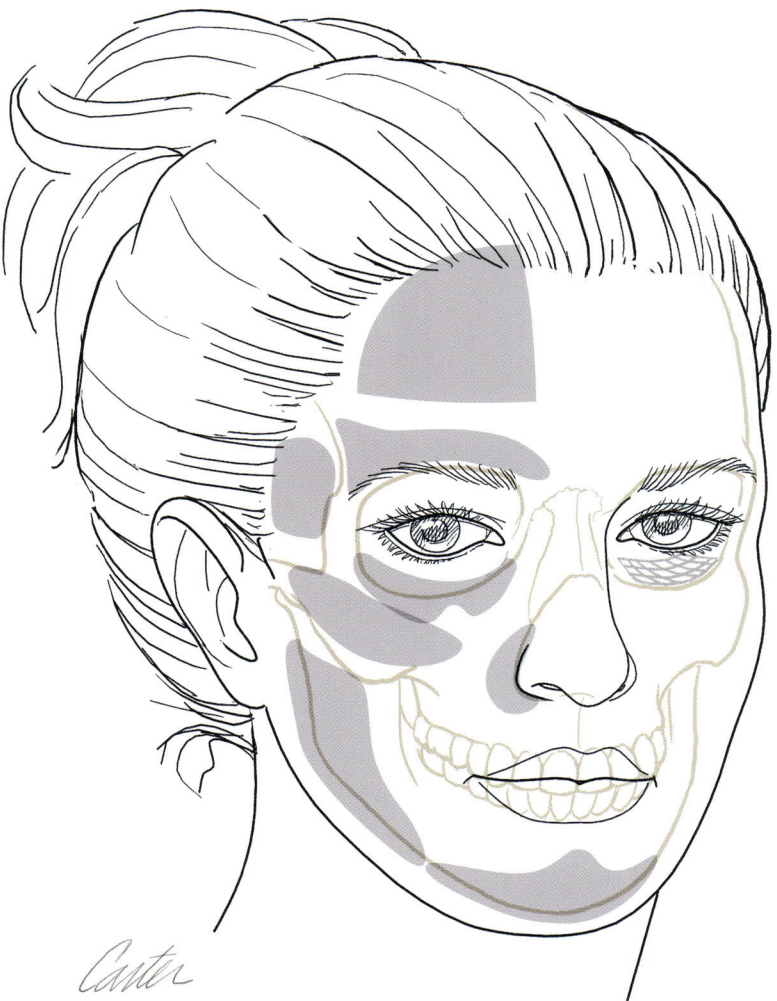

Carter

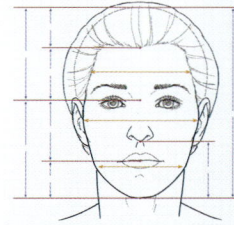

Chapter 1

Indications, evaluation, and planning

The size and shape of the facial skeleton are fundamental determinants of the facial appearance. Small asymmetries in skeletal morphology can be noticeable, and small changes through surgical intervention can be powerful.

Conceptually, autogenous bone would be the best material to restore or improve the craniofacial skeleton, because it has the potential to be revascularized and then incorporated into the facial skeleton. In time, it could be biologically indistinguishable from the adjacent native skeleton. Practically, the use of autogenous bone is limited. The morbidity, time, and hospital costs associated with autogenous bone graft harvest can be significant. Furthermore, the inevitable resorption and the poor handling characteristics of autogenous bone grafts also limit the quality and predictability of the aesthetic result. With the exception of interposition grafts used to reconstruct segmental load-bearing defects of the maxilla and mandible, the majority of craniofacial skeleton replacement, and particularly facial skeleton augmentation, is done with alloplastic implants. A diagrammatic survey of the alloplastic implants used for facial skeletal reconstruction and enhancement is presented in Figure 1.1.

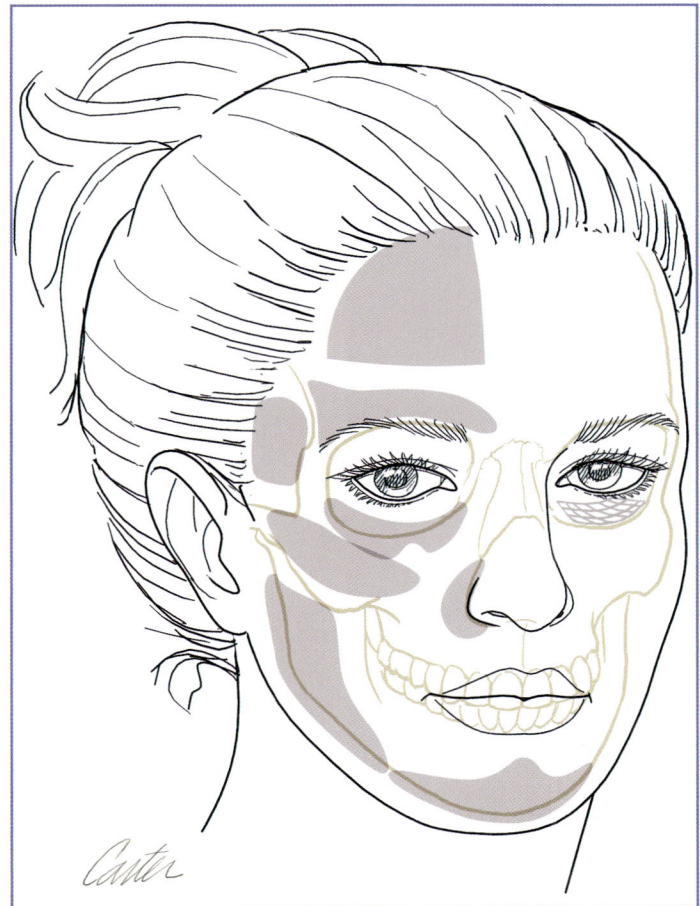

Figure 1.1 A diagrammatic survey of the alloplastic implants used for facial skeletal reconstruction and enhancement.

INDICATIONS

Facial skeleton augmentation

Patients with normal, deficient, and surgically altered or traumatically deformed anatomy may all benefit from implant augmentation of their craniofacial skeleton.

Most often, facial skeletal augmentation is done to enhance facial appearance in patients whose skeletal relationships are considered within the normal range. They want more definition and angularity to their appearance. Other patients desire to 'balance' their facial dimensions. The woman in Figure 1.2 underwent malar augmentation to provide angularity to her midface, and chin augmentation to balance her profile.

Craniofacial deformities that are disfiguring and are of functional consequence to vision, breathing, and mastication usually require skeletal osteotomies and rearrangement as treatment. Less severe midface and mandibular hypoplasia are common facial skeletal variants. In patients with these morphologies, occlusion is normal or has been compensated by orthodontics. These patients have neither respiratory nor ocular compromise. In skeletally deficient patients

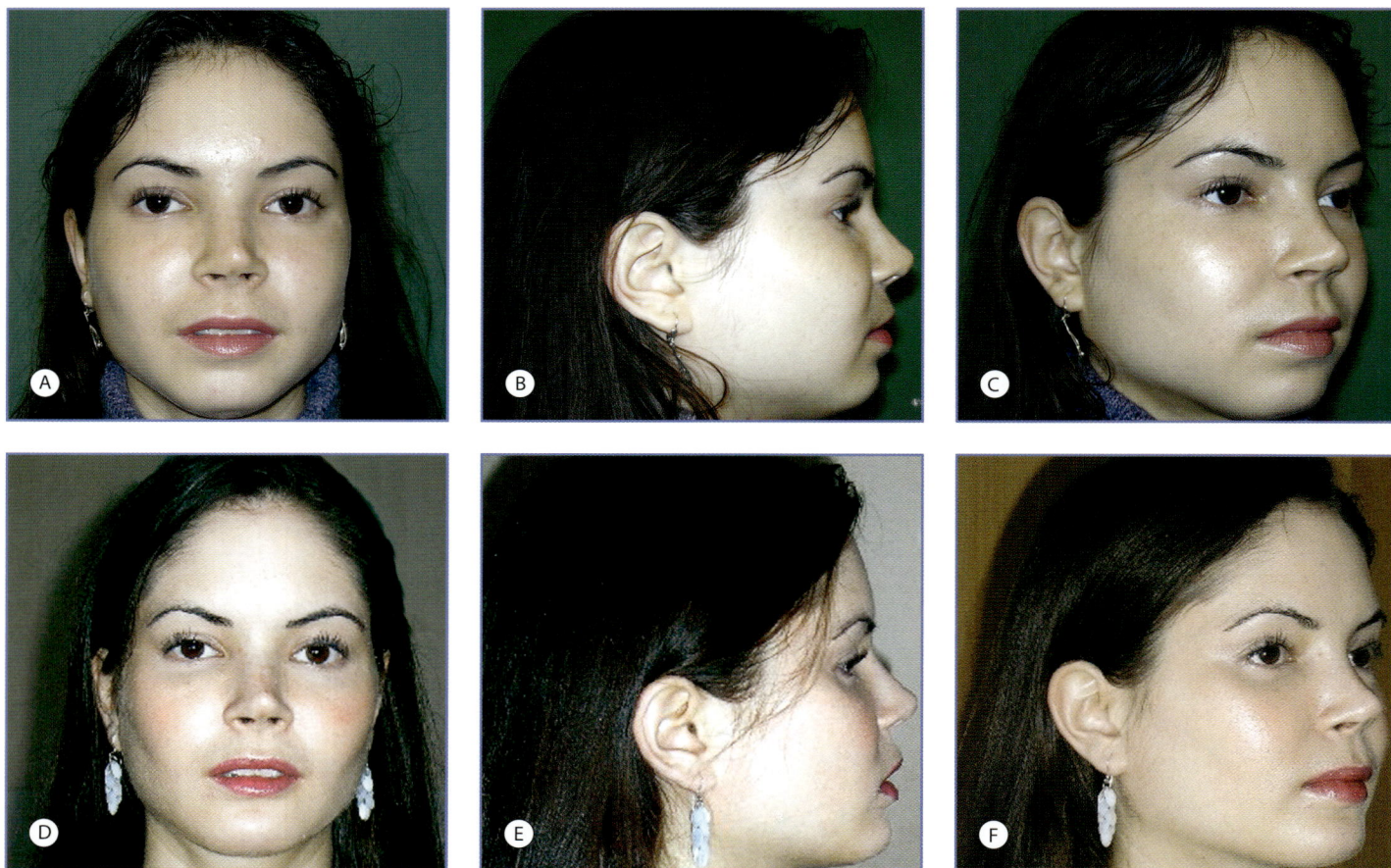

Figure 1.2 A 24-year-old woman underwent malar augmentation, chin augmentation, and submental lipectomy. (**A–C**) Preoperative frontal, lateral, and oblique views. (**D–F**) Postoperative frontal, lateral, and oblique views.

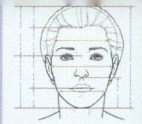

whose occlusion is normal or has been previously normalized by orthodontics, skeletal repositioning would necessitate additional orthodontic tooth movement. Such a treatment plan is time-consuming, costly, and potentially morbid. It is therefore appealing to few patients. In these patients, the appearance of skeletal osteotomies and rearrangements can be simulated through the use of facial implants. Diagrammatic representations of how implant surgery can mimic the appearance of skeletal osteotomies are shown in Figures 1.3 and 1.4. Figure 1.5 shows a patient who underwent multiple implant correction of his midface and mandibular deficiencies.

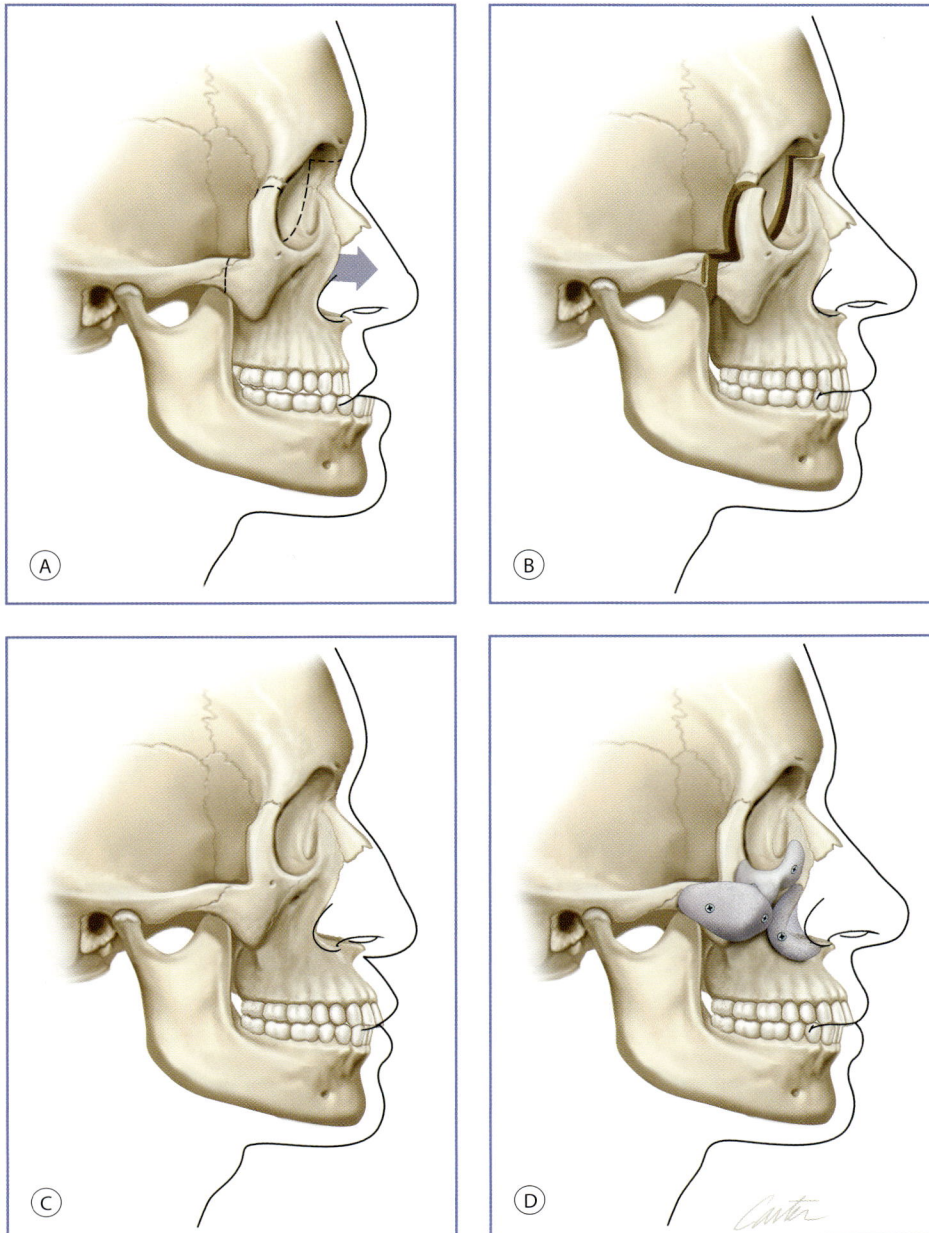

Figure 1.3 How multiple implant augmentation of the midface skeleton can simulate the visual appearance of LeFort III osteotomy and advancement without altering dental occlusion. (A) Midface concavity and class 3 malocclusion. (B) Osteotomy and advancement at the LeFort III level provide midface projection and class I occlusion. (C) Midface concavity and class I occlusion. (D) Multiple midface implants provide the visual effect of LeFort III osteotomy and advancement but do not alter occlusion.

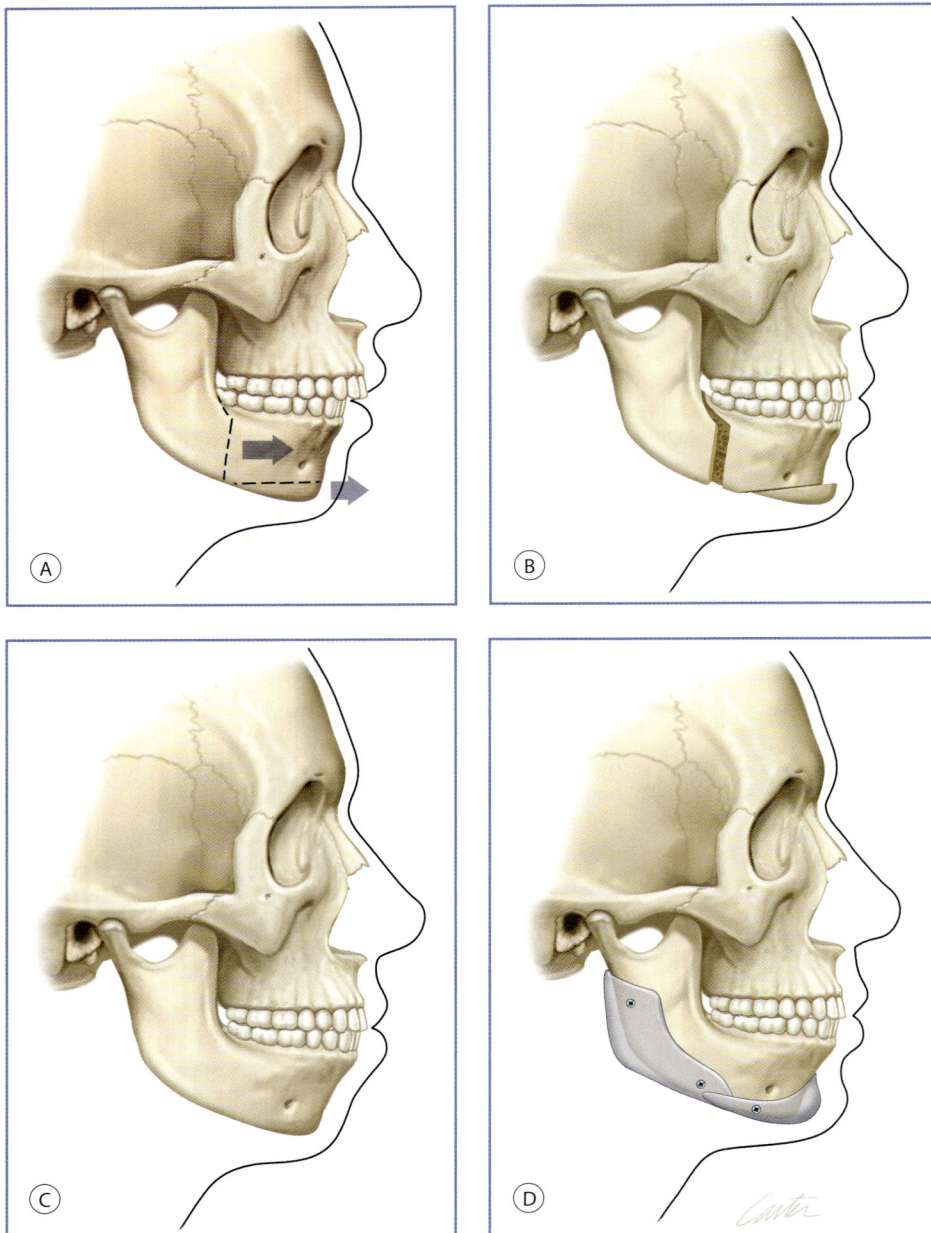

Figure 1.4 (**A**) Mandibular deficiency with class 2 malocclusion. (**B**) After sagittal split osteotomy with horizontal osteotomy advancement of the chin to increase chin projection. Note that the occlusion has been corrected from class II to class I. (**C**) Mandibular deficiency with class I occlusion. (**D**) The visual effect of sagittal split osteotomy and horizontal osteotomy of the chin with advancement has been simulated with mandible and chin implants. Note that the class I occlusion is unchanged. Notice also that the border regularities inherent with skeletal osteotomies are avoided when implants are used.

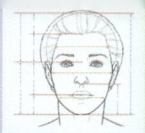

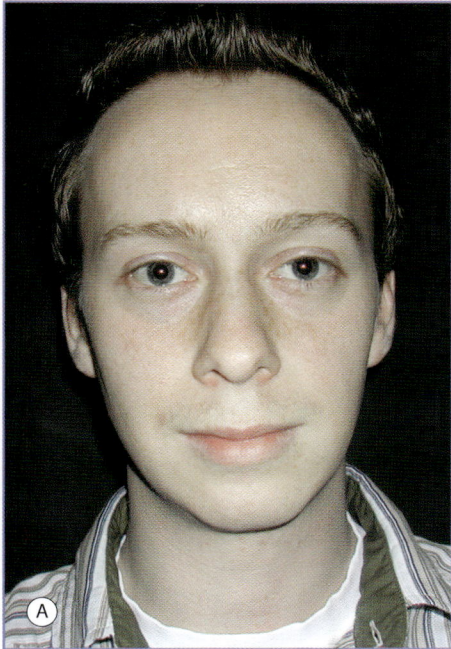

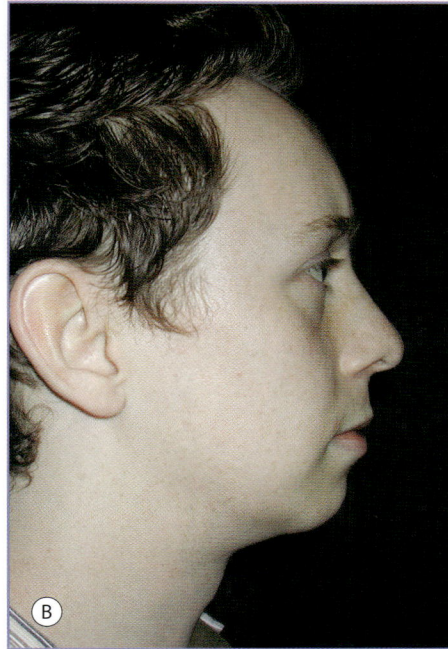

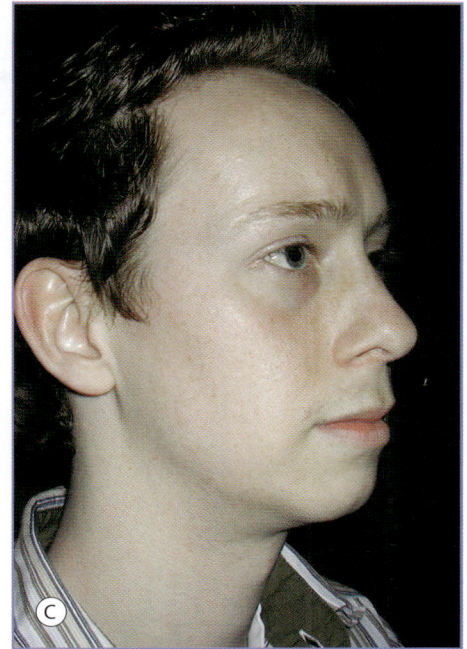

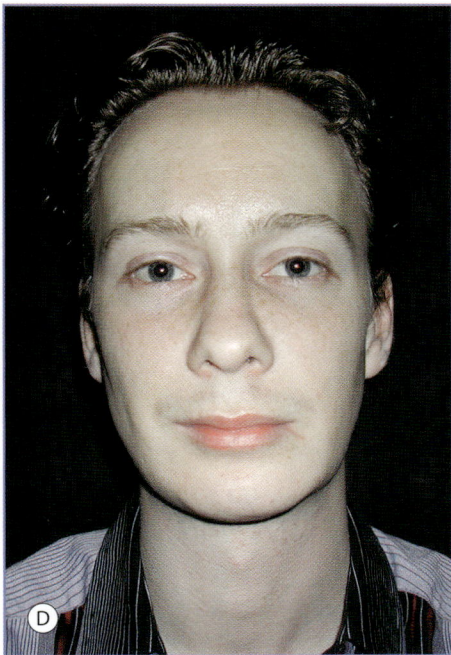

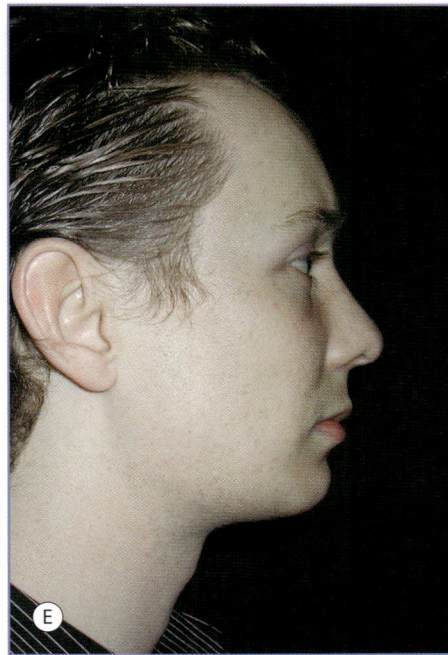

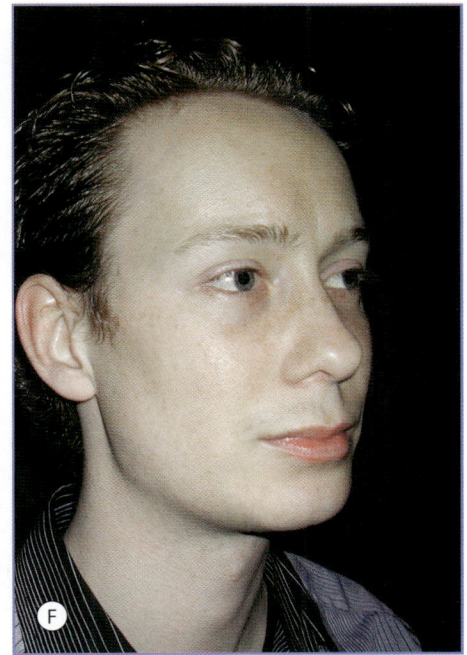

Figure 1.5 A 24-year-old man underwent infraorbital rim, paranasal, and medial malar augmentation to correct midface deficiency. He also underwent mandibular and chin augmentation. (**A–C**) Preoperative frontal, lateral, and oblique views. (**D–F**) Postoperative frontal, lateral, and oblique views.

Patients with craniofacial syndrome microforms and those with previously corrected syndromic deficiencies can often benefit from implant augmentation. Figure 1.6 shows a patient with Treacher Collins syndrome whose orbitomalar area was reconstructed with implants. Onlay rib grafts, placed when she was a teenager, had resorbed.

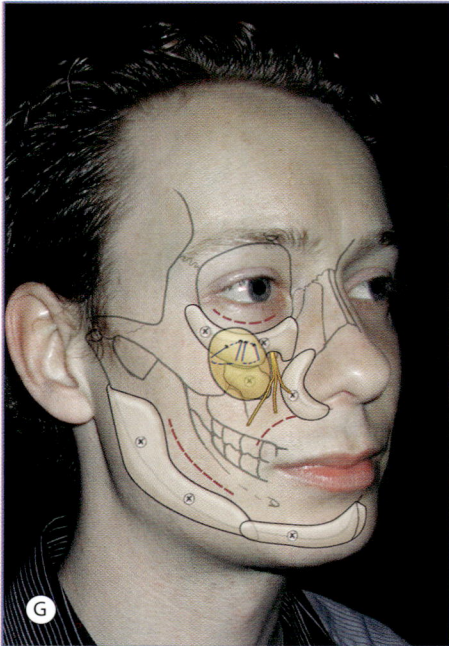

Figure 1.5 (*Cont'd*) (**G**) Diagrammatical representation of operation.

Figure 1.6 A 35-year-old woman with malar and lateral orbital deficiency due to Treacher Collins syndrome underwent reconstruction after silicone implants placed during her teenaged years had been removed to treat infection. Rib grafts had resorbed. Reconstruction was performed with custom-carved porous polyethylene implants that were fixed with metal screws. Surgery was performed through bicoronal, intraoral, and transconjunctival incisions. In addition, lateral canthopexies and a sliding advancement genioplasty were performed. (**A**) Preoperative and (**B**) postoperative frontal views. (**C**) Preoperative and (**D**) 2-year postoperative lateral views. (From Yaremchuk 2003,[11] with permission.)

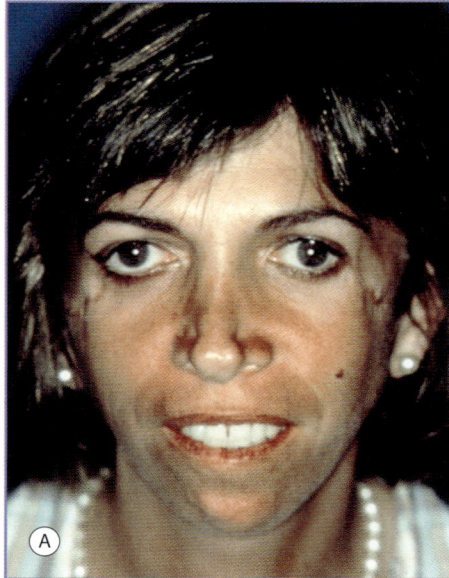

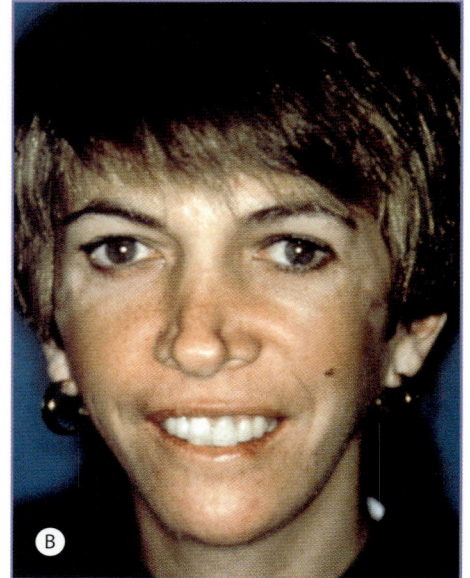

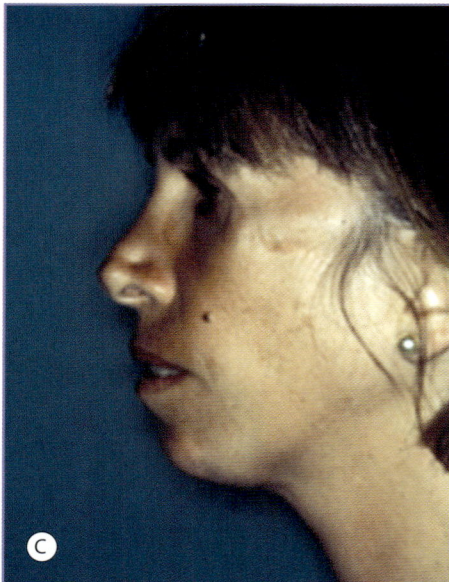

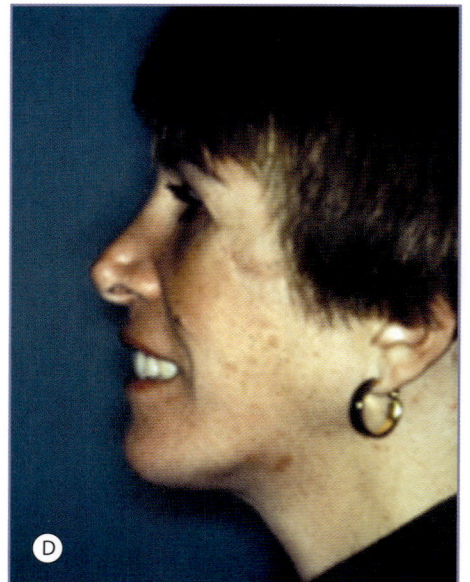

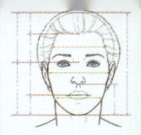

Figure 1.7 shows a 30-year-old woman with Stickler syndrome who had undergone monobloc facial advancement surgery as a child. Forehead contour and supraorbital rim–globe relationships were improved with an acrylic onlay cranioplasty.

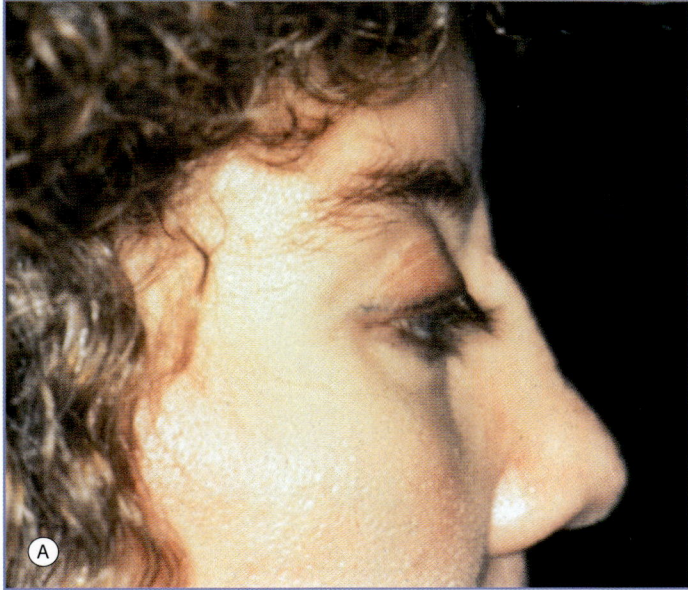

Figure 1.7 A 30-year-old woman with Stickler syndrome had undergone monobloc facial advancement surgery as a child. Forehead contour and supraorbital rim–globe relationships were improved with an acrylic onlay cranioplasty. A porous polyethylene implant was used to augment the radix and nasal dorsum. An orbital decompression was also performed. (**A**) Preoperative lateral view. (**B**) The 1-year postoperative lateral view.

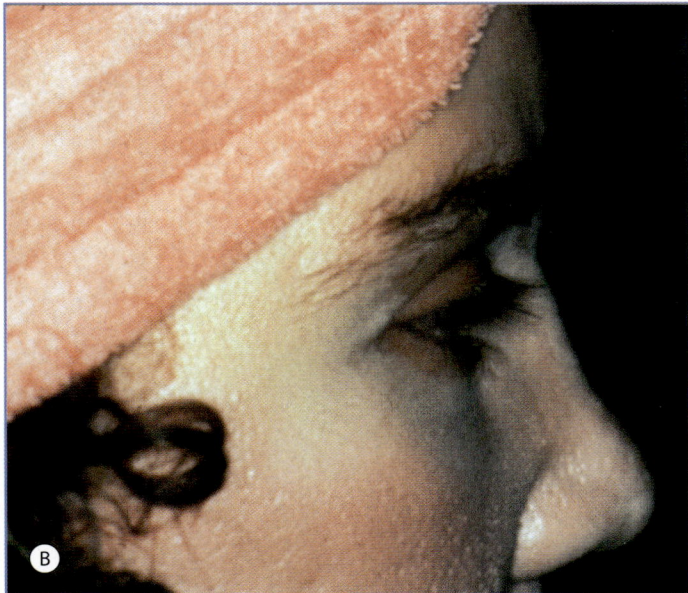

Posttraumatic and postablative deformities may also benefit from alloplastic implant reconstruction (Fig. 1.8).

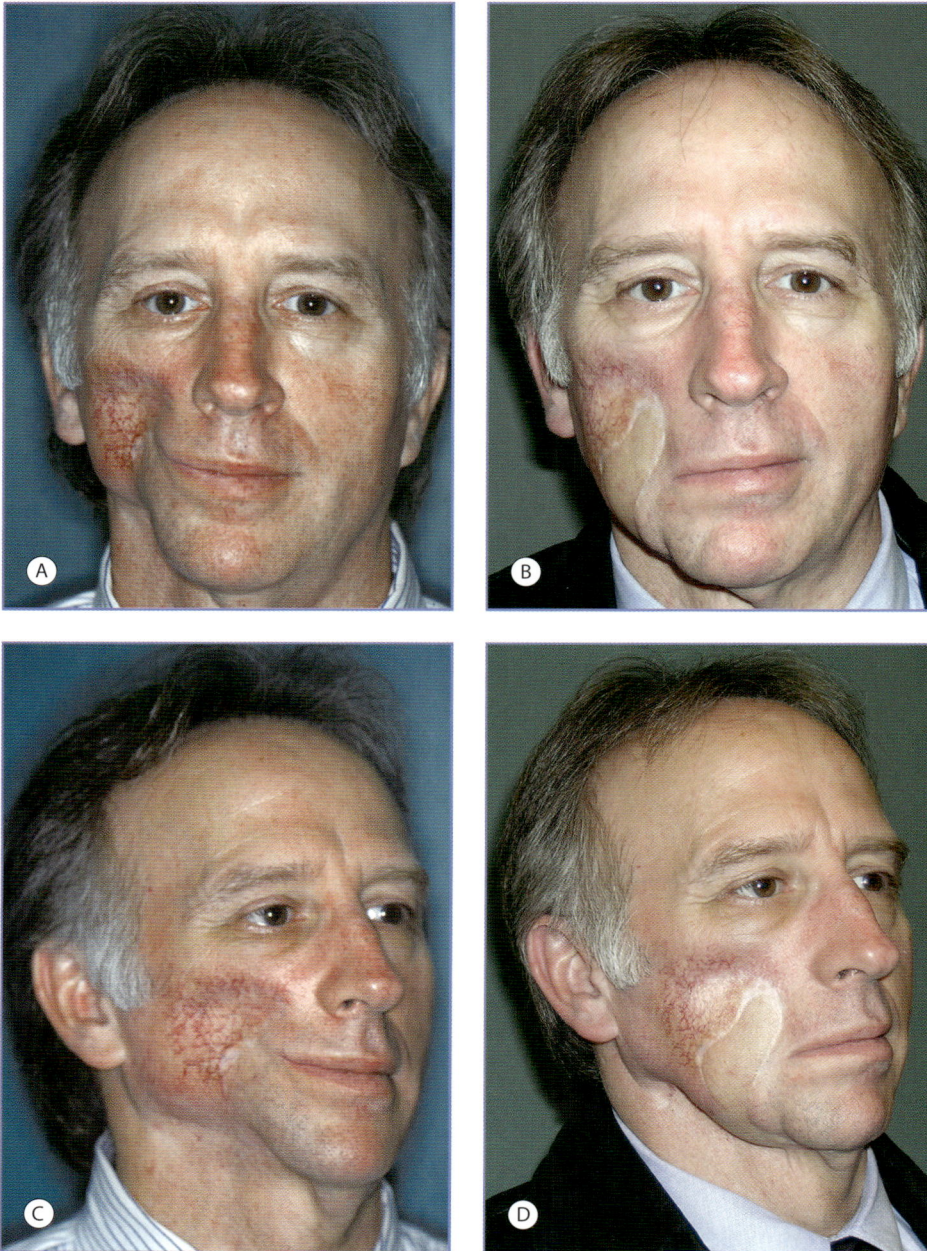

Figure 1.8 A 48-year-old man had undergone multiple excisions of a recurrent basosquamous carcinoma of the right cheek. Surgeries included partial maxillectomy, parotidectomy, and border mandibulectomy. The area was irradiated. The mandibular border defect was reconstructed with a porous polyethylene implant. The soft tissue defect was reconstructed with a radial forearm free flap. (**A**) Preoperative and (**B**) 2-year postoperative frontal views. (**C**) Preoperative and (**D**) 2-year postoperative oblique views.

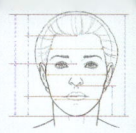

Facial skeleton replacement

Indications for alloplastic replacement of the craniofacial skeleton are limited. These areas must be non-load bearing and protected from sinus exposure. Replacement in load-bearing areas inevitably leads to micromotion at the implant–bone interface, with bone erosion and subsequent implant extrusion. Implants that are chronically exposed to the sinuses are inevitably contaminated with bacteria and lost to infection. Portions of the cranial vault and internal orbit are the areas reliably replaced by alloplastic implants.

Figure 1.9 shows a 40-year-old woman who underwent lateral malar and arch resection for malignancy. Reconstruction was done with porous polyethylene implants fixed with plates and screws (Fig. 1.10).

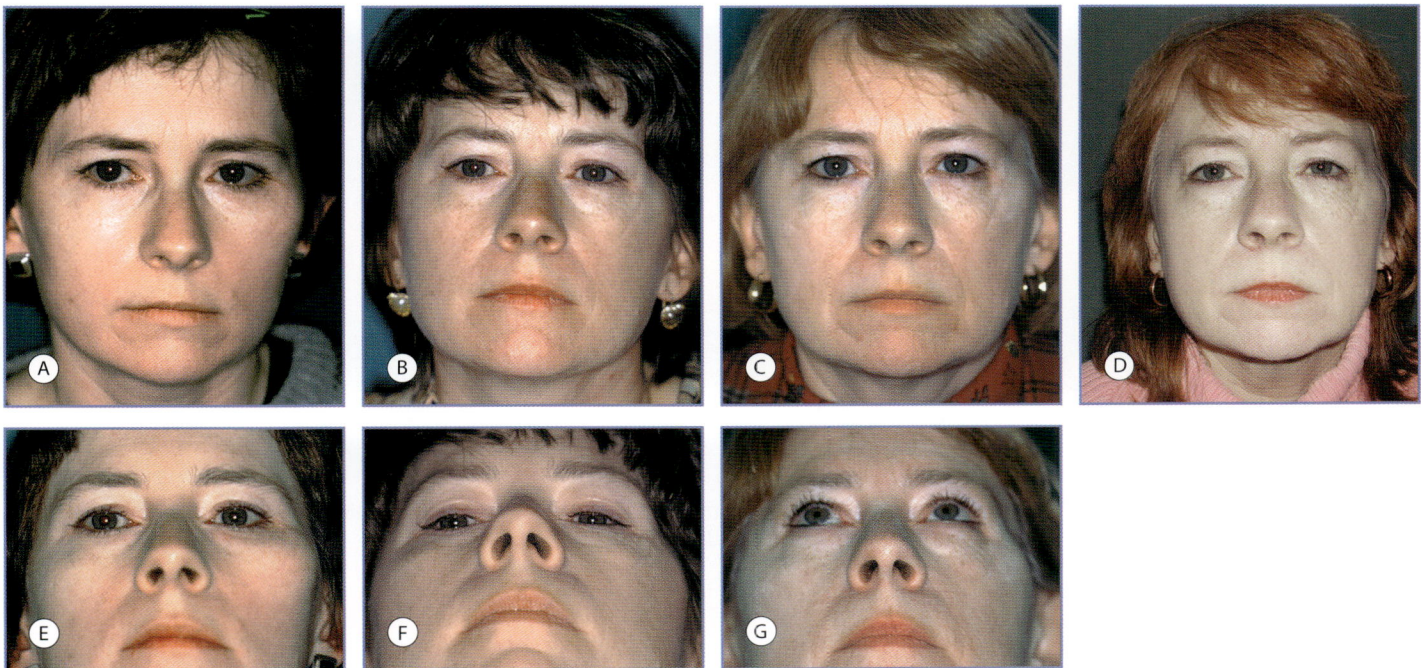

Figure 1.9 A 40-year-old woman who was referred with a chondromyxoid fibroma of the zygoma. The patient was treated with radical removal of the involved facial skeleton and immediate reconstruction with porous polyethylene implants stabilized with plates and screws. The patient remains tumor-free and symptom-free 14 years after the reconstructive operation. Frontal views (**A**) preoperatively, (**B**) 1 year postoperatively, (**C**) 10 years postoperatively, and (**D**) 14 years postoperatively. A worm's eye view of the patient (**E**) before the operation, (**F**) 1 year after the operation, and (**G**) 10 years after the operation. *(From Carr et al. 1992,[1] with permission.)*

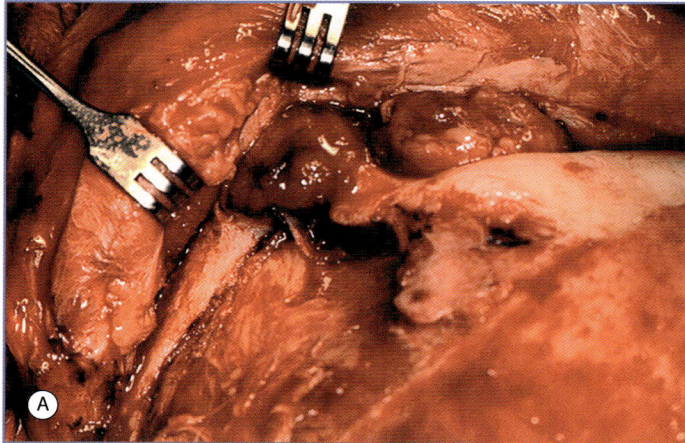

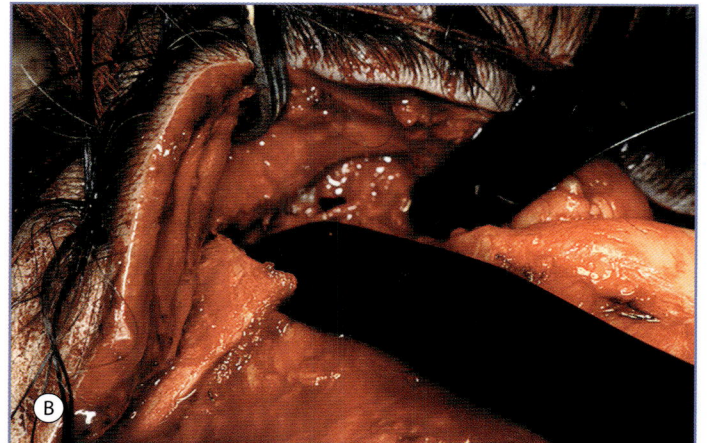

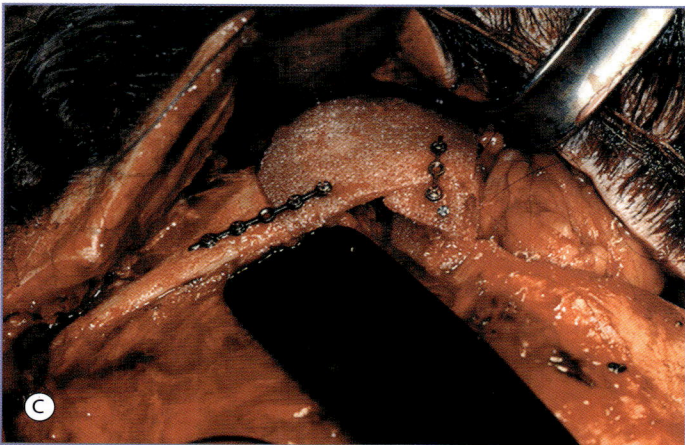

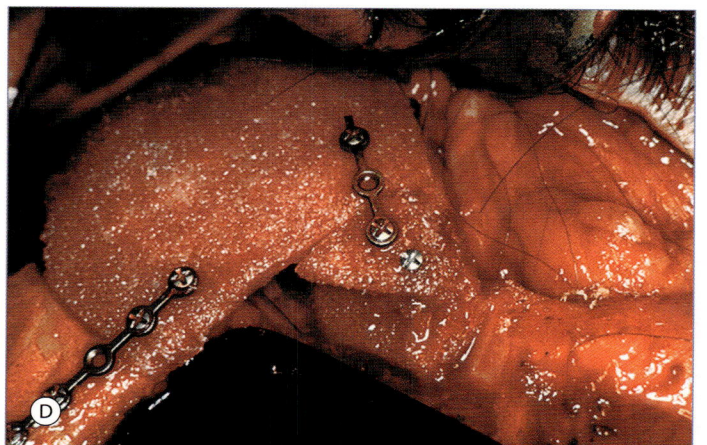

Figure 1.10 Intraoperative views from the coronal approach of the operation with the results shown in Figure 1.9. (**A**) Tumor before removal. (**B**) After removal. (**C**) After reconstruction. (**D**) Close-up of reconstruction.

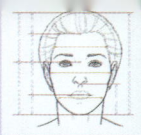

Skeletal versus soft tissue augmentation

Plastic surgery's past decade is notable for its recognition that aging is accompanied by facial soft tissue atrophy. Facial rejuvenative surgery is no longer one of simple excising and tightening. The value of soft tissue repositioning and augmentation have been recognized and exploited. Unfortunately, because the ultimate expression of skeletal or soft tissue structure is reflected on the skin's surface, some surgeons have used this as a justification for the equivalence and interchangeability of soft and hard tissue augmentation. For example, malar skeletal implants are used to restore cheek fullness, while fat grafts are used to create malar prominence. Up to a millimeter or so, the visual effect of either augmentation modality may be equivalent, depending on the thickness of the overlying soft tissue envelope. However, beyond a minimal augmentation, the visual effects of these modalities are markedly different. This is easily conceptualized when envisioning large augmentations. A large implant placed on the malar bone will make the cheek project more, making the face more defined and angular, and therefore making the face appear thinner and more skeletal (Fig. 1.11). Implanting fat into the cheeks will also make the cheek project more; however, the face will appear increasingly round and therefore less defined and less angular (Fig. 1.12).

PEARL

Soft tissue augmentation does not provide the same visual effect as skeletal augmentation, and vice versa.

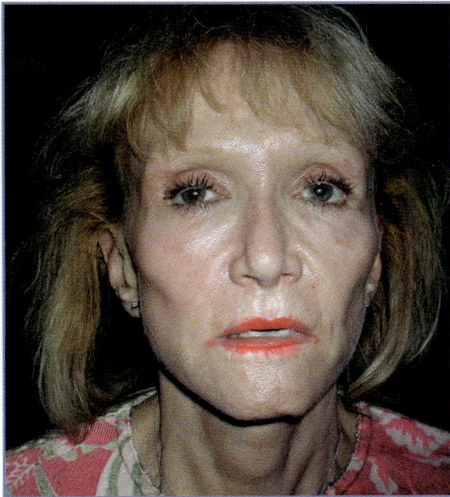

Figure 1.11 A 64-year-old woman had previous malar implant surgery, upper and lower lid blepharoplasty, and rhytidectomy as rejuvenative procedures. The large implant created an overly prominent skeletal contour.

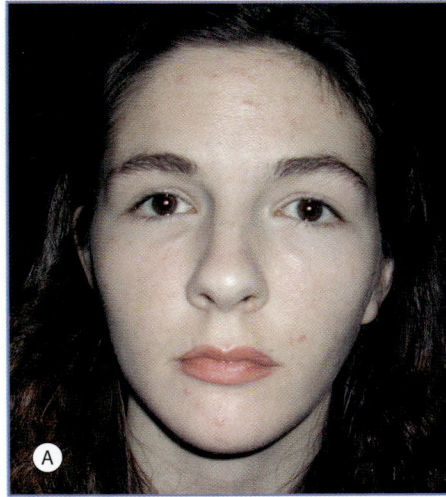

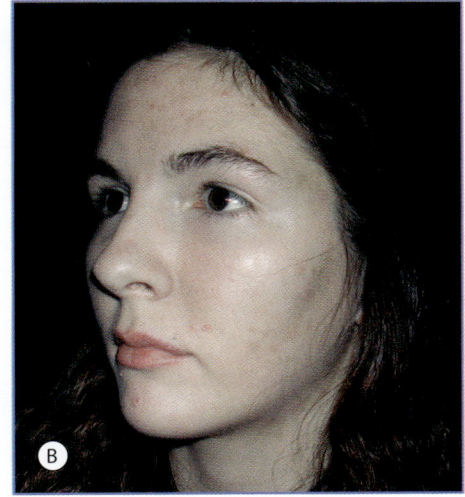

Figure 1.12 A 30-year-old woman had undergone fat grafting of the malar midface area. Fat grafting in this young woman obliterated skeletal definition. (**A**) Frontal and (**B**) oblique views.

PREOPERATIVE EVALUATION

Physical examination

Physical examination is the most important element of preoperative assessment and planning for both reconstructive and cosmetic procedures. Reviewing life size photographs with the patient can be helpful when discussing aesthetic concerns and goals.

All faces are asymmetric. Asymmetries are usually subtle but, with sufficient scrutiny, detectable (Fig. 1.13). Their recognition preoperatively is important to both the surgeon and the patient. The patient's asymmetry should be pointed out during the preoperative consultation so that the patient can anticipate asymmetry in the postoperative result.

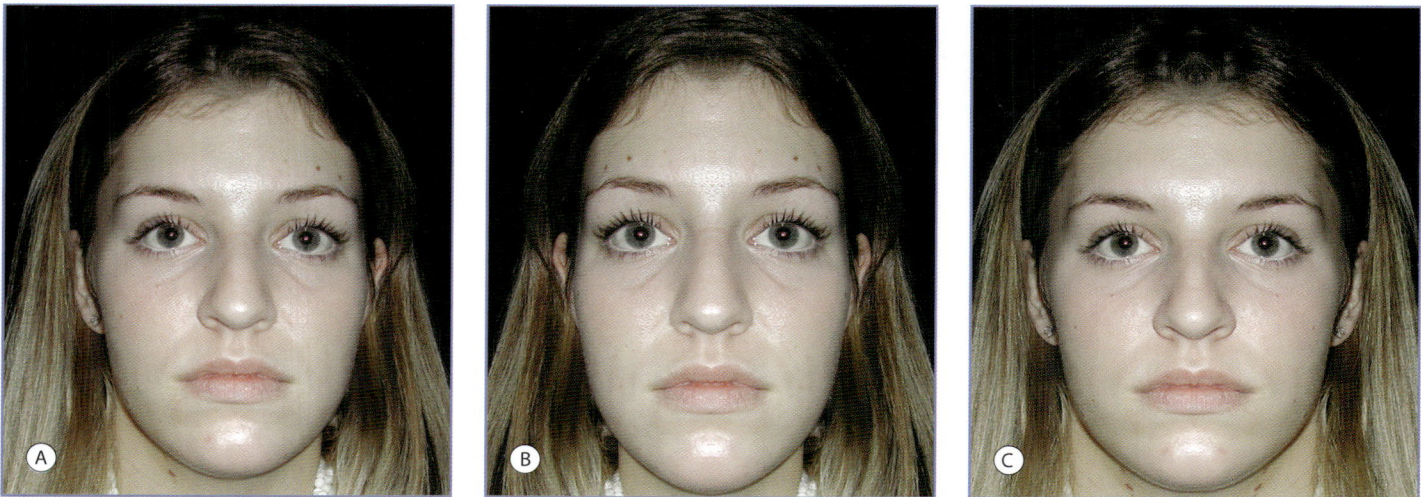

Figure 1.13 To demonstrate the asymmetry in a 'normal' face, a photograph has been manipulated to create three separate images. (**A**) Frontal view of a 20-year-old woman presenting for rhinoplasty. (**B**) Composite created by joining the left side of the face with its mirror image. (**C**) Composite created by joining the right side of the face with its mirror image.

As asymmetries become more severe, it is important to recognize that they are more complex than relative skeletal deficiencies or excesses. Rather, they reflect three-dimensional differences that are most easily conceptualized as twists of the facial skeleton.

Radiologic examination

Most aesthetic procedures are not done without preoperative radiologic assessment. In general, the size and position of the implant are largely aesthetic judgments. Cephalometric x-rays are most often used for planning chin and mandibular augmentation surgery. These studies define skeletal dimensions and asymmetries as well as the thickness of the chin pad.

Whereas preoperative radiologic examination is uncommon for purely aesthetic surgery, computed tomography (CT) evaluation is almost routine for reconstructive procedures. CT scans provide the ability to view the skeleton in different planes and, through computer manipulation, in three dimensions. CT imaging provides digitized information that can be transferred to design software. This can be used to create life-sized models and custom implants. Models are helpful in planning surgery for skeletal deformities and asymmetries (Fig. 1.14).

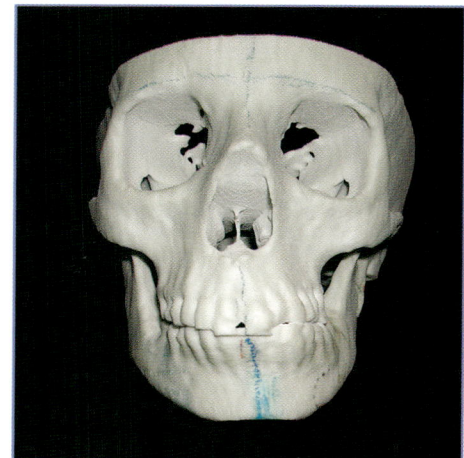

Figure 1.14 Computed tomography data were used to fabricate a skull model in planning surgery for a patient with facial asymmetry.

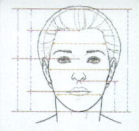

The use of custom implants is an efficient technique to reconstruct cranial defects (Fig. 1.15).

PREOPERATIVE PLANNING

For most reconstructive problems, surgery is performed to return the involved area to its original appearance or, if that is not possible, to one that is symmetric and accepted as normal. When alloplastic implants are used to make the face more attractive, the aesthetic goal is more arbitrary. Because implant augmentation of the facial skeleton results in measurable changes in facial dimensions and proportion, it is intuitively attractive and appropriate to use facial measurements to evaluate the face and to guide surgery.

Mathematical ideals

In his book on Leonardo da Vinci's anatomical drawings, Martin Clayton explained how mathematic ideals influenced classical and Renaissance artists in their perception and depiction of the human body.[2] The ancient Greeks observed that musical notes created by strings whose lengths were in simple numeric ratios were intrinsically pleasing. They extended this concept to spatial intervals and established the concept that harmonic ratios were intrinsically 'right' and thus fundamental to the structure of the universe.

In the first century BC, Vitruvius adapted the proportional concept to the human body. He proposed that the body should be divisible into equal parts, and that all its units should be expressible in terms of that unit or fractions of the whole. His treatise *De architectura*, which described his proportional system, was one of the few classical texts that survived to the Renaissance, and it became highly influential in the thinking of artists and scholars of that time, including Leonardo da Vinci. Early in his career, Leonardo adopted many of Vitruvius' ratios. Most of us today associate Leonardo's anatomical drawings with his rendition of Vitruvius' ideal proportions for the human body (*c*.1490–2), whereby 'the body when standing with arms stretched fits into a square and, with all limbs splayed, into a circle centered on the navel' (Fig. 1.16).

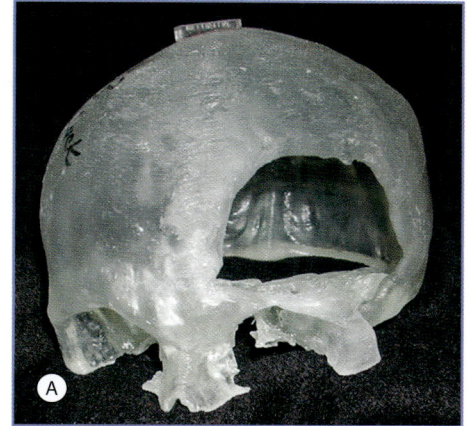

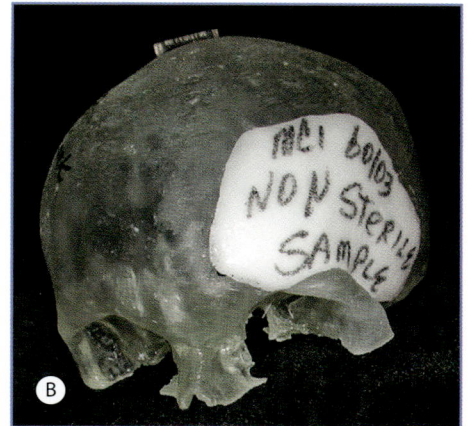

Figure 1.15 Skull model and custom implant obtained from three-dimensional computed tomography scan data.

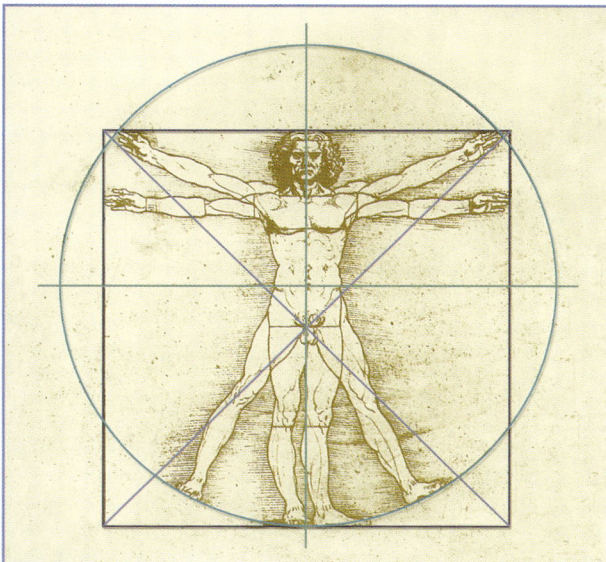

Figure 1.16 Leonardo's rendition of Vitruvius' ideal proportions for the human body (*c*.1490–2), whereby 'the body when standing with arms stretched fits into a square and, with all limbs splayed, into a circle centered on the navel'. Leonardo later realized after studying human cadavers that the human body does not conform to these proportions.

Leonardo soon found limitations in the use of proportions to depict the human form. By 1500, he abandoned the idea of a single canon of ideal proportion to describe the human body. In the winter of 1510, he collaborated with the professor of anatomy at the University of Pavia, Marcantonio della Torre. This relation provided Leonardo access to human material, allowing him to depict human structure with great accuracy. As Leonardo learned human anatomy, he realized that the use of ideal proportions thwarted its accurate depiction. He used proportion as a tool to help describe its form and function rather than as an end in itself.

Although usually referenced in texts discussing facial skeletal augmentation, neoclassical canons have a limited role in surgical evaluation and planning because, similar to what Leonardo found, they are based on idealizations. When the dimensions of normal males and females were evaluated objectively and compared with these artistic ideals, it was found that some theoretic proportions are one of many variations found in healthy normal individuals, or those determined more attractive than normal individuals, and some are never found (Fig. 1.17).[3,4] The neoclassical canons do not allow for facial dimensions known to differ with sex and age. Most of these canons of proportion, for example that the width of the upper face is equal to five eye widths, are interesting but hold for few individuals and cannot be obtained surgically or, if obtainable, only with extremely sophisticated craniofacial procedures.

Researchers from various disciplines have emphasized the difficulties with mathematically defining a beautiful face. For example, the orthodontist Ricketts has pointed out that although the ratio phi, equal to 1.1618 and known as the divine proportion, may be seen in many biologic forms and its approximation may characterize certain relations of the normal human face, it does not distinguish beautiful from plain.[5] The psychologist Etcoff analyzed human beauty and its impact on society in a book that is subtitled *The Science of Beauty*. She also found that the perception of beauty could not be defined by mathematical formulae. The summary of her analysis of mathematic ideals to human beauty was, 'For scientists in this century, the key to understanding human beauty is in our biology not in mathematics'.[6]

Because neither the normal nor the beautiful face can be defined by mathematic ideals, we have found it more useful to use the anthropometric measurements of normal persons, rather than neoclassical canons, to guide our gestalt for the selection of implants for facial skeletal augmentation.

25.0%

25.0%

25.0%

25.0%

(A)

21.1%

24.3%

26.5%

26.9%

(B)

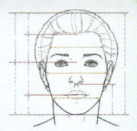

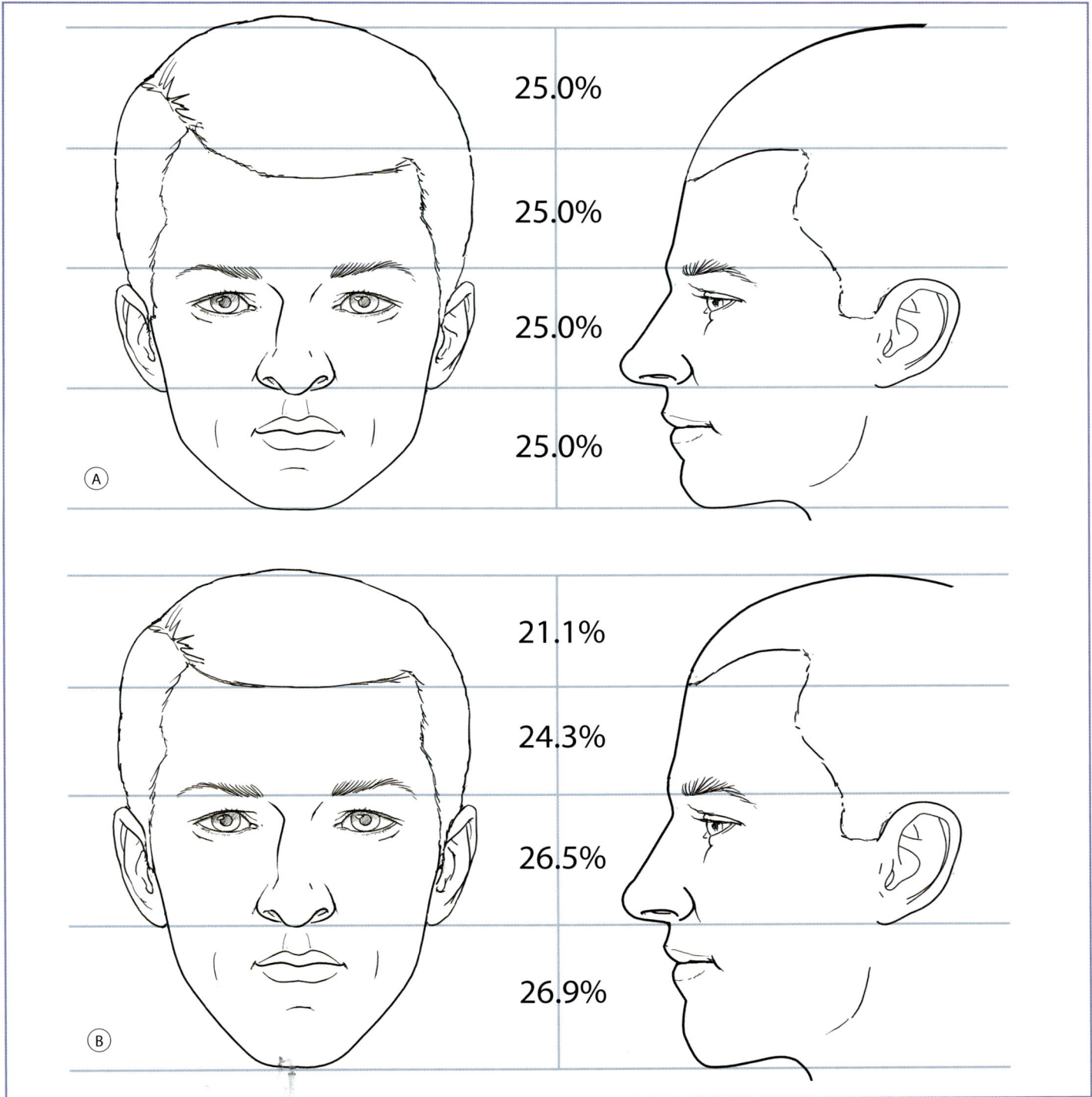

Figure 1.17 A comparison of young adult faces constructed from neoclassical canons (**A**) and from anthropometric measurements (**B**). (**A**) Frontal and lateral views of the young adult face constructed with the help of the neoclassical canons. The head and face have five equal vertical sections and four equal horizontal sections. The nose width equals the eye fissure width and the interocular distance. (**B**) Frontal and lateral views of the average young North American white person's head and face constructed with mean measurements of both sexes. In general, these measurements are different from the idealized ones shown in (**A**). *(From Farkas et al. 1985,[3] with permission.)*

Facial anthropometrics

Leslie Farkas, a medical anthropologist, has accumulated large numbers of precise, reproducible surface measurements of various population groups of both sexes.[7] These data define normative values, as well as gender and ethnic differences, in facial measurements and proportions. The anthropometric data used in this book come from measurements made in a large group of young North American white adult men and women.[7] Similar information is available for Asian and African people and certain other groups.[8–10]

Anthropometric landmarks, measurements, and inclinations are useful for planning implant and other craniofacial surgery. Table 1.1 lists anthropometric landmarks (landmarks used in craniofacial anthropometry and radiographic cephalometry may have the same name but not the same anatomical location), while Table 1.2 lists measurements and inclinations. These are diagrammed in Figures 1.18 through 1.20.

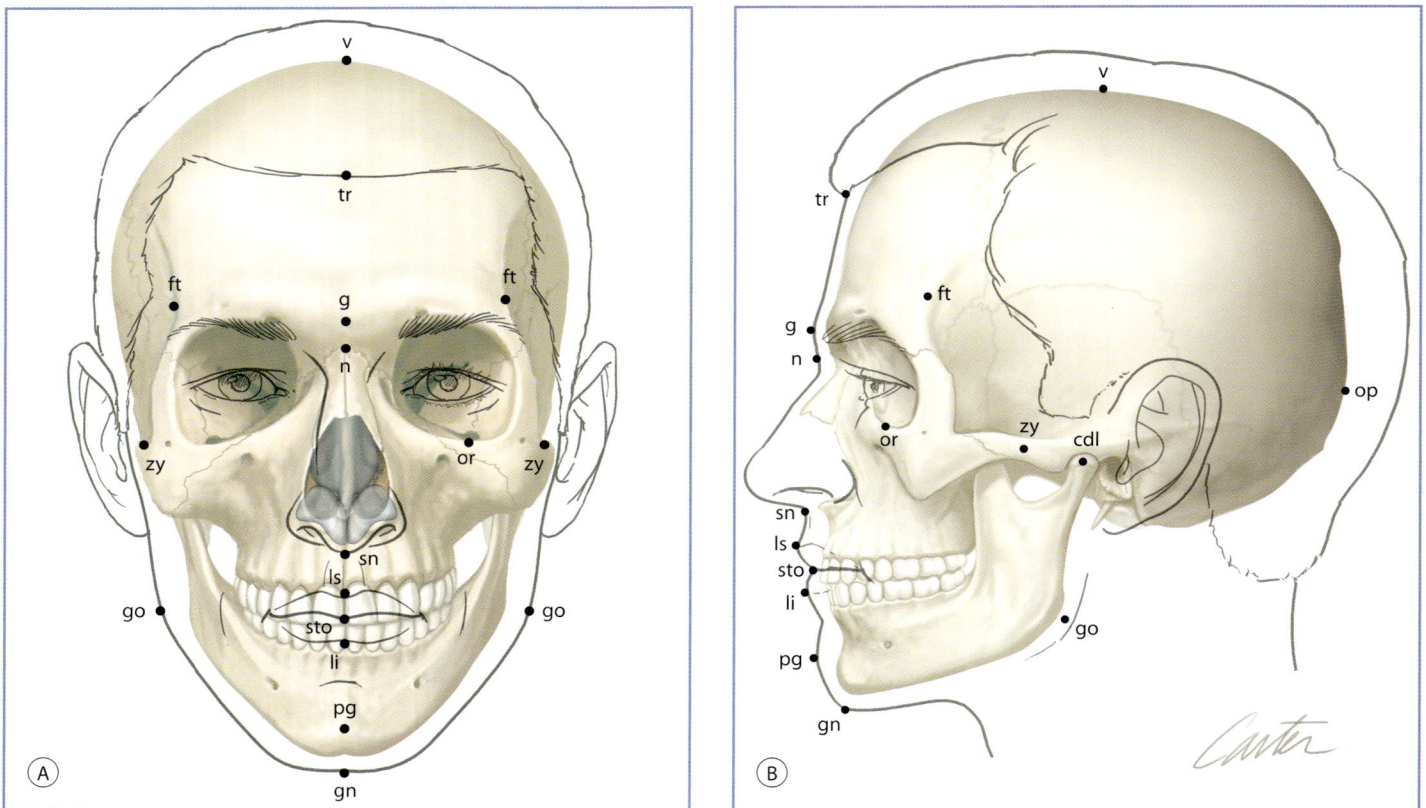

Figure 1.18 Anthropometric landmarks relevant to implant surgery. See Table 1.1 for definitions. The schematic drawings show the surface landmarks in relation to the underlying facial skeleton. (**A**) Frontal. (**B**) Lateral. op, opisthocranion.

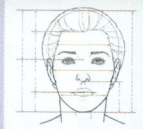

Anthropometric landmarks useful for evaluating the face	
Landmark (abbreviation[a])	Notes
Craniofacial complex	
Vertex (v)	The highest point of the head when the head is oriented in the Frankfort horizontal.
Glabella (g)	The most prominent midline point between the eyebrows. It is identical to the bony glabella on the frontal bone.
Fronto temporale (ft)	The point on each side of the forehead, laterally from the elevation of the linea temporalis. It approximately corresponds with the tail of the eyebrow.
Zygion (zy)	The most lateral point of each zygomatic arch.
Gonion (go)	The most lateral point on the mandibular angle close to the bony gonion.
Pogonion (pg)	The most anterior midpoint of the chin. It is located on the skin surface in front of the identical bony landmark of the mandible.
Menton (or gnathion) (gn)	The lowest median landmark on the lower border of the mandible. It is the lowest point on the face used in measuring facial height. It is identical to the bony gnathion.
Condylion laterale (cdl)	The most lateral point on the surface of the condyle of the mandible.
Trichion (tr)	The point on the hairline in the midline of the forehead.
Orbits	
Endocanthion (en)	The point on the inner commissure of the eye fissure.
Exocanthion (ex)	The point at the outer commissure of the eye fissure.
Center point of the pupil (p)	Determined with the head in the rest position and the patient looking straight ahead.
Orbitale (or)	The lowest point on the lower margin of each orbit. It is identical to the bony orbitale.
Palpebral superius (ps)	The highest point in the midportion of the margin of each upper lid.
Palpebral inferius (pi)	The lowest point in the midportion of the margin of each lower lid.
Orbitale superius (os)	In young adults, it is the highest point on the lower border of the eyebrow. It is close to the highest bony point of the upper margin of the bony orbit.
Superciliare (sci)	The highest point on the upper border in the midportion of each eyebrow.
Nose	
Nasion (n)	The point in the midline of both the nasal root and the nasal suture. It is identical to the bony nasion.
Subnasale (sn)	The midpoint of the angle at the columella base where the lower border of the nasal septum and the surface of the upper lip meet. It is not identical to the bony subnasion.
Lips and mouth	
Labiale superius (ls)	The midpoint of the vermilion of the upper lip.
Labiale inferius (li)	The midpoint of the vermilion of the lower lip.
Stomion (sto)	The imaginary point at the intersection of the vertical facial midline and the horizontal labial fissure.

[a]Abbreviations used in Table 1.2 and Figures 1.18–1.21.
(After Farkas et al. 1994[7].)

Table 1.1 Anthropometric landmarks useful for evaluating the face

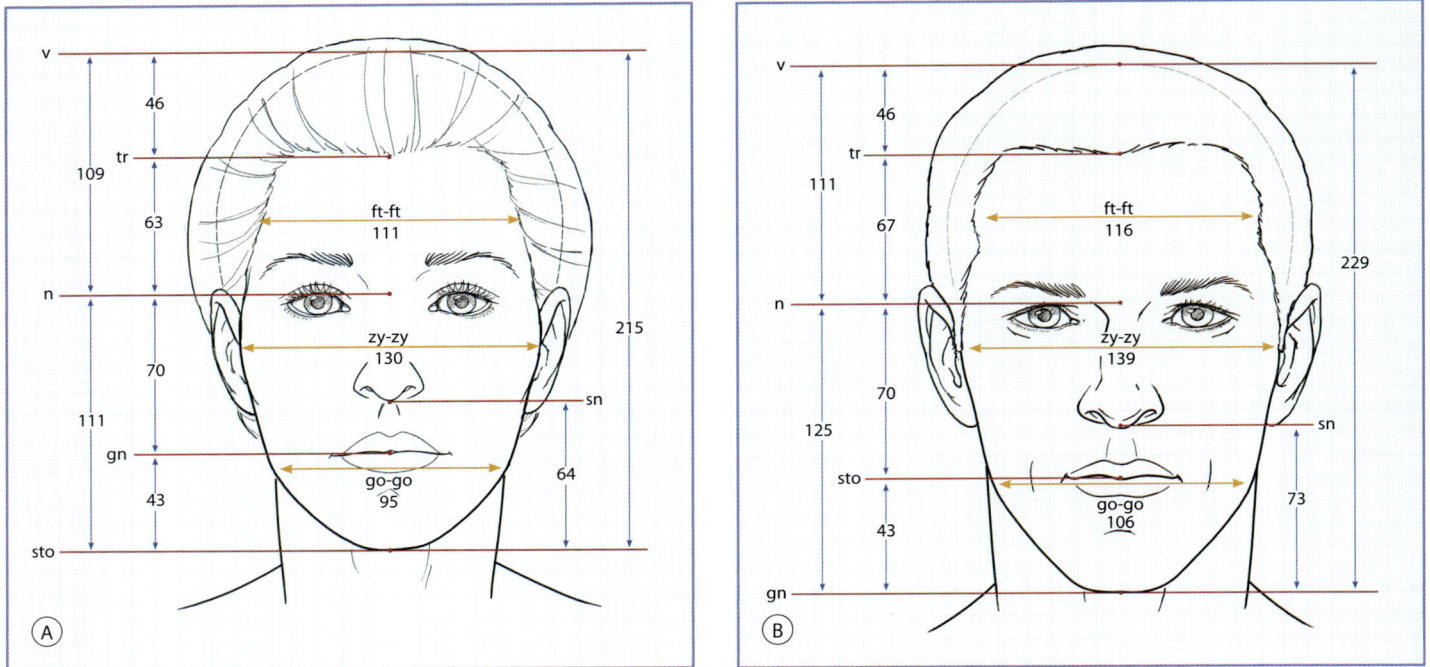

Figure 1.19 Frontal view of (**A**) female and (**B**) male faces drawn from average anthropometric measurements for 21-year-old North American white persons. See Table 1.1 for definitions.

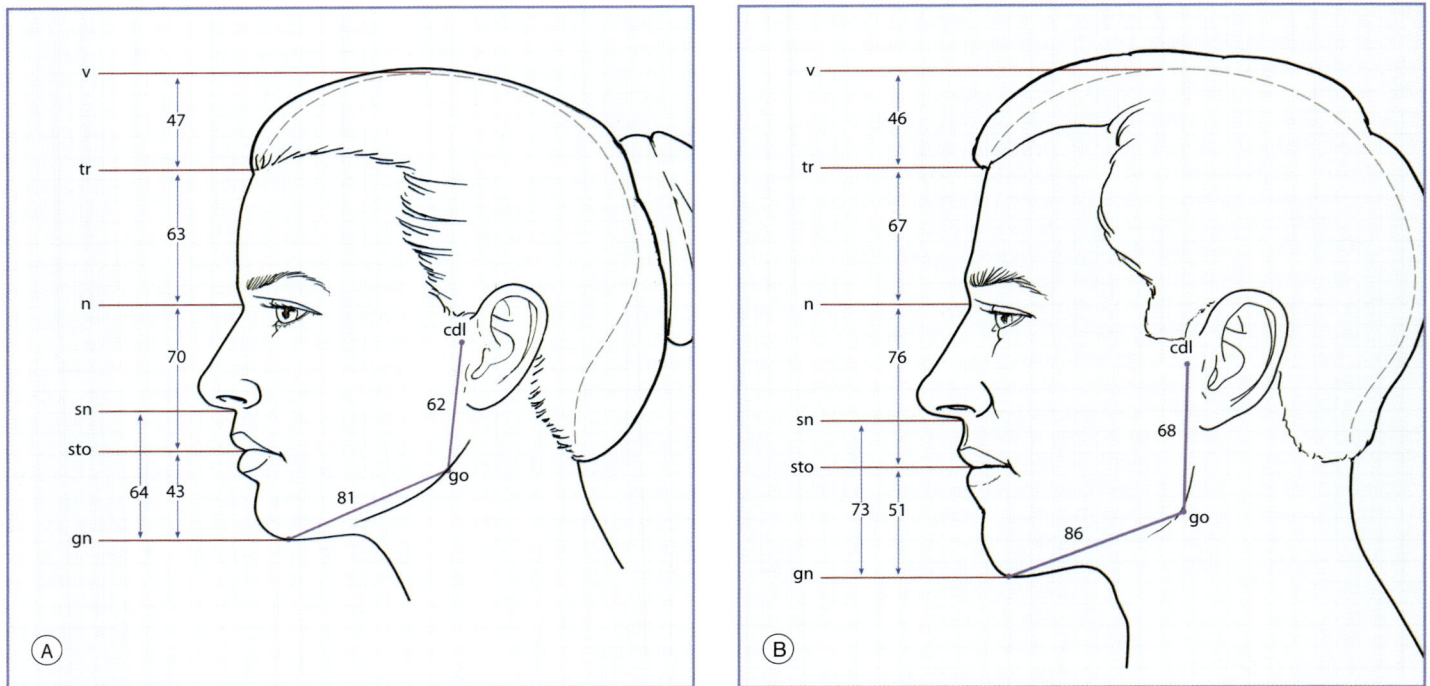

Figure 1.20 Lateral view of (**A**) female and (**B**) male faces drawn from average anthropometric measurements for 21-year-old North American white persons. See Table 1.1 for definitions.

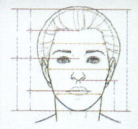

Craniofacial complex measurements useful for evaluating the face				
	Measurement	Facial area	Male	Female
			Height (mm)	
Single linear frontal	v–gn	Upper, middle, and lower face	229 ± 7	215 ± 8
	v–n	Upper face	111 ± 7	109 ± 6
	v–tr	Hair-bearing scalp	46 ± 9	47 ± 8
	tr–n	Forehead	67 ± 8	63 ± 6
	n–gn	Middle and lower face	125 ± 6	111 ± 5
	n–sto	Middle face	76 ± 4	70 ± 3
	sn–gn	Lower face	73 ± 5	64 ± 4
	sto–gn	Mandible	51 ± 4	43 ± 3
Single paired frontal	go–cdl	Mandibular ramus	68 ± 5	62 ± 5
	go–gn	Mandibular body	86 ± 5	81 ± 4
			Width (mm)	
Single linear frontal	ft–ft	Forehead	116 ± 5	111 ± 4
	zy–zy	Midface	139 ± 5	130 ± 5
	go–go	Lower face	106 ± 7	95 ± 5
			Profile (°)	
Single angular lateral (measured from the vertical)	tr–g	Forehead	−10 ± 4	−6 ± 5
	g–sn	Middle face	2 ± 3	2 ± 3
	g–ls	Middle face (Leiber's line)	1 ± 4	2 ± 3
	sn–pg	Lower face	−11 ± 5	−13 ± 5
	li–pg	Mandible	−15 ± 7	−19 ± 7
	g–pg	General	−3 ± 3	−4 ± 3
(After Farkas et al. 1994,[7] with permission.)				

Table 1.2 Craniofacial complex measurements useful for evaluating the face

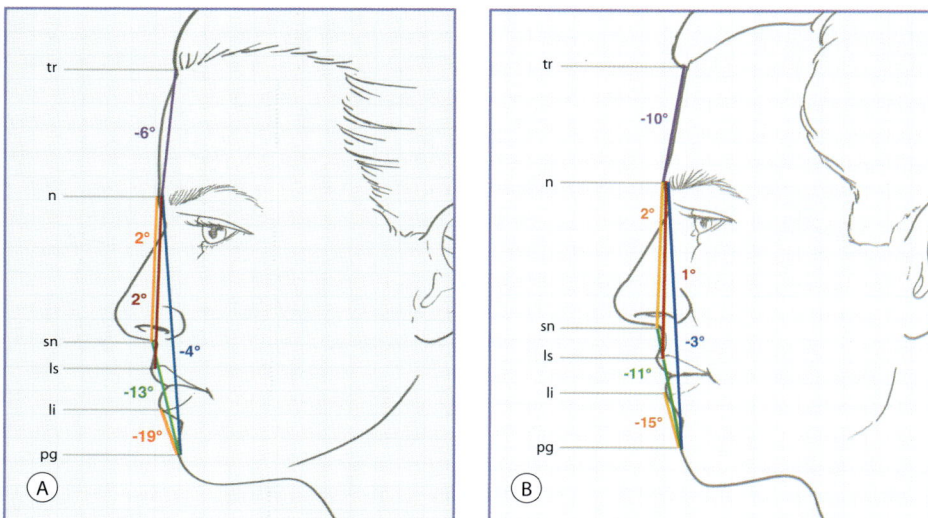

Figure 1.21 Lateral views of (**A**) female and (**B**) male faces drawn from average anthropometric measurements for 21-year-old North American white persons, showing profile inclinations. See Table 1.1 for definitions.

These objective data identify the sexual dimorphism in human faces. On average, all facial measurements are greater in men than in women. In addition, the relations between measurements differ in men and women. These differences are pronounced in the lower third of the face. The bigonial distance (go-go) is the transverse facial dimension that has the greatest difference between the sexes. In other words, the lower one-third of women's faces tends to be absolutely and relatively narrower than that of men. Gender-related differences have implications for surgical planning. For example, if a normally dimensioned male mandible is augmented in the transverse dimension, it may be perceived as stronger. However, if a normally dimensioned female mandible is augmented, it may be perceived as masculine.

Anthropometric data aid facial evaluation and surgical planning by describing normal facial measurements and relations. With this framework, the status of the patient is more easily understood and the goals of surgery defined.

Its small dimensions and complex configuration make millimeter differences and changes noticeable and significant in the face. For these reasons, it is important to know the average or 'normal' dimensions of the face and its component features. Implants that are too large create unnatural contours that relate poorly to other areas of the face. Inappropriate implants may therefore upset the balance of the face. Facial implants must be appropriately sized, shaped, and positioned to be effective.

REFERENCES

1. Carr NJ, Rosenberg AE, Yaremchuk MJ. Chondromyxoid fibroma of the zygoma. J Craniofac Surg 1992; 3(4):217–222.
2. Clayton M. Leonardo da Vinci—the divine and the grotesque. London: Royal Collection Enterprises; 2002.
3. Farkas L, Hreczko TA, Kolar JC, et al. Vertical and horizontal proportions of the face in young adult North American Caucasians: revision of neoclassical canons. Plast Reconstr Surg 1985; 75(3):328–338.
4. Farkas LG, Kolar JC. Anthropometrics and art in the aesthetics of women's faces. Clin Plast Surg 1987; 14(4):599–616.
5. Ricketts RM. Divine proportions in facial esthetics. Clin Plast Surg 1982; 9(4):401–422.
6. Etcoff N. Survival of the prettiest. New York: Anchor Books; 2000.
7. Farkas LG, Hreczko TA, Katic MJ. Appendix A. Craniofacial norms in North American Caucasians from birth (one year) to young adulthood. In: Farkas LG, ed. Anthropometry of the head and face. 2nd edn. New York: Raven Press; 1994.
8. Farkas LG, Ngim RCK, Lee ST. Appendix B. Craniofacial norms in 6-, 12-, and 18-year-old Chinese subjects. In: Farkas LG, ed. Anthropometry of the head and face. 2nd edn. New York: Raven Press; 1994.
9. Farkas LG, Venkatadri G, Gubbi AV. Appendix C. Craniofacial norms in young adult African-Americans. In: Farkas LG, ed. Anthropometry of the head and face. 2nd edn. New York: Raven Press; 1994.
10. Farkas LG, Katic MJ, Forrest CR. International anthropometric study of facial morphology in various ethnic groups/races. J Craniofac Surg 2005; 16:615–646.
11. Yaremchuk MJ. Facial skeletal reconstruction using porous polyethylene implants. Plast Reconstr Surg 2003; 111(6):1818–1827.

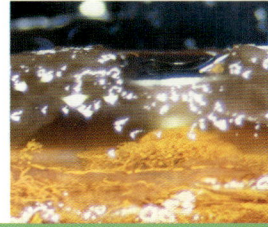

Chapter 2

Implant materials

The craniofacial skeleton is reconstructed with both autogenous bone and alloplastic implants. Alloplastic implants are used only as onlay grafts to the native skeleton to improve facial contour. They are also used to replace missing portions of the non-load-bearing cranial vault and internal orbit. Autogenous bone may also be used for these purposes, but most often it is used to replace segmental, load-bearing defects of the facial skeleton. Virtually all aesthetic facial skeletal augmentation as well as cranial vault replacement is done with alloplastic materials. Three basic categories of alloplastic materials are used in facial reconstruction. Polymers and ceramics are used to replace or augment bone. Metals are used as fixation or support devices.

BONE

Autogenous bone has long been considered the standard material to restore or improve the craniofacial skeleton, because it has the potential to be revascularized and then assimilated into the facial skeleton. In time, it could be biologically indistinguishable from the adjacent native skeleton. These attributes make it ideal and the only material available to reliably reconstruct segmental load-bearing defects of the facial skeleton. When used as an onlay graft, these attributes lead to graft resorption and unreliable augmentation of the facial skeleton.

Factors that impact result

Clinical experience and laboratory investigation have revealed that the fate of non-vascularized onlay bone grafts placed in the craniofacial skeleton depends on three interrelated factors: the architecture of the graft, its revascularization, and the recipient site.

Graft architecture and revascularization

Onlay grafts harvested from the calvarium are superior to graft harvested from the iliac crest in volume maintenance.[1–8] This difference was initially attributed to the embryonic origin of the graft, prompting use of the terms *membranous* and *endochondral* grafts as opposed to the anatomical terms *calvarial* and *iliac crest* grafts. Kusiak et al. reported from the University of Pennsylvania Plastic Surgery Laboratories that calvarial bone grafts become revascularized earlier than iliac grafts, and attributed this volume maintenance to their early revascularization.[1] However, this explanation was questioned when Lin et al.[7] and Sullivan et al.[8] reported more extensive revascularization in iliac crest grafts.

I participated in Kant Lin's study[7] during my craniofacial fellowship at the University of Pennsylvania. Lin evaluated the volume persistence of calvarial and iliac crest grafts fixed to the rabbit snout with lag screws (Fig. 2.1). While reviewing histologic sections during that study, we noted that early revascularization of the grafts occurred only in the cancellous portion of both grafts. In fact, it appeared that the cortical portion of both grafts acted as a mechanical barrier to ingrowing blood vessels (Fig. 2.2). This observation prompted Neil Chen's study at the Massachusetts General Hospital a few years later.[9]

Using a model similar to Lin's,[7] Chen et al.[9] also evaluated the volume persistence of calvarial and iliac crest grafts fixed to the rabbit snout with lag screws. In addition, he correlated graft revascularization and graft resorption with graft architecture in the cortical and cancellous regions of both calvarial

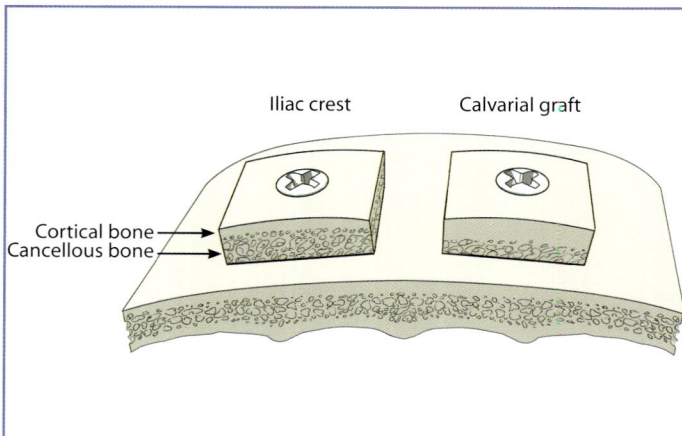

Figure 2.1 Placement of iliac crest and calvarial onlay bone grafts on the snout of the rabbit.

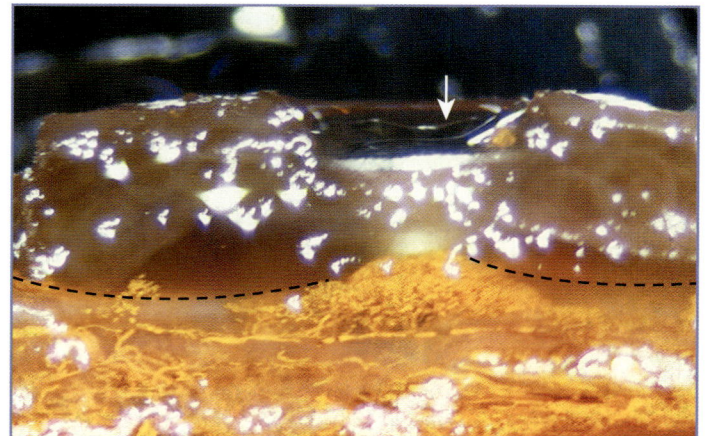

Figure 2.2 Latex vascular cast injection of 6-week onlay bone graft harvested from the calvarium and fixed to the snout of its rabbit host with a lag screw (× 5). Arrow points to lag screw. Broken line separates cortical layer (above) from cancellous layer (below). Note that the vessels (yellow dye) penetrate only the cancellous portions of the graft. (From Chen et al. 1994,[9] with permission.)

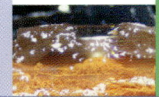

and iliac grafts. Revascularization was evaluated using latex vascular cast injection, while osteoclastic activity was evaluated using a tartrate-resistant acid phosphatase stain. As expected, he found that at 70 days the calvarial grafts demonstrated greater volume maintenance than the iliac bone (72% versus 32%, $P < 0.025$). He found significantly greater revascularization and osteoclastic activity in the cancellous portion of both the calvarial and iliac crest bone grafts by the 10th day after onlay grafting. Minimal activities were present in the cortical bone (Figs 2.3 and 2.4). Because calvarial grafts contain more cortical bone, the superior volume maintenance can be understood by the influence of bone architecture on revascularization and resorption. Cortical bone is more slowly revascularized, and therefore less available to osteoclastic activity. The amount of cortical bone in an onlay graft determines its volume maintenance. The importance of graft architecture, as opposed to its embryologic origin, to the volume persistence of onlay bone grafts has been supported in later studies by Gosain.[10,11]

PEARL

The revascularization of onlay bone grafts makes them susceptible to osteoclast activity and hence resorption with volume loss.

PEARL

Because cortical bone is less easily revascularized than cancellous bone, onlay grafts with proportionately more cortical bone (e.g. calvarial grafts) will maintain their volume longer than grafts with proportionately more cancellous bone (e.g. iliac grafts).

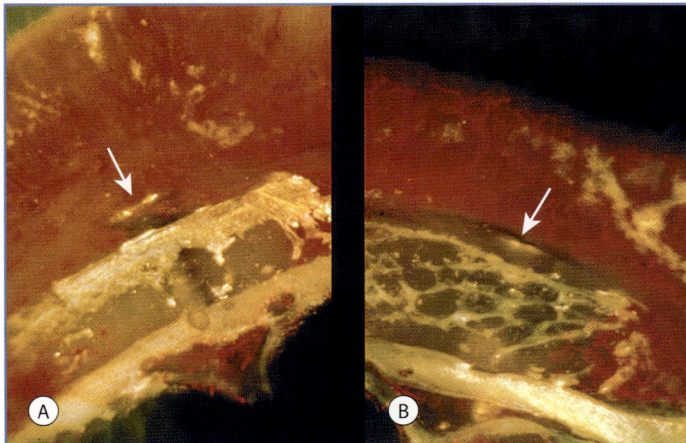

Figure 2.3 Latex vascular cast injection of (**A**) the 10-day calvarial graft and (**B**) the 10-day iliac crest graft (× 10). The orientation is similar to that shown in Figure 2.1. Arrows point to lag screws. Note that the blood vessels (red dye) penetrate only the cancellous portions of the graft. (From Chen et al. 1994,[9] with permission.)

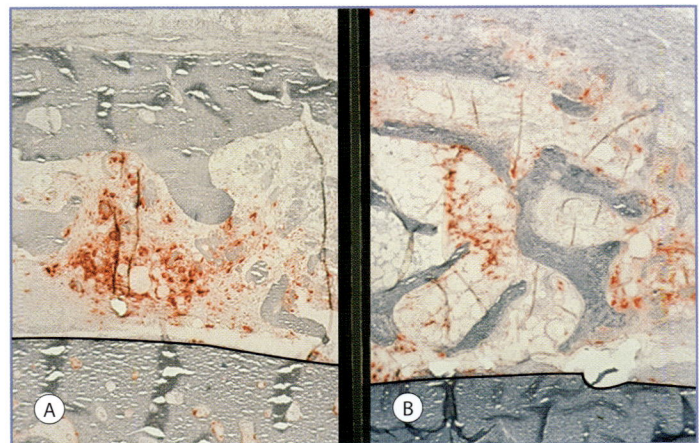

Figure 2.4 Tartrate-resistant acid phosphatase (TRAP) histochemical stain of the osteoclastic activity of 10-day (**A**) calvarial and (**B**) iliac crest grafts (both × 50). There was significant osteoclastic activity (red dye) in the cancellous areas of the grafts but minimal activity in the cortex. Solid line separates onlay graft from snout. TRAP stain penetration mimics that of vascular penetration shown in Figure 2.3. (From Chen et al. 1994,[9] with permission.)

Rigid fixation

Chen's study also explained the observation of others that rigid fixation improves graft volume maintenance.[3,6,7] Lag screw fixation obliterates the gap between the graft and the recipient bed, and therefore may reduce neovascularization of the graft at this interface. Rigid fixation may therefore improve the volume maintenance of onlay bone grafts by limiting, rather than facilitating, revascularization of the graft.[9]

Recipient site

The volume maintenance of a bone graft depends on where it is placed. Zins et al. originally proposed that bone grafts placed in depository fields on the growing facial skeleton would have improved volume maintenance.[12] Gosain et al., using an adult animal model, recently found complete or near complete resorption of onlay bone grafts over 1 year (despite the use of rigid fixation and irrespective of their depository or resorptive recipient beds).[13] Rather than its embryologic role in facial growth, the recipient site impacts the fate of a bone graft by the functional stresses it places on the graft. These stresses are determined by regional musculoskeletal forces and by deforming forces of the overlying soft tissue envelope.

The description of this phenomenon is attributed to the German anatomist Julius Wolff and has long been referred to as Wolff's law. It was described for the axial skeleton but is equally applicable to the craniofacial skeleton. When used as an interposition or inlay graft to fill a defect in a location with significant musculoskeletal forces acting on it, for example the mandible, functional stresses will result in the graft's eventual remodeling into a size and shape similar to the segment it is replacing. When the bone replaced provides a more protective function with little stress on it, for example the cranial vault, the graft loses volume due to osteolysis, as well as revascularization and osteoclastic resorption. Similarly, the volume persistence of onlay bone grafts will be determined by the musculoskeletal forces working on them and the deforming forces of the overlying soft tissue envelope.

In summary, the fate of an onlay bone graft is unpredictable[13] but depends on its revascularization and factors that impact its subsequent remodeling. If a bone graft does not become revascularized, it acts like a sequestrum, which remains inert and can maintain its volume indefinitely.[14] This realization prompted my use of certain alloplastic materials to replace or augment the facial skeleton. The use of alloplastic materials also has the advantage of avoiding the morbidity, time, and cost associated with autogenous graft harvest.

> **PEARL**
>
> After a bone graft is revascularized, its volume will be determined by functional stresses.

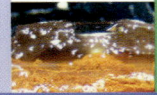

ALLOPLASTIC MATERIALS

Virtually all aesthetic facial skeletal augmentation is done with alloplastic materials. The use of synthetic material avoids donor area morbidity while vastly simplifying the procedure in terms of time and complexity. Implant materials used for facial skeletal augmentation are biocompatible; that is, they have an acceptable reaction between the material and the host. In general, the host has little or no enzymatic ability to degrade the implant, with the result that the implant tends to maintain its volume and shape. Likewise, the implant has a minimal and predictable effect on the host tissue that surrounds it. This type of relationship is an advantage over the use of autogenous bone or cartilage which, when revascularized, will be remodeled to varying degrees, thereby changing volume and shape.

The alloplastic implants presently used for facial reconstruction have not shown any toxic effects on the host.[15] The host responds to these materials by forming a fibrous capsule around the implant, which is the body's way of isolating the implant from the host. The most important implant characteristic that determines the nature of the encapsulation is the implant's surface characteristics. Smooth implants result in the formation of smooth-walled capsules (Fig. 2.5). Porous implants allow varying degrees of soft tissue ingrowth, which results in a less dense capsule (Fig. 2.6).

Animal studies have demonstrated that implant pore sizes of more than 100 μm encourage tissue ingrowth.[16–18] Pore sizes of less than 100 μm limit tissue ingrowth, wherea materials with large pore sizes (>300 μm) have drawbacks associated with material breakdown.[19,20] It is a clinical observation that porous implants, as a result of fibrous tissue ingrowth, have less tendency to erode underlying bone, to migrate, due to soft tissue mechanical forces, and perhaps to be less susceptible to infection when challenged with an inoculum of bacteria.

PEARL

The surface characteristics of an implant influence the surrounding soft tissue response to the implant. Smooth-surfaced implants induce denser capsule formation than porous implants.

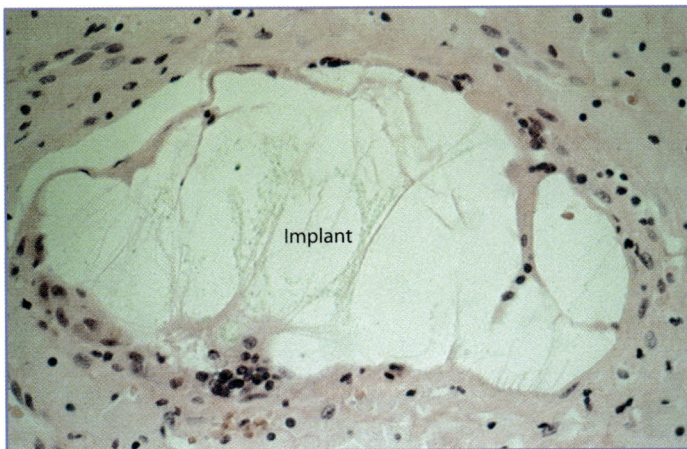

Figure 2.5 Connective tissue forming a capsule around a smooth-surfaced polymethylmethacrylate implant (original magnification, × 400; hematoxylin and eosin stain). (From Rubin and Yaremchuk 1997,[15] with permission.)

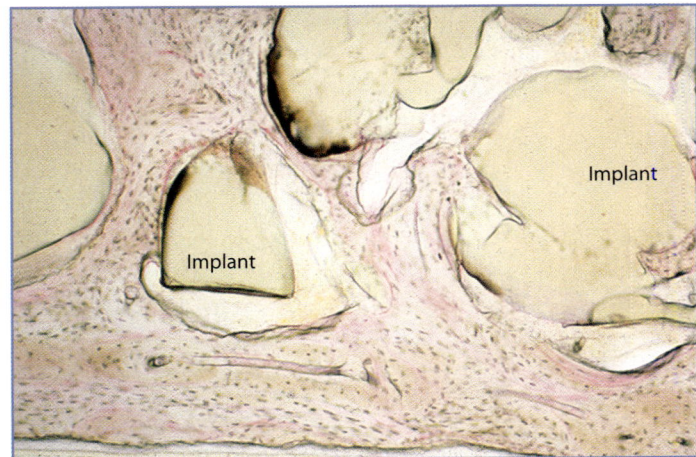

Figure 2.6 Tissue ingrowth into a porous polyethylene implant (original magnification, × 100; hematoxylin and eosin stain). (From Rubin and Yaremchuk 1997,[15] with permission.)

Three basic categories of alloplastic materials are used in facial reconstruction. Polymers and ceramics are used to replace or augment bone. Metals are used as fixation or support devices.

Metals

The three types of metals currently used as fixation devices are stainless steel, cobalt–chromium alloy (Vitallium), and titanium (either pure titanium or as an alloy with aluminum and vanadium). Titanium has largely replaced the other two metals for craniofacial use because of its high strength and reduced artifact on computed tomography and magnetic resonance imaging studies.[21–23]

Polymers

Polymers are long molecules composed of repeating subunits. Structure of the subunit, chain length, and cross-links all determine the physical properties of the material. Eppley has summarized the attributes of these materials.[24]

Polysiloxane (silicone)

Polysiloxane is a polymer created from interlinking silicone and oxygen [$S_1O(CH_3)_2$] with methyl side groups, and as such is the only non-carbon chain polymer used in medical implantation. Solid silicone or the silicone rubber used for facial implants is a vulcanized form of polysiloxane.

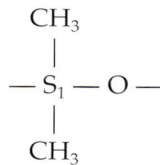

$$\begin{array}{c} CH_3 \\ | \\ - S_1 - O - \\ | \\ CH_3 \end{array}$$

Solid silicone has the following advantages: it can be sterilized by steam or irradiation, it can be carved with either a pair of scissors or a scalpel, and it can be stabilized with a screw or a suture. Because it is smooth, it can be removed quite easily. Disadvantages include the tendency to cause resorption of the bone underlying it, particularly when used to augment the chin; the potential to migrate if not fixed; and the potential for its fibrous capsule to be visible when placed under a thin soft tissue cover. Figure 2.7 shows examples of silicone malar and chin implants.

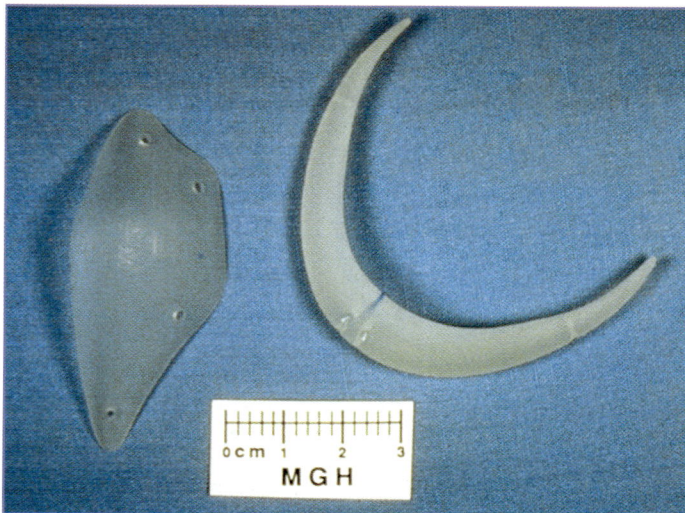

Figure 2.7 Examples of silicone malar (left) and chin (right) implants. These implants have a smooth surface and are relatively flexible, depending on the thickness of the implant.

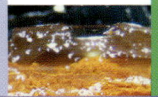

Polytetrafluoroethylene

Polytetrafluoroethylene (PTFE), Gore-Tex (W.L. Gore, Flagstaff, Arizona), has a carbon-ethylene backbone to which are attached four fluorine molecules.

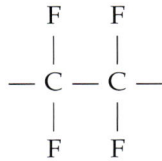

$$
\begin{array}{c}
FF \\
|| \\
-\,C\,-\,C\,- \\
|| \\
FF
\end{array}
$$

It is very chemically stable, has a non-adherent surface and, because it is not cross-linked, is very flexible. There is extensive experience with the use of this material for vascular prostheses, soft tissue patches, and sutures. A variety of preformed implants are available for both subdermal and subperiosteal placement. Preformed implants are made with a pore size between 10 and 30 μm, which allows for some soft tissue ingrowth. However, it is smooth enough to be maneuvered easily through soft tissues. This material can be fixed to underlying structures with sutures or screws. It is easily sterilized. Figure 2.8 shows examples of PTFE implants.

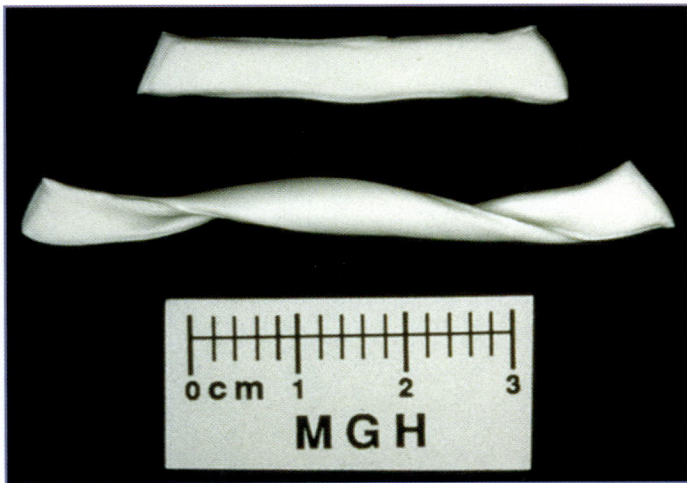

Figure 2.8 Examples of polytetrafluoroethylene (Gore-Tex) implants. These implants are the softest and most flexible of the commonly used facial implants. For this reason, some surgeons use them to augment soft tissue contours. Their small pore size allows minimal surface ingrowth of soft tissues.

Acrylic

Acrylic is used in cranioplasty procedures for filling full-thickness cranial defects, or in forehead-contouring procedures. Acrylic biomaterials are made from polymerized esters of either acrylic or methyl acrylic acids (methylmethacrylate). Acrylic implants have smooth surfaces, are strong, and are inflexible.

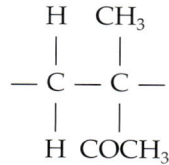

$$
\begin{array}{ccc}
\mathrm{H} & & \mathrm{CH_3} \\
| & & | \\
-\mathrm{C} & - & \mathrm{C}- \\
| & & | \\
\mathrm{H} & & \mathrm{COCH_3}
\end{array}
$$

The most commonly used material for skull reconstruction is polymethylmethacrylate (PMMA). PMMA is radiolucent and therefore does not affect postoperative imaging. It is unaffected by temperature and is strong. When used for full-thickness defects, it can fill intracranial dead space—a problem with bone cranioplasty. When used as an onlay, bony overcorrection can compensate for overlying soft tissue deficiencies, resulting in a smooth skin surface contour. Because it is encapsulated by the host rather than incorporated by surrounding soft tissues, PMMA is believed by some to be more susceptible to infection and late complications. Cranioplasty kits are available that contain a single dose of 30 g of powdered polymer and 17 mL of liquid monomer. The elements are mixed with a spatula in a bowl. Doughing time varies with the temperature and is about 5 min at 22°C (72°F). Figure 2.9 shows the liquid monomer and powdered polymer prior to mixing.

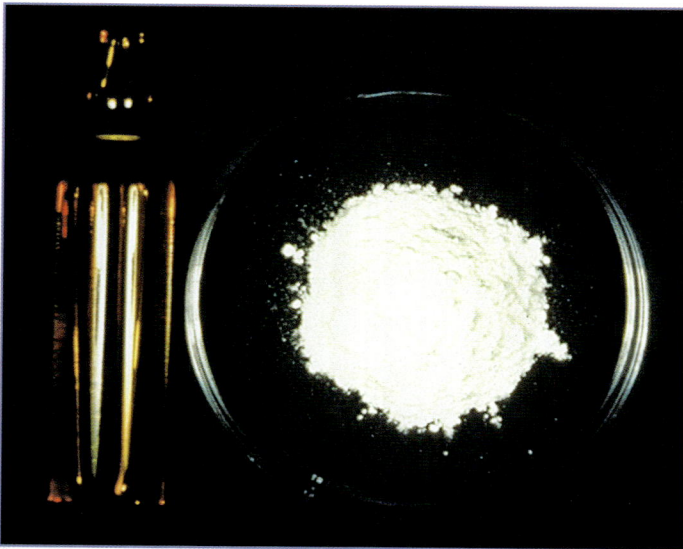

Figure 2.9 Example of a polymethylmethacrylate cranioplasty kit, with the liquid monomer on the left and the powdered polymer on the right. The implants resulting after polymerization are smooth, hard, and strong.

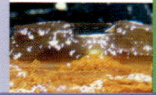

Polyethylene

Polyethylene is a simple carbon chain of ethylene monomer. The high-density, porous variety —Medpor (Porex, Fairburn, Georgia)—is used for facial implants because of its higher tensile strength.

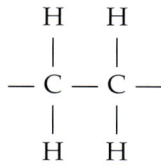

$$-\;\overset{\displaystyle H}{\underset{\displaystyle H}{\overset{|}{\underset{|}{C}}}}\;-\;\overset{\displaystyle H}{\underset{\displaystyle H}{\overset{|}{\underset{|}{C}}}}\;-$$

Polyethylene, although chemically similar to PTFE, has a much firmer consistency, resisting material compression while still permitting some flexibility. In addition to being firmer than PTFE, it has an intramaterial porosity between 125 and 250 μm, which allows more extensive fibrous ingrowth than with Gore-Tex. The porosity of Medpor has both advantages and disadvantages. The advantages of porous polyethylene include its tendency to allow extensive soft tissue ingrowth, thereby lessening its tendency to migrate and to erode underlying bone. Its firm consistency allows it to be easily fixed with screws and contoured with a scalpel or power equipment without fragmenting. However, its porosity causes soft tissue to adhere to it, making placement more difficult and requiring larger pockets to be made than with smoother implants. The soft tissue ingrowth also makes implant removal more difficult than with smooth-surfaced implants.

Polyethylene is the implant material of choice for this author. A porous polyethylene implant is shown in Figure 2.10.

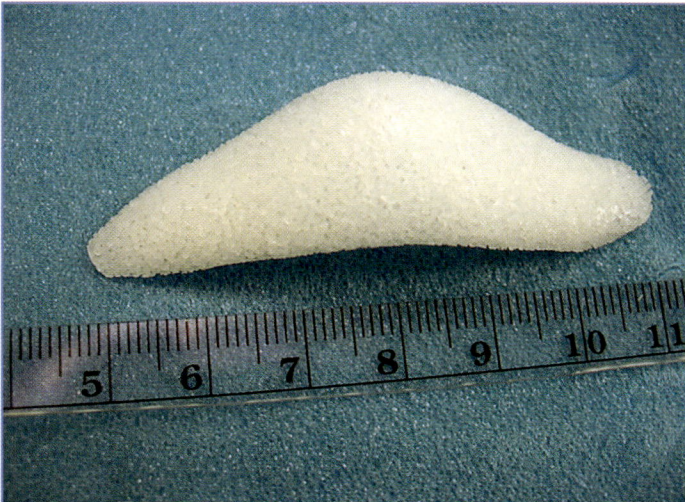

Figure 2.10 Example of a porous polyethylene (Medpor) implant. These implants are bendable, depending on their thickness, and are adaptable to the facial skeleton. They have a pore size that allows some soft tissue ingrowth.

Polymethylmethacrylate–polyhydroxylethylmethacrylate

HTR (Walter Lorenz Surgical, Inc., Jacksonville, Florida) derives its name from the acronym for hard tissue replacement. It is a porous composite of PMMA and polyhydroxylethylmethacrylate that allows some soft tissue ingrowth. A calcium hydroxide coating imparts a negative surface charge to encourage bony ingrowth and deter adhesion of bacteria to the implant.[25] Unlike Gore-Tex and Medpor, HTR is not flexible. Examples of HTR implants are shown in Figure 2.11.

Ceramics

Ceramic materials are usually heated to high temperatures (sintered) to fuse their crystal-like components.

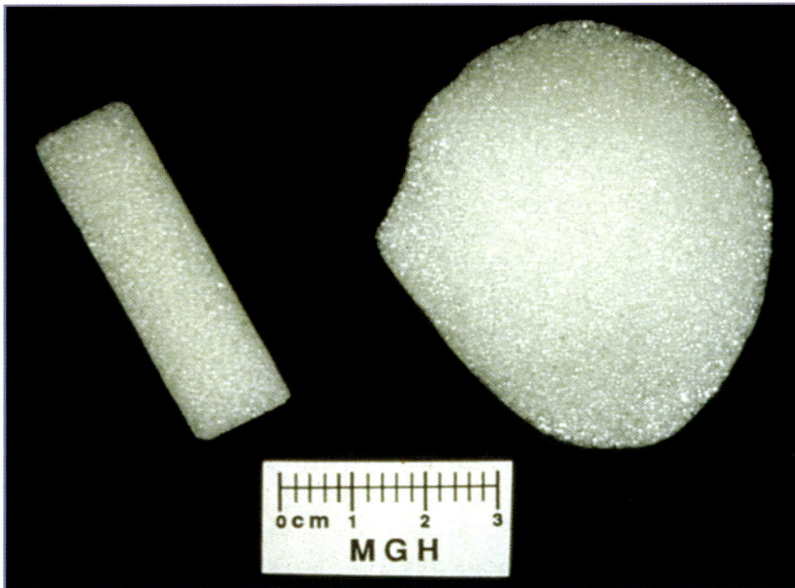

Figure 2.11 Examples of HTR implants. These implants are rigid. They have a pore size that allows some soft tissue ingrowth.

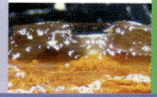

Hydroxyapatite

The ceramic material most commonly used in craniofacial surgery is hydroxyapatite. Hydroxyapatite is a calcium phosphate salt found as a major component of bone matrix. Dense hydroxyapatite can be produced synthetically. Porous hydroxyapatite can be entirely synthetic, or formed by chemically converting the naturally porous calcium carbonate skeleton of marine coral.

Unlike the other biomaterials presented in this chapter, which have no osteo-activity, calcium phosphates have the theoretic advantage of being osteoinductive and osteoconductive. Osteoinduction is the ability of the biomaterial to initiate osteogenesis without ingrowth from adjacent bone. Osteoconduction is the ability for the biomaterial to act as a bridge for the ingrowth of bone from an adjacent osseous bed. These attributes have been shown experimentally[26,27] but have not demonstrated clinical relevance in the craniofacial skeleton.

Porous hydroxyapatite is available as granules for injection and as blocks. The blocks are brittle. Although hydroxyapatite is osteoactive and has the potential to be replaced by bone, this has been an inconsistent clinical finding. A hydroxyapatite block is shown in Figure 2.12.

Hydroxyapatite is also available in a cement paste that has been advocated as a material to be used for cranioplasty. The cement paste has an advantage over the ceramic form in that it can be shaped during surgery. To date, there is no histologic evidence of significant bone ingrowth or resorption of this material in humans over a follow-up period of up to 3 years.[24] These findings are consistent with results from animal studies.[28,29]

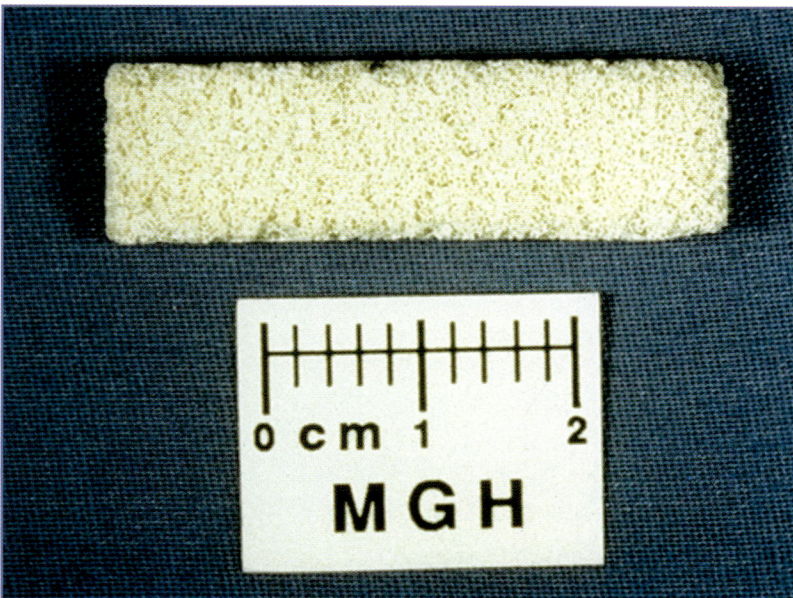

Figure 2.12 Example of a hydroxyapatite block. These implants are brittle.

AUTHOR'S PREFERRED IMPLANT MATERIALS

All the facial implant materials described in the above section have chemical composition and biostability providing appropriate biocompatibility for clinical use. This author has personal experience with all these materials. It is my preference to use titanium fixation devices because, unlike stainless steel and Vitallium, titanium causes little artifact distortion on computed tomography and magnetic resonance images.[21–23] I have used PMMA for cranioplasty because it is strong, is stable, and can conform to any required contour. It is my preference to perform facial skeletal implant augmentation with porous polyethylene because of its handling and surface characteristics. The rationale for the use of this material is expanded below.

Porous polyethylene (Medpor) is firm and flexible. It is easily carved with a scalpel or contoured with a rasp or motorized burr. It can be immobilized with sutures or, with my preference, screws. It can be molded to the external contours of the skeleton by heating it in water, although I prefer not to take advantage of this attribute.

The favorable biocompatibility of this implant material can also be attributed to its porous surface. Porous polyethylene has pores of sufficient size to allow fibrous tissue ingrowth and relative host incorporation, as opposed to the host encapsulation observed with smooth-surfaced implants. Porous polyethylene has a continuous system of inner connecting pores approximately 100–250 µm in diameter. Animal studies have demonstrated that pore sizes of more than 100 µm encourage tissue ingrowth.[16,30] Pore sizes of less than 100 µm limit the extent of tissue ingrowth, whereas materials with large pore sizes have drawbacks associated with material breakdown.[18–20]

Clinical specimens demonstrated rapid ingrowth of fibrous tissue after human implantation. Rather than the dense connective tissue capsules observed with smooth-surfaced implants, porous polyethylene implants exhibited a thin connective tissue membrane that was contiguous with the ingrown tissue.[31] It was noted during revisional operations that fibrous tissue ingrowth was sufficient to result in bleeding when the implants were modified in situ with a scalpel, and in certain circumstances ingrowth exhibited sufficient vascularity to allow skin grafts to be placed directly over the implant.[31]

Fibrous tissue ingrowth improves the biocompatibility of porous implants because it limits their movement. Movement is an essential factor in determining the host response to an implant.[20] Because the host foreign body reaction encapsulates smooth-surfaced implants, a smooth implant never binds to the host bed and therefore is predisposed to move. Encapsulation of smooth implants and their subsequent predisposition to movement are directly or indirectly responsible for the majority of the late complications observed with smooth implants. These complications include the tendency of smooth implants placed in the orbital floor to migrate and distort the eyelids;[32–35] cause hemorrhage;[36–40] obstruct the lacrimal system;[41,42] or erode into the maxillary sinus, acting as a nidus for infection.[43,44] The rapid tissue ingrowth and mucosalization of porous polyethylene implants, as observed in animal studies designed to stimulate orbital floor reconstruction,[45] immobilizes these implants, which explains why these complications have not been reported with the use of porous polyethylene.

When used to augment the chin, smooth silicone implants are known to cause significant bone resorption, which is attributed to implant motion caused by the overlying mentalis muscle.[46,47] Although it is usually not clinically apparent, bone resorption accompanying silicone chin implantation may be severe enough to result in tooth root erosion among patients with excessive mentalis muscle contraction.[48] I believe that smooth implant migration is the reason for implant malpositioning in certain clinical instances. Animal studies have demonstrated that porous implants result in less bone resorption than do smooth implants.[49] Bikhazi and Van Antwerp, in a prospective cephalometric study of five patients undergoing chin augmentation with porous polyethylene implants, did not observe bone resorption beneath the implants.[50] When I removed cheek implants at 6 months, and chin and mandibular implants at 1 year, the erosion was barely perceptible.

MORBIDITY AND COMPLICATIONS ASSOCIATED WITH ALLOPLASTIC IMPLANTS

General considerations
Carcinogenicity and systemic disease
The induction of malignancy or injury to organs or organ systems is a potential concern of foreign materials implanted into the human body. Clinical observation suggests that the risk of cancer with metal or polymer implant devices is extremely low. An English language literature review conducted in 1997 revealed only one case of a tumor associated with a facial implant.[15] The histology of this tumor showed squamous cell cancer rather than sarcoma, making the implant–tumor connection less clear.

Implanted metals are known to corrode and release metal ions.[51–57] Accumulation of metal ions has been found adjacent to metal fixation devices.[51,52] The corrosion process can result in a local fibroblastic tissue reaction[53,54] that has been implicated in implant failure in long bone fixation devices.[55,56] Postmortem studies have found accumulations of metal productions in regional lymph nodes, liver, and spleen.[57] Despite the documented spread of degradable products from metal implants, no direct association between implant corrosion products and systemic disease has been drawn.[15]

There are scant data to support a connection between polymer implants and carcinogenicity or systemic disease. Five cases of sarcoma associated with Dacron vascular prostheses (latency 6 months to 5 years) appear in the literature.[58,59] No cases of cancer have been reported in association with the polymer craniofacial implants.

The large clinical experience of breast augmentation provides the best information supporting a lack of correlation between connective tissue disease and silicone implant material. Gabriel et al. investigated the risk of connective tissue disease in 749 women with breast implants observed for an average of 7.8 years.[60] In another study, Sanchez-Guerrero et al. studied 1183 members of the Nurse Health Study Cohort with breast implants observed for an average of 9.9 years.[61] Both studies found no increased risk for connective tissue diseases after silicone breast augmentation.

Hypersensitivity

An uncommon reaction to metal implants is a type 4 (cell-mediated) hyper-sensitivity reaction resulting in pain, non-union of bone, and overlying dermatitis. This has been reported with Vitallium[62,63] and stainless steel,[64–66] and suggested for titanium.[67–69] In maxillofacial use, hypersensitivity reactions have been noted with the use of stainless steel wire[70,71] and plates.[72] Sensitivity is often confirmed by patch testing, and removal of the implant resulted in resolution of symptoms in all reports.

True hypersensitivity reactions to prefabricated polymer implants are almost unheard of. The free monomer of PMMA, however, has been noted to cause asthmatic reactions in operating room staff during surgical procedures. A high concentration of vaporized monomer during the curing process can affect sensitized individuals, especially if the room is not properly ventilated.[73]

Specific implant complications

We reviewed nearly 200 clinical studies reporting series of patients with implantable biomaterials in the face.[15] Studies that failed to provide information concerning both the total number of patients and the specific number of complications encountered were excluded. Complication rates were then extracted from the remaining papers and entered into a computer database. The data were tabulated, and weighted averages by sampling size were calculated for different complications of materials used in various applications. Wherever possible, complication rates from studies describing use of a single material at various sites were separated by implant site. Case reports describing less common complications were collected for discussion but not included in the database or in data tabulations. Only complications related to the implant material itself were included in the data analysis. Poor outcomes relating closely to surgical technique were excluded from the list of implant-related compli-cations. Examples are hematoma, nerve injury, overcorrection of enophthalmos, and placement of improperly sized malar implants. Similarly, patient requests for implant removal because of dissatisfaction or fear of harboring foreign material were also excluded.

The list of designated implant-related complications used for data analysis included infection, fistula, exposure, extrusion, displacement, implant fracture, seroma, persistent edema, prominence, pain, inflammatory reaction, hardware loosening, hypersensitivity, and neoplasm. The last two items on this list occur with sufficient rarity as to not play a significant role in analysis of data from these clinical studies. Moreover, certain complications arising by a similar process were grouped together for simplicity; these include infection/fistula and exposure/extrusion. It is difficult to attribute many of the complications listed above solely to the implant material itself. There is much overlap between surgical technique, host response, and potential toxicity of the implant. For example, widely differing perioperative antibiotic regimens combined with varying attention to aspects of technique can influence infection rates for a given material and site. The incidence of displacement of an implant can be influenced by variation in the method of mechanical fixation. One can also argue that pain and prominence are often due to technical factors. Nevertheless, we attempted to exclude those complications obviously due to surgical technique and include those for which the characteristics of the material could play an important role.

Studies assessing polymeric and ceramic implants at mixed sites

Polymers have been used as an implant material in plastic surgery for many decades. One of the longest retrospective studies on the use of polyethylene is a 32-year experience published by Rubin.[74] He reported an 89% success rate from mixed implant sites including malar, nose, mandible, skull, and orbital floor. This study attests to the long-term stability of implantable devices. His custom-made dense polyethylene implants have no modern commercial equivalent, however, and data from this work were not tabulated with results from other studies using standard porous polyethylene devices.

Silicone has been a widely used implant material. Seven studies, describing 239 patients,[75–81] reveal an infection rate of 3.8% and an exposure/extrusion rate of 2.9% for mixed facial implant sites. Porous polyethylene enjoyed a much lower infection rate (0.9%) and almost no displacement.[82–85] Hydroxyapatite had a favorable infection rate of 2.7%, but also carried a 2% incidence of prominence.[86–89] Expanded PTFE had an infection rate of 2.2%.[90–92] Overall, the infection rate for polymeric and ceramic implants at mixed sites was 3.0% in 939 patients reviewed. These data are summarized in Table 2.1.

Complication rates for polymer and ceramic materials at mixed sites						
	Implant material					
	Silicone	Porous polyethylene	Proplast	Hydroxyapatite	Expanded PTFE	Overall
No. of studies reviewed	7	4	2	4	3	20
No. reporting follow-up time	6	3	2	4	2	17
Range of follow-up times	1 month–13 years	3 months–3 years	13 months–6 years	6 months–5 years	Up to 30 months	–
No. reporting no implant-related complications	2	1	1	1	0	5
Total number of patients	239	216	41	150	273	919
Average complication rates (%)						
Infection	3.8	0.9	14.6	2.7	2.2	3.0
Exposure/extrusion	2.9	0.5	0	0	0.7	1.2
Displacement	4.6	0	0	3.3	0	1.7
Seroma	0	0.9	0	0	0	<0.5
Persistent edema	0.8	0	0	0	0	<0.5
Prominence	0	0	0	2.0	0	<0.5
Inflammatory reaction	0	0	0	0	1.8	0.5
Implants removed due to implant-related complications	11.7	0.5	14.6	1.3	1.8	4.6

PTFE, polytetrafluoroethylene.
(After Rubin and Yaremchuk 1997,[15] with permission.)

Table 2.1 Complication rates for polymer and ceramic materials at mixed sites

Clinical series and case reports can provide useful information about factors that contribute to morbidity with implants. Implant composition is one such factor. Given that several biomaterials are well tolerated in the human body, the actual chemical structure of an implant is important only to the degree that it influences the consistency and surface characteristics of the finished device. For example, porous forms of polyethylene and PTFE are extruded from the orbital floor much less frequently than smooth-surfaced nylon implants. The ingrowth of tissue helps fix the porous implant in place. Moreover, experimental data suggest that the presence of host defenses within the implant can decrease the risk of infections.

Implant site is clearly related to morbidity. Complication rates are lowest in the chin and malar regions, and highest in the nose and ear, where the soft tissue cover is thin and often under tension from the implanted device (Fig. 2.13).

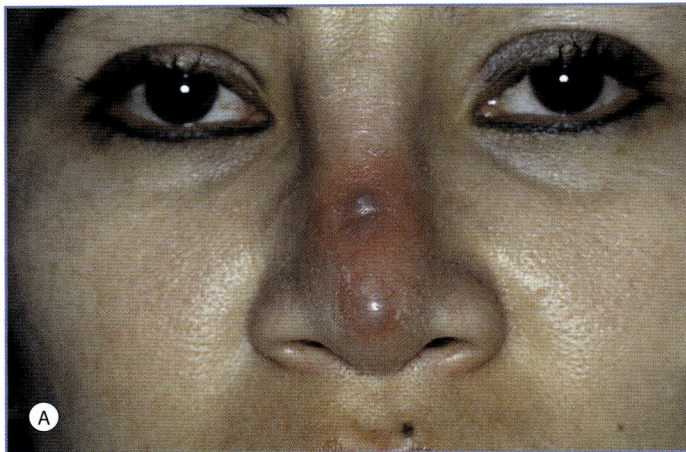

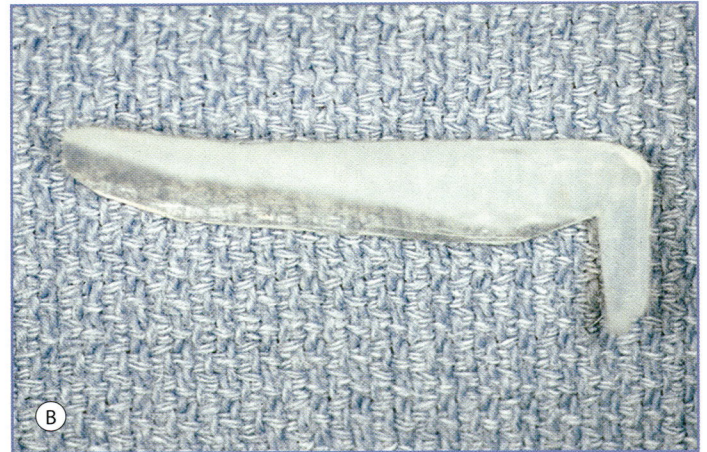

Figure 2.13 Clinical example of a large alloplastic nasal implant creating tension on the overlying soft tissues, resulting in erosion of the soft tissues and extrusion of the implant. This not uncommon scenario grounds the argument that alloplastic implants are inappropriate for use in the face. This complication reflects an error in judgment by the surgeon rather than a fundamental problem in the material properties of the implant. (**A**) Appearance at presentation. (**B**) The implant after removal.

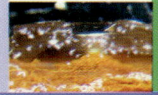

Limitations of clinical series

One striking feature of clinical studies reporting on the use of biomaterials is the variation in follow-up times. Nearly all studies observe patients through the early postoperative period, but early results may mean little for implants placed under load or beneath a thin soft tissue cover.

Using the body of literature to understand implant complications has limitations. First, one must assume that complication rates published in the literature reflect the actual experiences of most surgeons. This may not be true. Some clinicians may be reluctant to publish a series with poor results. In addition, patients with implant failures may be treated by other physicians while being lost to follow-up by the primary surgeon. The importance of careful follow-up and accurate reporting by surgeons cannot be overstressed. Second, one must be cautious when comparing data on implant complications averaged from a number of retrospective studies. This type of analysis suggests trends in complication rates with different materials at different sites, but is not a truly accurate way of comparing materials. Adequate comparison of implant materials would require prospective studies that control for surgical technique, patient selection, and follow-up time. The data derived in this review are most useful when the number of patients in each group is large, and when great differences in complication rates are seen between groups. For example, an infection rate of 1.4% for all chin implants becomes meaningful when it is based on reports encompassing over 2000 patients.

Personal experience with porous polyethylene implants

In 2003, I reported my personal experience with porous implants used for facial skeletal reconstruction.[93] This was based on an experience with 162 patients operated on over an 11-year period (1990–2001). In this series, no implants were extruded or migrated, formed clinically apparent capsules, or caused symptoms attributable to bioincompatibility. The overall reoperation rate was 10% ($n = 16$), which included operations to remove implants because of acute infection (2%, $n = 3$) or late infection (1%, $n = 1$), or to remove implants causing displeasing contours (2%, $n = 3$).

When reviewing the subsequent 200 patients since that report, there have been three patients with implant-related infections. Two of these patients presented after previous implant surgery that had failed because of infection. The third patient was HIV-positive. Implants are susceptible to bacterial colonization and infection.

The presence of a foreign body decreases the minimal infecting dose of *Staphylococcus aureus* in an animal model, due to impaired bacterial clearance.[94,95] If microorganisms are not eliminated rapidly from an implant surface, they will adhere to the implant initially by non-specific physical forces and then by the formation of biofilms characterized by clustering together in an extracellular matrix attached to the implant.[96] Biofilms protect bacteria from host defenses and antibiotics.

Only aggressive debridement and long-term suppressive therapy have been effective in treating orthopedic implant-related infections. This approach is usually not appropriate in facial implant patients, because both debridement and chronic infection may be deforming in this appearance-conscious population. Because antibiotic treatment alone is usually not successful, facial implant-related infections are treated by implant removal and appropriate wound care. Implants may be replaced in 6–12 months.

There have been no materials-related problems during the ensuing period. This experience is similar to that of others.[97–107]

REFERENCES

1. Kusiak JF, Zins JE, Whitaker LA. The early revascularization of membranous bone. Plast Reconstr Surg 1985; 76(4):510–516.
2. Zins JE, Whitaker LA. Membranous versus endochondral bone: implications for craniofacial reconstruction. Plast Reconstr Surg 1983; 72(6):778–785.
3. LaTrenta GS, McCarthy JG, Breitbart AS, et al. The role of rigid fixation in bone-graft augmentation of the craniofacial skeleton. Plast Reconstr Surg 1989; 84(4):578–588.
4. Phillips JH, Rahn BA. Fixation effects on membranous and endochondral onlay bone graft revascularization and bone deposition. Plast Reconstr Surg 1990; 85(6):891–897.
5. Hardesty RA, Marsh JL. Craniofacial onlay bone grafting: a prospective evaluation of graft morphology, orientation and embryonic origin. Plast Reconstr Surg 1990; 85(1):5–14.
6. Phillips JH, Rahn BA. Fixation effects on membranous and endochondral onlay bone-graft resorption. Plast Reconstr Surg 1988; 82(5):872–877.
7. Lin KY, Bartlett SP, Yaremchuk MJ, et al. The effect of rigid fixation on the survival of onlay bone grafts: an experimental study. Plast Reconstr Surg 1990; 86(3):449–456.
8. Sullivan WG, Szwajkun PR. Revascularization of cranial versus iliac crest bone grafts in the rat. Plast Reconstr Surg 1991; 87(6):1105–1109.
9. Chen NT, Glowacki J, Bucky LP, et al. The roles of revascularization and resorption on the endurance of craniofacial onlay bone grafts in the rabbit. Plast Reconstr Surg 1994; 93(4):714–722.
10. Gosain AK, Persing JA. Symposium: biomaterials in the face—benefits and risks. J Craniofac Surg 1999; 10(5):404–414.
11. Gosain AK. Biomaterials in facial reconstruction. Oper Tech Plast Reconstr Surg 2003; 9:23.
12. Zins JE, Kusiak JF, Whitaker LA, et al. The influence of recipient site on bone grafts to the face. Plast Reconstr Surg 1984; 73(3):371–381.
13. Gosain AK, Riordan PA, Song L, et al. A 1-year study of hydroxyapatite-derived biomaterials in an adult sheep model: III. Comparison with autogenous bone graft for facial augmentation. Plast Reconstr Surg 2005; 116(4):1044–1052.
14. Albreksson T. Repair of bone grafts. A vital microscopic and histological investigation in the rabbit. Scand J Plast Reconstr Surg 1980; 14(1):1–12.
15. Rubin JP, Yaremchuk MJ. Complications and toxicities of implantable biomaterials used in facial reconstructive and aesthetic surgery: a comprehensive review of the literature. Plast Reconstr Surg 1997; 100(5):1336–1353.
16. Klawitter JJ, Bagwell JG, Weinstein AM, et al. An evaluation of bone growth into porous high density polyethylene. J Biomed Mater Res 1976; 10(2):311–323.
17. Spector M, Flemming WW, Sauer BW. Early tissue infiltrates in porous polyethylene implants into bone: a scanning electron microscope study. J Biomed Mater Res 1975; 9(5):537–542.
18. Spector M, Harmon SL, Kreutner A. Characteristics of tissue ingrowth into Proplast and porous polyethylene implants in bone. J Biomed Mater Res 1979; 13(5):677–692.
19. Berghaus A, Mulch G, Handrock M. Porous polyethylene and Proplast: their behavior in a bony bed. Arch Otorhinolaryngol 1984; 240:115–123.
20. Maas CS, Merwin GE, Wilson J, et al. Comparison of biomaterials for facial bone augmentation. Arch Otolaryngol Head Neck Surg 1990; 116(5):551–556.
21. Fiala TGS, Paige KT, Davis TL, et al. Comparison of artifact from craniomaxillofacial internal fixation devices: magnetic resonance imaging. Plast Reconstr Surg 1994; 93(4):725–731.
22. Saxe AW, Doppman JL, Brennan MF. Use of titanium surgical clips to avoid artifacts seen on computed tomography. Arch Surg 1982; 117(7):978–979.
23. Fiala TGS, Novelline RA, Yaremchuk MJ. Comparison of CT imaging artifacts from craniomaxillofacial internal fixation devices. Plast Reconstr Surg 1993; 92(7):1227–1232.
24. Eppley BL. Alloplastic implantation. Plast Reconstr Surg 1999; 104(6):1761–1783.
25. Eppley BL, Sadove AM, German RZ. Evaluation of HTR polymer as a craniomaxillofacial graft material. Plast Reconstr Surg 1990; 86(6):1085–1092.
26. Chiroff R, White E, Weber J. Tissue ingrowth of Replamineform implants. J Biomed Mater Res 1975; 9(4):29–45.
27. Gosain AK, Song L, Riordan P, et al. Part I: a 1-year study of osteoinduction in hydroxyapatite-derived biomaterials in an adult sheep model. Plast Reconstr Surg 2002; 109(2):619–630.

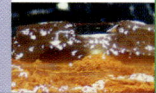

28. Gosain AK. Biomaterials for reconstruction of the cranial vault. Plast Reconstr Surg 2005; 116(2):663–666.
29. Holmes R, Halger H. Porous hydroxyapatite as a bone graft substitute in cranial reconstruction: a histometric study. Plast Reconstr Surg 1988; 81(5):662–671.
30. Spector M, Flemming WR, Sauer BW. Early tissue infiltrate in porous polyethylene implants into bone: a scanning electron microscope study. J Biomed Mater Res 1975; 9(5):537–542.
31. Wellisz T, Kanel G, Anooshian RV. Characteristics of the tissue's response to Medpor porous polyethylene implants in the human facial skeleton. J Long Term Eff Med Implants 1993; 3:223.
32. Wolfe SA. Correction of a persistent lower eyelid deformity caused by a displaced orbital floor implant. Ann Plast Surg 1979; 2(5):448–451.
33. Hoffman S. Loss of a silastic chin implant following a dental infection. Ann Plast Surg 1981; 7(6):484–486.
34. Wolfe SA. Correction of a lower eyelid deformity caused by multiple extrusions of alloplastic orbital floor implants. Plast Reconstr Surg 1981; 68(3):429–432.
35. Brown AE, Banks P. Late extrusion of alloplastic orbital floor implants. Br J Oral Maxillofac Surg 1981; 68:429.
36. Mauriello JA Jr, Flanagan JC, Peyster RG. An unusual late complication of orbital floor fracture repair. Ophthalmology 1984; 91(1):102–107.
37. Davis RM. Late orbital implant migration. Ann Ophthalmol 1986; 18(6):223–224.
38. Loftfield K, Jordan DR, Fowler J, et al. Orbital cyst formation associated with Gelfilm use. Ophthal Plast Reconstr Surg 1987; 3(3):187–191.
39. Sutula FC, Palu RN. Delayed chocolate cyst after blowout fracture. Ophthal Plast Reconstr Surg 1991; 7(4):267–268.
40. Marks MW, Yeatts RP. Hemorrhagic cysts of the orbit as a long-term complication of prosthetic orbital floor implant. Plast Reconstr Surg 1994; 93(4):856–859.
41. Kohn R, Romano PE, Puklin JE. Lacrimal obstruction after migration of orbital floor implant. Am J Ophthalmol 1976; 82(6):934–936.
42. Mauriello JA Jr, Fiore PM, Kotch M. Dacryocystitis: late complication of orbital floor fracture repair with implant. Ophthalmology 1987; 94(3):248–250.
43. Anderson MF. Sinusitis related to use of foreign materials to treat orbital floor injuries. Report of two cases. J Oral Surg 1967; 25:182.
44. Peak J, Haria S, Sleeman D. Facial pain due to a displaced orbital floor implant: report of case. J Oral Maxillofac Surg 1992; 50(11):1234–1235.
45. Dougherty WR, Wellisz T. The natural history of alloplastic implants and orbital floor reconstruction: an animal model. J Craniofac Surg 1994; 5(1):26–32.
46. Robinson M. Bone resorption under plastic chin implants. Arch Otolaryngol 1972; 95:30.
47. Friedland JA, Coccaro PJ, Converse JM. Retrospective cephalometric analysis of mandibular bone absorption under silicone rubber chin implants. Plast Reconstr Surg 1976; 57(2):144–151.
48. Matarasso A, Elias AC, Elias RL. Labial incompetence: a marker for progressive bone resorption in silastic chin augmentation. Plast Reconstr Surg 1996; 98(6):1007–1014.
49. Wellisz T, Lawrence M, Jazayeri MA, et al. The effects of alloplastic onlays on bone in the rabbit mandible. Plast Reconstr Surg 1995; 96(4):957–963.
50. Bikhazi HB, Van Antwerp R. The use of Medpor in cosmetic and reconstructive surgery: experimental and clinical evidence. In: Stucker FJ, ed. Plastic and reconstructive surgery of the head and neck. St. Louis: Mosby; 1990:271–273.
51. Schliephake H, Lehmann H, Kunz U, et al. Ultrastructural findings in soft tissues adjacent to titanium plates used in jaw fracture treatment. Int J Oral Maxillofac Surg 1993; 22(1):20–25.
52. Rosenberg A, Gratz KW, Sailer HF. Should titanium miniplates be removed after bone healing is complete? Int J Oral Maxillofac Surg 1993; 22(3):185–188.
53. Swann M. Malignant soft-tissue tumor at the site of a total hip replacement. J Bone Joint Surg Br 1984; 66(5):629–631.
54. Thomas KA, Cook SD, Haring AF, et al. Tissue reaction to implant corrosion in 38 internal fixation devices. Orthopedics 1988; 11(3):441–451.
55. Byrne JE, Lovasko JH, Laskin DM. Corrosion of metal fracture fixation appliances. J Oral Surg 1973; 31(8):639–645.
56. Cohen J, Wulff J. Clinical failure caused by corrosion of a Vitallium plate. J Bone Joint Surg Am 1972; 54(3):617–628.
57. Case CP, Langkamer VG, James C, et al. Wide-spread dissemination of metal debris from implants. J Bone Joint Surg Br 1994; 76(5):701–712.
58. Herrmann J, Kanhouwa S, Kelley R, et al. Fibrosarcoma of the thigh associated with a prosthetic vascular graft. N Engl J Med 1971; 284(2):91.

59. Burns W, Kanhouwa S, Tillman L, et al. Fibrosarcoma occurring at the site of a plastic vascular graft. Cancer 1972; 29(1):66–72.

60. Gabriel SE, O'Fallon WM, Kurland LT, et al. Risk of connective-tissue diseases and other disorders after breast implantation. N Engl J Med 1994; 330(24):1697–1702.

61. Sanchez-Guerrero J, Colditz G, Karlson E, et al. Silicon breast implants and the risk of connective tissue diseases and symptoms. N Engl J Med 1995; 332(25):1666–1670.

62. McKenzie A, Aitken C, Ridsdill-Smith R. Urticaria after insertion of Smith–Petersen Vitallium nail. Br Med J 1967; 4:36.

63. Halpin DS. An unusual reaction in muscle in association with a Vitallium plate: a report of possible metal hypersensitivity. J Bone Joint Surg Br 1975; 57(4):451–453.

64. Barranco V, Solomon H. Eczematous dermatitis from nickel. JAMA 1972; 220(9):1244.

65. Barranco V, Solomon, H. Eczematous dermatitis caused by internal exposure to nickel. South Med J 1974; 66:447.

66. Cramer M, Lucht U. Metal sensitivity in patients treated for tibial fractures with plates of stainless steel. Acta Orthop Scand 1977; 348:245.

67. Lalor PA, Revell PA, Gray AB, et al. Sensitivity to titanium: a cause of implant failure? J Bone Joint Surg Br 1991; 73(1):25–28.

68. Lalor PA, Gray AB, Wright S, et al. Contact sensitivity to titanium in a hip prosthesis? Contact Dermatitis 1990; 23(3):193–194.

69. Abdallah H, Balsara RK, O'Riordan AC. Pacemaker contact sensitivity: clinical recognition and management. Ann Thorac Surg 1994; 57(4):1017–1018.

70. Schriver WR, Schereff RH, Domnitz JM, et al. Allergic rezones to stainless steel wire. Oral Surg Oral Med Oral Pathol 1976; 42(5):578–581.

71. Guyuron B, Lasa CI Jr. Reaction to stainless steel wire following orthognathic surgery. Plast Reconstr Surg 1992; 89(3):540–542.

72. Roed-Petersen B, Roed-Petersen J, Jorgensen KD. Nickel allergy and osteomyelitis in a patient with metal osteosynthesis of a jaw fracture. Contact Dermatitis 1979; 5(2):108–112.

73. Pickering CAC, Bainbridge D, Birtwistle IH, et al. Occupational asthma due to methyl methacrylate in an orthopaedic theatre sister. Br Med J 1986; 292:1362.

74. Rubin L, Rubin LR. Polyethylene as a bone and cartilage substitute: a 32-year retrospective. In: Rubin L, ed. Biomaterials in reconstructive surgery. St. Louis: Mosby; 1983:474–493.

75. Davis P, Jones S. The complications of silastic implants: experience with 137 consecutive cases. Br J Plast Surg 1971; 24(4):405–411.

76. Habal M, Chalian V. Experience with prefabricated silicone implants for reconstruction in facially deformed patients. J Prosthet Dent 1974; 32(3):292–299.

77. Lash H, Apfelberg DB, Lavey EB, et al. Custom-fabricated silicone implants for contour restoration. Ann Plast Surg 1979; 2(2):97–102.

78. Laub DR, Sohn W, Lash H, et al. Accurate reconstruction of traumatic bony contour defects of periorbital area with prefabricated silastic. J Trauma 1970; 10(6):472–480.

79. Mohler LR, Porterfield HW, Ferraro JW. Custom implants for reconstruction of craniofacial defects. Arch Surg 1976; 111:452.

80. Wilkinson T, Iglesias J. Room temperature vulcanizing silastic in facial contour reconstruction. J Trauma 1975; 15(6):479–482.

81. Raval P, Schaff NG. Custom fabricated silicone rubber implants for tissue augmentation: a review. J Prosthet Dent 1981; 45(4):432–434.

82. Berghaus A. Porous polyethylene in reconstructive head and neck surgery. Arch Otolaryngol 1985; 111:154.

83. Romano J, Iliff N, Manson P. Use of Medpor porous polyethylene implants in 140 patients with facial fracture. J Craniofac Surg 1993; 4(3):142–147.

84. Wellisz T, Dougherty W, Gross J. Craniofacial applications for the Medpor porous polyethylene flex-block implant. J Craniofac Surg 1992; 3(2):101–107.

85. Yaremchuk MJ, Sims D, Casanova R, et al. Long term follow up of expanded polyethylene implants for aesthetic and reconstructive facial skeletal surgery. Presented at the 6th International Congress of Craniofacial Surgery, Saint Tropez, France, October 21–24, 1995.

86. Byrd H, Hobar P, Shewmake K. Augmentation of the craniofacial skeleton with porous hydroxyapatite granules. Plast Reconstr Surg 1993; 91(1):15–22.

87. Papacharalambous S, Anastasoff K. Natural coral skeleton used as onlay graft for contour augmentation of the face. Int J Oral Maxillofac Surg 1993; 22(5):260–264.

88. Salyer KE, Hall CD. Porous hydroxyapatite as an onlay bone-graft substitute for maxillofacial surgery. Plast Reconstr Surg 1989; 84(2):236–244.

89. Rosen HM, Ackerman JL. Porous block hydroxyapatite in orthognathic surgery. Angle Orthod 1991; 61(3):185–191.

90. Mole B. The use of Gore-Tex in aesthetic surgery of the face. Plast Reconstr Surg 1992; 90(2):200–206.

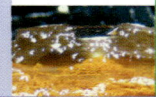

91. Lassus C. Expanded PTFE in the treatment of facial wrinkles. Aesthetic Plast Surg 1991; 15(2):167–174.
92. Cisneros JL, Singla R. Intradermal augmentation with expanded polytetrafluoroethylene (Gore-Tex) for facial lines and wrinkles. J Dermatol Surg Oncol 1993; 19(6):539–542.
93. Yaremchuk MJ. Facial skeletal reconstruction using porous polyethylene implants. Plast Reconstr Surg 2003; 111(6):1818–1827.
94. Zimmerli W, Trampuz A, Ochsnr PE. Prosthetic joint infections. N Engl J Med 2004; 351(16):1645–1654.
95. Zimmerli W, Waldvogel FA, Vaudaux P, et al. Pathogenesis of foreign body infection: description and characteristics of an animal model. J Infect Dis 1982; 146(4):487–497.
96. Costerton JW, Stewart PS, Greenberg EP. Bacterial biofilms: a common cause of persistent infections. Science 1999; 284:1318–1322.
97. Lacey M, Antonyshyn O. Use of porous high-density polyethylene implants in temporal contour reconstruction. J Craniofac Surg 1993; 4(2):74–78.
98. Wellisz T, Dougherty W. The role of alloplastic skeletal modification in the reconstruction of facial burns. Ann Plast Surg 1993; 30(6):531–536.
99. Rubin PAD, Bilyk JR, Shore JW. Orbital reconstruction using porous polyethylene sheets. Ophthalmology 1994; 101(1):1697–1708.
100. Couldwell WT, Chen TC, Weiss MH, et al. Cranioplasty with Medpor porous polyethylene Flexblock implant. J Neurosurg 1994; 81(3):483–486.
101. Frodel JL, Lee S. The use of high-density polyethylene implants in facial deformities. Arch Otolaryngol Head Neck Surg 1998; 124(11):1219–1223.
102. Turegun M, Sengezer M, Guler M. Reconstruction of saddle nose deformity using porous polyethylene implants. Aesthetic Plast Surg 1998; 22(1):38–41.
103. Romo T III, Sclafani AP, Sabini P. Use of porous high-density polyethylene in revision rhinoplasty and in the platyrrhine nose. Aesthetic Plast Surg 1998; 22:221.
104. Choi JC, Fleming JC, Aitken PA, et al. Porous polyethylene channel implants: a modified porous polyethylene sheet implant designed for repairs of large and complex orbital wall fractures. Ophthal Plast Reconstr Surg 1999; 15(1):56–66.
105. Niechajev I. Porous polyethylene implants for nasal reconstruction: clinical and histologic studies. Aesthetic Plast Surg 1999; 23(6):395–402.
106. Janecka IP. New reconstructive technologies in skull base surgery: role of titanium mesh and porous polyethylene. Arch Otolaryngol Head Neck Surg 2000; 126(3):396–401.
107. Ng SG, Madill SA, Inkster CF, et al. Medpor porous polyethylene implants in orbital blowout fracture repair. Eye 2001; 15:578–582.

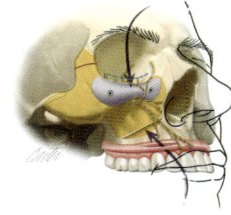

Chapter 3

Operative technique for facial skeletal augmentation

This chapter presents the basic steps of the author's operative technique of implant augmentation of the facial skeleton.

ANESTHESIA AND PREPARATION

Although not mandatory, most operations are performed with the patient under general endotracheal anesthesia or, when intraoral incisions are used, nasotracheal anesthesia. Because most operations employ intraoral incisions, this approach allows optimum preparation of the operative site and control of the airway (Fig. 3.1). The operative field is infiltrated with a solution containing adrenaline (epinephrine) (1:200 000) to minimize bleeding. Both the skin and the oral mucosa are prepared with a povidone–iodine solution.

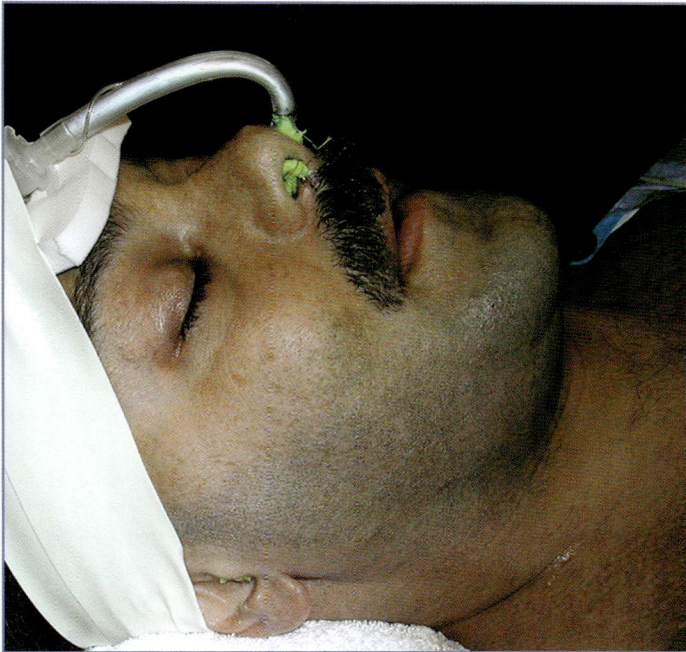

Figure 3.1 General anesthesia using nasotracheal intubation is ideal for midface and mandible augmentation. The airway is protected and controlled. A panoramic view of the operative area is provided.

INCISIONS

Incisions are borrowed from craniofacial and aesthetic surgery (Fig. 3.2).

Coronal incisions are used to place implants in the frontal and temporal areas. Transconjunctival retroseptal incisions are used to access the infraorbital rim and internal orbit. The lateral extent of the lower lid blepharoplasty incision provides access to the lateral orbit and zygomatic arch. This small cutaneous incision leaves an inconspicuous scar. Intraoral incisions are used to augment the midface as well as the mandibular body and ramus. Intraoral incisions are made with a generous labial cuff to allow watertight mucosal closure. Chin area augmentation is performed through submental incisions. Placement of incisions directly over implants is avoided.

Cephalosporins are administered perioperatively. I neither impregnate the implant with an antibiotic solution nor irrigate the operative site prior to wound closure with an antibiotic solution.

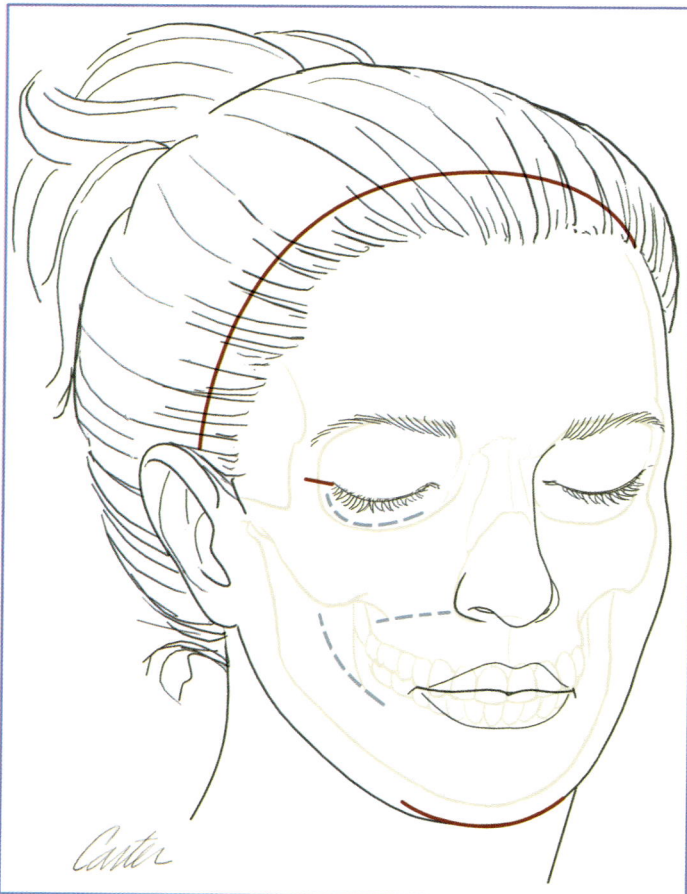

Figure 3.2 Incisions used to access the facial skeleton according to anatomical location. These include the bicoronal incision, the lateral extent of the lower lid blepharoplasty incision, and the submental incision (solid lines), as well as the transconjunctival retroseptal and intraoral labial sulcus incisions (broken lines).

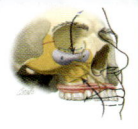

EXPOSURE

Wide subperiosteal exposure is important for several reasons. It allows accurate identification of the area to be augmented; important adjacent structures, such as the infraorbital nerve, thereby preventing their iatrogenic damage; and landmarks for orientation and hence symmetric implant positioning. Wide exposure also allows easy access for screw immobilization of the implant and its final in-place contouring. The resultant soft tissue mobilization also allows tension-free closure of the access incision (Fig. 3.3). This technique differs significantly from tradition, whereby dissection of only the area to be augmented was advocated. The resultant small pocket was intended to prevent postoperative implant migration. A limited dissection is possible for placement of smooth-surfaced implants but is not possible for the placement of porous implants to which soft tissues tend to adhere (like Velcro), making placement difficult.

PEARL

Wide subperiosteal exposure of the area to be augmented optimizes accuracy of implant placement.

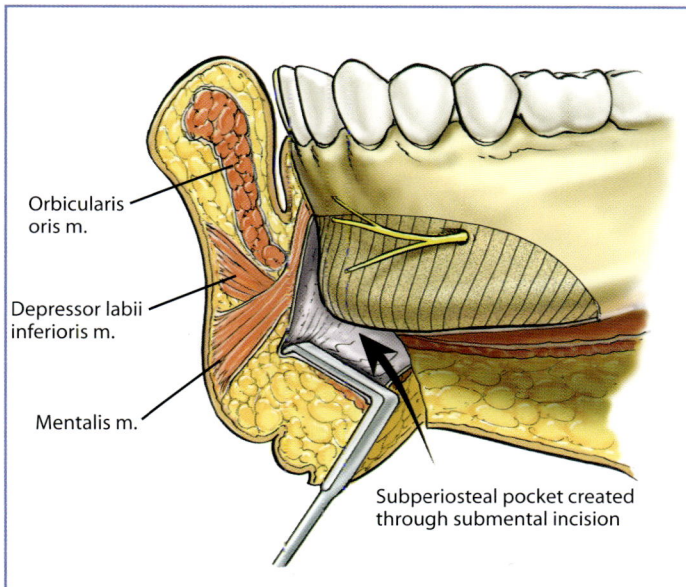

Figure 3.3 Surgical access to the chin and anterior mandibular border. A submental skin and subcutaneous incision is telescoped over the chin. The striped area denotes the area of subperiosteal dissection. Note that a pocket larger than the implant is dissected to allow ease of implant insertion and to provide a panoramic view of the area to be augmented.

IMPLANT SELECTION

I prefer porous polyethylene implants (Medpor; Porex, Fairburn, Georgia) to augment the facial skeleton.

Porous polyethylene is firm and flexible. It is easily carved with a scalpel, or contoured with a rasp or motorized burr. It can be immobilized with sutures or, with my preference, screws. It can be molded to the external contours of the skeleton by heating it in water, although I prefer not to take advantage of this attribute.

The favorable biocompatibility of this implant material can also be attributed to its porous surface. Porous polyethylene has pores of sufficient size to allow fibrous tissue ingrowth and relative host incorporation, as opposed to the host encapsulation observed with smooth-surfaced implants. Porous polyethylene has a continuous system of inner connecting pores approximately 100–250 μm in diameter. Animal studies have demonstrated that pore sizes of more than 100 μm encourage tissue ingrowth.[1,2] Pore sizes of less than 100 μm limit the extent of tissue ingrowth, whereas materials with large pore sizes have drawbacks associated with material breakdown.[3–5]

Clinical specimens demonstrated rapid ingrowth of fibrous tissue after human implantation. Rather than the dense connective tissue capsules observed with smooth-surfaced implants, porous polyethylene implants exhibited a thin connective tissue membrane that was contiguous with the ingrown tissue.[5] It was noted during revisional operations that fibrous tissues ingrowth was sufficient to result in bleeding when the implants were modified in situ with a scalpel, and in certain circumstances ingrowth exhibited sufficient vascularity to allow skin grafts to be placed directly over the implant.[5]

Fibrous tissue ingrowth improves the biocompatibility of porous implants because it limits their movement. Movement is an essential factor in determining the host response to an implant.[6] Because the host foreign body reaction encapsulates smooth-surfaced implants, a smooth implant never binds to the host bed and therefore is predisposed to move. Encapsulation of smooth implants and their subsequent predisposition to movement are directly or indirectly responsible for the majority of the late complications observed with smooth implants.[7–20]

When used to augment the chin, smooth silicone implants are known to cause significant bone resorption, which is attributed to implant motion caused by the overlying mentalis muscle.[21,22] Although it is usually not clinically apparent, bone resorption accompanying silicone chin implantation may be severe enough to result in tooth root erosion among patients with excessive mentalis muscle contraction.[23] I believe that smooth implant migration is the reason for implant malpositioning in certain clinical instances. Animal studies have demonstrated that porous implants result in less bone resorption than do smooth implants.[24] Bikhazi and Van Antwerp, in a prospective cephalometric study of five patients undergoing chin augmentation with porous polyethylene implants, did not observe bone resorption beneath the implants.[25] When I removed cheek implants at 6 months, and chin and mandibular implants at 1 year, the erosion was barely perceptible.

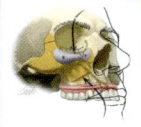

The use of porous implants has been criticized; unlike smooth implants, they require wider exposure for positioning and are more difficult to remove.[26] Personal preference and the 'learning curve' have made both these problems less significant for me. Wider exposure has been demonstrated to result in more accurate implant positioning. Because the initial augmentation has been considered accurate for the majority of patients, revisional surgical procedures have been infrequent. When porous polyethylene implants require removal, dissection directly on the implant minimizes adjacent soft tissue trauma. The absence of a thick fibrous capsule allows the soft tissues to collapse, permitting restoration of the preimplantation contour. This is not always the case after silicone implant removal.[27]

It is important to note that the manufacturer provides multiple implant shapes and sizes intended for specific anatomical areas. It is unusual for me to use an implant without changing its contour (reducing it) to meet the needs of the specific situation (Fig. 3.4).

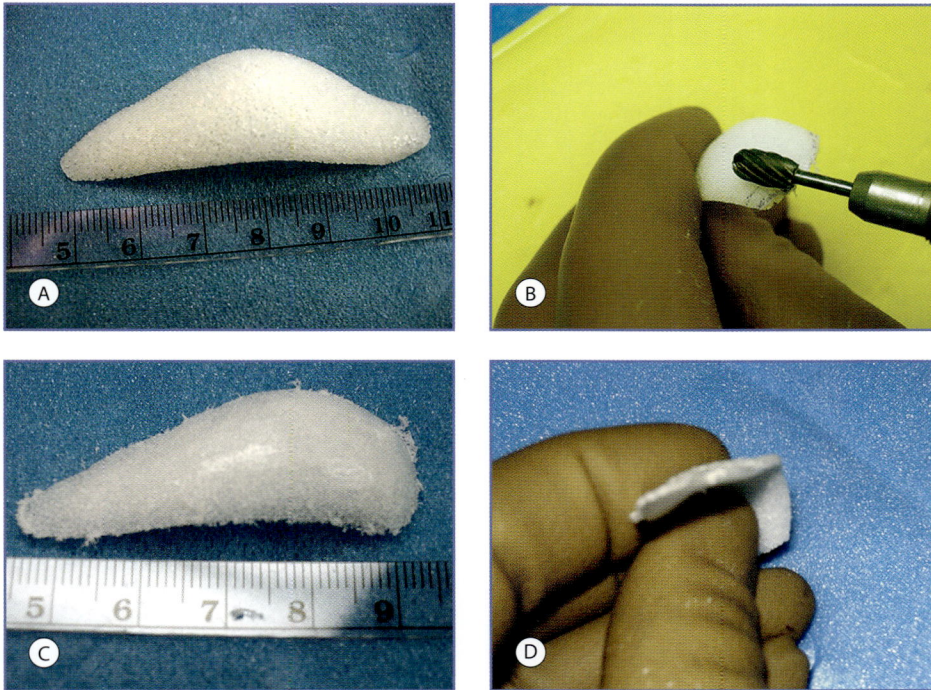

Figure 3.4 A porous polyethylene implant is contoured with a high-speed burr. This maneuver customizes the implant to meet the specific needs of the patient. Tapering the edges of the implant provides an imperceptible transition between the implant and the native skeleton. (**A**) Implant before modification. (**B**) Implant being modified with a high-speed burr. (**C**) Appearance of implant after modification. (**D**) End-on view of implant after modification. The tapered edge will provide an imperceptible transition between the implant and the native skeleton.

49

SCREW FIXATION

Screw fixation of the implant to the skeleton provides both practical and theoretic advantages. Screw fixation prevents movement of the implant, which adds precision as well as early and late predictability to the result. Theoretically, the elimination of implant motion should hasten fibrous incorporation while minimizing capsule formation and underlying bone resorption. By applying the implant to the skeleton, screw fixation eliminates any gaps between the implant and the recipient bed.

Gaps are potential sites for hematoma or seroma accumulation. Gaps also result in an effective increase in augmentation. For example, a 2-mm gap between the recipient bed and the posterior surface of a 5-mm implant would produce an augmentation equivalent to a 7-mm implant whose posterior surface was applied directly to the anterior surface of the skeleton (Figs 3.5 and 3.6).

PEARL

Screw fixation not only prevents implant movement but also obliterates gaps between the implant and the native skeleton. Gaps result in unanticipated increase in implant augmentation.

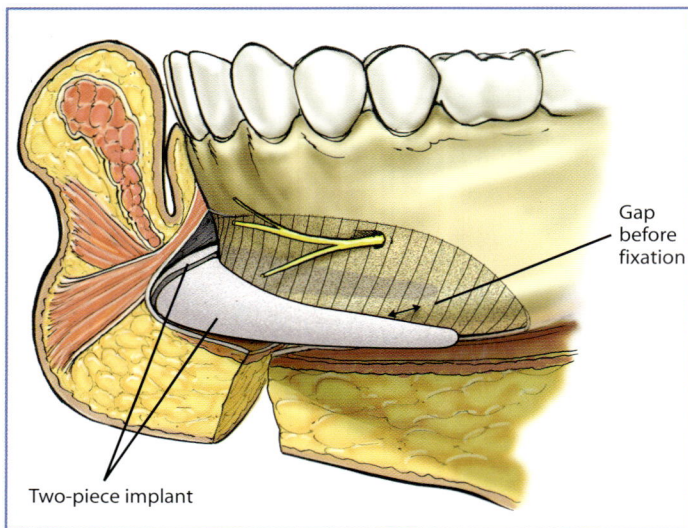

Two-piece implant

Gap before fixation

Figure 3.5 A two-piece porous polyethylene implant placed in a subperiosteal pocket. The two-piece design allows the lateral extension of the implant to follow the inclination of the mandible border. Note that, because the contour of the posterior surface of the implant does not mimic the contour of the anterior surface of the mandible, there is a gap between the mandible and the implant.

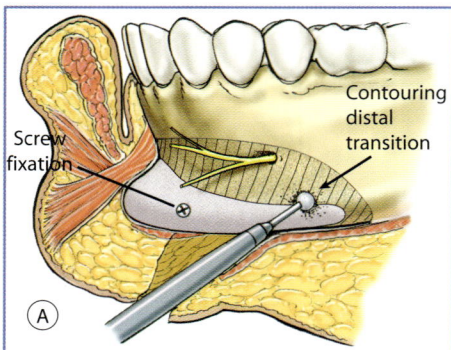

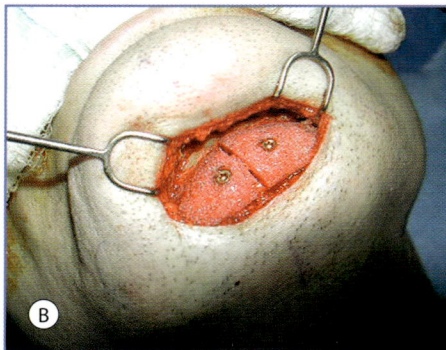

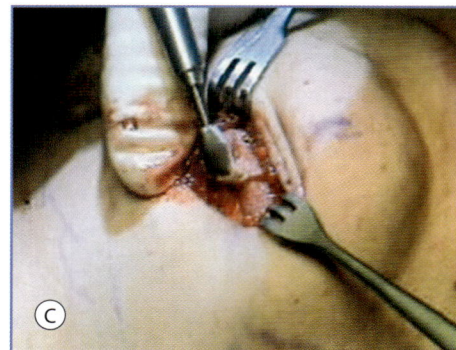

Screw fixation

Contouring distal transition

Figure 3.6 Screw fixation of the implant to the mandible prevents implant movement and eliminates gaps between the implant and the anterior surface of the mandible. Screw fixation also allows in-place contouring of the implant to ensure desired contour and an imperceptible implant–skeleton transition. (**A**) In-place contouring of an implant fixed to the mandible with titanium screws. (**B**) Clinical photograph of chin implant immobilized with screws. (**C**) Clinical photograph of screw-immobilized chin implant being contoured with a high-speed burr. The inferior border is being reduced to ensure proper vertical height of the chin.

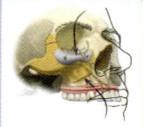

Screw immobilization of the implant allows in-place contouring of the implant at the recipient site. This final adjustment can be performed with a scalpel, rasp, or high-speed burr. It facilitates the custom carving of the implant, in terms of required gross contour, and can allow creation of a clinically imperceptible transition between the implant and the recipient skeleton (Fig. 3.6).

The above-described approach for the patient's skeletal augmentation can be considered an extension of the evolution of facial skeletal reconstruction in the 1980s. At that time, extended open reduction and the rigid internal fixation of facial skeletal fractures became the standard of care in North America. This more extensive surgery allowed better restoration of the skeletal anatomy. In this case, wide subperiosteal exposure and rigid fixation of porous implants allows more accurate alteration of the facial skeletal anatomy. In my personal experience, both techniques required a learning curve but, once obtained, I would not consider returning to previous methods of reconstruction.

PERSONAL EXPERIENCE

In 2003, I reported my personal experience with porous implants used for facial skeletal reconstruction.[28] This report was based on an experience with 162 patients operated on over an 11-year period (1990–2001). In this series, no implants were extruded or migrated, formed clinically apparent capsules, or caused symptoms attributable to bioincompatibility. The overall reoperation rate was 10% ($n = 16$), which included operations to remove implants because of acute infection (2%, $n = 3$) or late infection (1%, $n = 1$), and to remove implants causing displeasing contours (2%, $n = 3$). When reviewing the subsequent 200 patients since that report, there have been three patients with implant-related infections. Two of these patients presented after previous implant surgery that had failed because of infection. The third patient was HIV-positive.

There have been no materials-related problems during the ensuing period, while the incidence of reoperation for contour improvement has been stable. This experience is similar to that of others who have reported their experience with significant follow-up for facial reconstruction using this material.[29–39]

REFERENCES

1. Klatwitter JJ, Bagwell JG, Weinstein AM, et al. An evaluation of bone growth into porous high density polyethylene. J Biomed Mater Res 1976; 10(2):311–323.
2. Spector M, Flemming WR, Sauer BW. Early tissue infiltrate in porous polyethylene implants into bone: a scanning electron microscope study. J Biomed Mater Res 1975; 9(5):537–542.
3. Spector M, Harmon SL, Kreutner A. Characteristics of tissue growth into Proplast and porous polyethylene implants in bone. J Biomed Mater Res 1979; 13(5):677–692.
4. Berghaus A, Mulch G, Handrock M. Porous polyethylene and Proplast: their behavior in a bony bed. Arch Otorhinolaryngol 1984; 240(2):115–123.
5. Maas CS, Merwin GE, Wilson J, et al. Comparison of biomaterials for facial bone augmentation. Arch Otolaryngol Head Neck Surg 1990; 116(5):551–556.
6. Wellisz T, Kanel G, Anooshian RV. Characteristics of the tissues response to Medpor porous polyethylene implants in the human facial skeleton. J Long Term Eff Med Implants 1993; 3:223.
7. Wolfe SA. Correction of a persistent lower eyelid deformity caused by a displaced orbital floor implant. Ann Plast Surg 1979; 2(5):448–451.
8. Hoffman S. Loss of a silastic chin implant following a dental infection. Ann Plast Surg 1981; 7(6):484–486.
9. Wolfe SA. Correction of a lower eyelid deformity caused by multiple extrusions of alloplastic orbital floor implants. Plast Reconstr Surg 1981; 68(3):429–432.

10. Brown AE, Banks P. Late extrusion of alloplastic orbital floor implants. Br J Oral Maxillofac Surg 1981; 68:429.
11. Mauriello JA Jr, Flanagan JC, Peyster RG. An unusual late complication of orbital floor fracture repair. Ophthalmology 1984; 91(1):102–107.
12. Davis RM. Late orbital implant migration. Ann Ophthalmol 1986; 18(6):223–224.
13. Loftield K, Jordan DR, Fowler J, et al. Orbital cyst formation associated with Gelfilm use. Ophthal Plast Reconstr Surg 1987; 3(3):187–191.
14. Sutula FC, Palu RN. Delayed chocolate cyst after blowout fracture. Ophthal Plast Reconstr Surg 1991; 7(4):267–268.
15. Marks MW, Yeatts RP. Hemorrhagic cysts of the orbit as a long-term complication of prosthetic orbital floor implant. Plast Reconstr Surg 1994; 93(4):856–859.
16. Kohn R, Romano PE, Puklin JE. Lacrimal obstruction after migration of orbital floor implant. Am J Ophthalmol 1976; 82(6):934–936.
17. Mauriello JA Jr, Fiore PM, Kotch M. Dacryocystitis: late complication of orbital floor fracture repair with implant. Ophthalmology 1987; 94(3):248–250.
18. Anderson MF. Sinusitis related to use of foreign materials to treat orbital floor injuries. Report of two cases. J Oral Surg 1967; 25(2):182–183.
19. Peak J, Haria S, Sleeman D. Facial pain due to a displaced orbital floor implant: report of case. J Oral Maxillofac Surg 1992; 50(11):1234–1235.
20. Dougherty WR, Wellisz T. The natural history of alloplastic implants and orbital floor reconstruction: an animal model. J Craniofac Surg 1994; 5(1):26–32.
21. Robinson M. Bone resorption under plastic chin implants. Arch Otolaryngol 1972; 95:30.
22. Friedland JA, Coccaro PJ, Converse JM. Retrospective cephalometric analysis of mandibular bone absorption under silicone rubber chin implants. Plast Reconstr Surg 1976; 57(2):144–151.
23. Matarasso A, Elias AC, Elias RL. Labial incompetence: a marker for progressive bone resorption in silastic chin augmentation. Plast Reconstr Surg 1996; 98(6):1007–1014.
24. Wellisz T, Lawrence M, Jazayeri MA, et al. The effects of alloplastic onlays on bone in the rabbit mandible. Plast Reconstr Surg 1995; 96(4):957–963.
25. Bikhazi HB, Van Antwerp R. The use of Medpor in cosmetic and reconstructive surgery: experimental and clinical evidence. In: Stucker FJ, ed. Plastic and reconstructive surgery of the head and neck. St. Louis: Mosby; 1990:271–273.
26. Terino EO. Alloplastic contouring in the malar–mid-face–middle third facial aesthetic unit. In: Terino EO, Flowers RS, eds. The art of alloplastic facial contouring. St. Louis: Mosby; 2000:79–96.
27. Cohen SR, Mardach OL, Kawamoto HK Jr. Chin disfigurement following removal of alloplastic chin implants. Plast Reconstr Surg 1991; 88(1):62–66.
28. Yaremchuk MJ. Facial skeletal reconstruction using porous polyethylene implants. Plast Reconstr Surg 2003; 111(6):1818–1827.
29. Lacey M, Antonyshyn O. Use of porous high-density polyethylene implants in temporal contour reconstruction. J Craniofac Surg 2003; 4(2):74–78.
30. Wellisz T, Dougherty W. The role of alloplastic skeletal modification in the reconstruction of facial burns. Ann Plast Surg 1993; 30(6):531–536.
31. Rubin PAD, Bilyk JR, Shore JW. Orbital reconstruction using porous polyethylene sheets. Ophthalmology 1994; 101(10):1697–1708.
32. Couldwell WT, Chen TC, Weiss MH, et al. Cranioplasty with Medpor porous polyethylene Flexblock implant. J Neurosurg 1994; 81(3):483–486.
33. Frodel JL, Lee S. The use of high-density polyethylene implants in facial deformities. Arch Otolaryngol Head Neck Surg 1998; 124(11):1219–1223.
34. Turegun M, Sengezer M, Guler M. Reconstruction of saddle nose deformity using porous polyethylene implants. Aesthetic Plast Surg 1998; 22(1):38–41.
35. Romo T III, Sclafani AP, Sabini P. Use of porous high-density polyethylene in revision rhinoplasty and in the platyrrhine nose. Aesthetic Plast Surg 1998; 22:221.
36. Choi JC, Fleming JC, Aitken PA, et al. Porous polyethylene channel implants: a modified porous polyethylene sheet implant designed for repairs of large and complex orbital wall fractures. Ophthal Plast Reconstr Surg 1999; 15(1):56–66.
37. Niechajev I. Porous polyethylene implants for nasal reconstruction: clinical and histologic studies. Aesthetic Plast Surg 1999; 23(6):395–402.
38. Janecka IP. New reconstructive technologies in skull base surgery: role of titanium mesh and porous polyethylene. Arch Otolaryngol Head Neck Surg 2000; 126(3):396–401.
39. Ng SG, Madill SA, Inkster CF, et al. Medpor porous polyethylene implants in orbital blowout fracture repair. Eye 2001; 15:578–582.

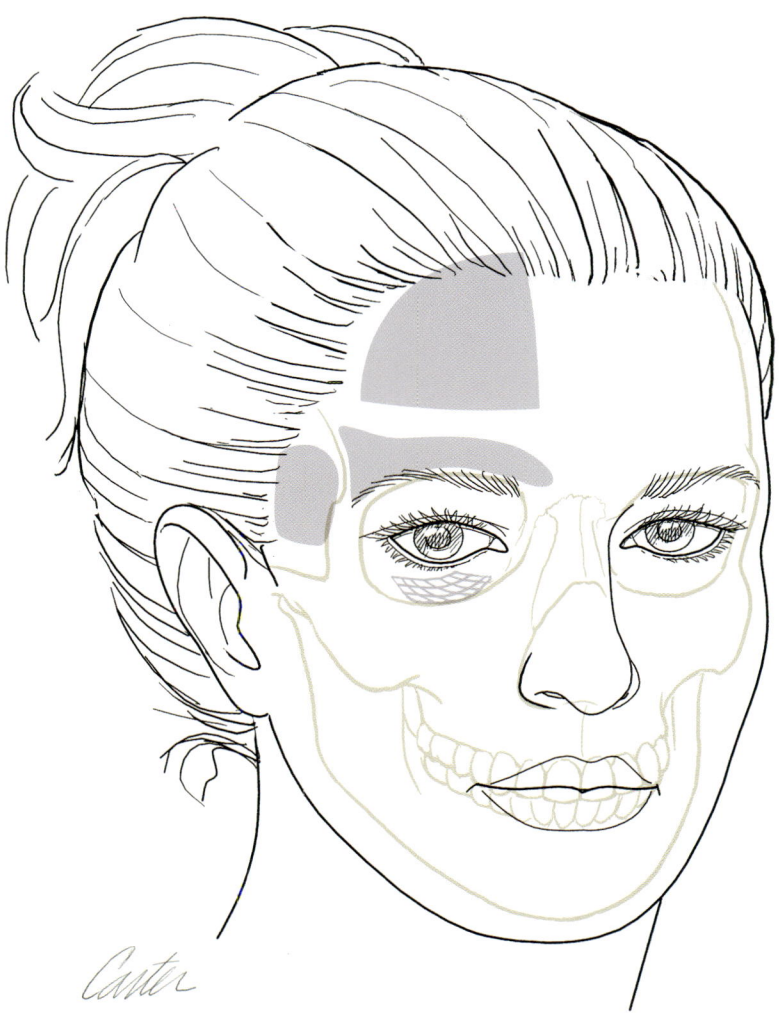

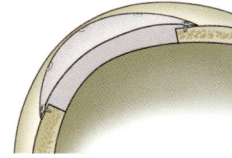

Chapter 4

Frontal bone and cranium

INDICATIONS FOR CRANIOPLASTY

The cranium is the part of the craniofacial skeleton that houses and protects the brain. The frontal bone is the major component of the anterior portion of the cranium, and is responsible for the appearance of the upper third of the face. Cranioplasty is usually performed to restore the integrity and appearance of the skull. This most often involves the reconstruction of full-thickness skeletal defects. Cranioplasty may also be performed to normalize or to improve the contours of the intact cranium, usually the frontal area, and hence the appearance of the upper third of the face.

Craniofacial deformities may be congenital or acquired. Significant congenital craniofacial deformities usually arise from premature suture fusion causing facial skeletal growth disturbances. The abnormal skull growth and morphology may compromise brain, visual, or respiratory function. Patients afflicted with these abnormalities usually require surgery in infancy or childhood. The surgery involves skeletal osteotomy and rearrangement to provide morphology compatible with brain expansion, as well as visual and respiratory function. Primary treatment of these deformities is outside the scope of this chapter.

This chapter does address treatment for those patients desiring improvement in their appearance and who have less severe, or microform variants of these congenital deformities resulting in contour abnormalities. These patients have their appearance improved with augmentation cranioplasty. Patients who have had previous treatment for major congenital, posttraumatic, or postablative deformities may benefit from onlay cranioplasty to refine the results of their previous treatment.

Acquired cranial bone deformities are usually full-thickness defects of the skull. In these situations, cranioplasty is done not only to normalize appearance but also, and more importantly, to provide protection for the brain. Cranial defects may result from bone loss after trauma. The most common etiology of full-thickness cranial defects is the infectious loss of a craniotomy flap created by the neurosurgeon to access the brain for neurosurgical treatment.

ANATOMY

Anthropometric data

The position and shape of the forehead are largely responsible for the appearance of the upper face. The important aesthetic variables are its inclination, its relation to the globes, and the relative prominence of its frontal sinus. The brows and the frontal hairline are surface landmarks that overlie the frontal area. Their shape and location also have a powerful impact on facial appearance.

Normal values for certain dimensions of the frontal area are presented in Figures 4.1–4.3.[1–3] The bitemporal distance or width of the upper face is similar in men and women (Fig. 4.1). Because men's heads and their features are, on average, larger than women's, this implies that the upper third of women's faces is relatively wide.

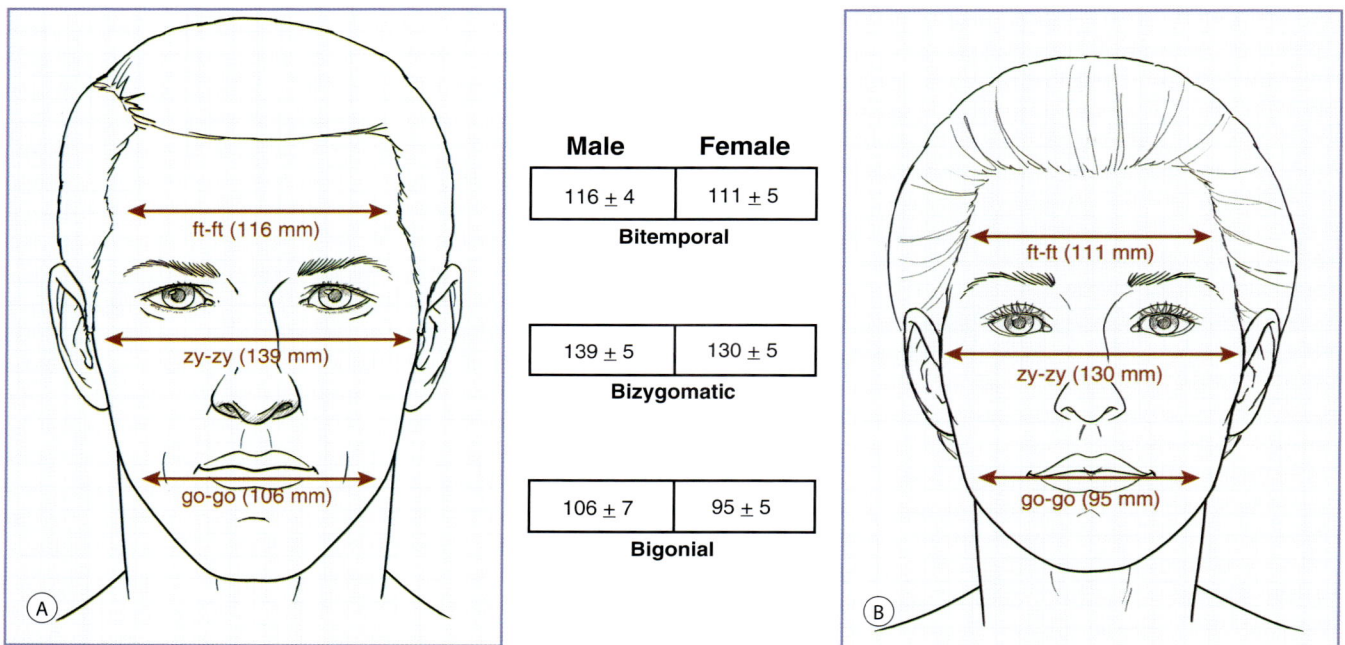

Male	Female
116 ± 4	111 ± 5
Bitemporal	
139 ± 5	130 ± 5
Bizygomatic	
106 ± 7	95 ± 5
Bigonial	

A: ft-ft (116 mm), zy-zy (139 mm), go-go (106 mm)

B: ft-ft (111 mm), zy-zy (130 mm), go-go (95 mm)

Figure 4.1 Normal values in millimeters for upper, middle, and lower facial width in (**A**) North American white adult men (ages 19–25) (*n* = 109) and (**B**) young adult women (*n* = 200).[1] Bitemporal distance (ft–ft) is measured from frontotemporal (ft) to frontotemporal, which is the point on each side of the forehead, laterally from the elevation of the linea temporalis. Bizygomatic distance (zy–zy) is measured from zygion (zy) to zygion, which is the most lateral point of each zygomatic arch. The bigonial distance (go–go) is measured from gonion (go) to gonion, which is the most lateral point of the mandibular angle close to the bony gonion. Because men's heads and their features are, on average, larger than women's, this implies that the upper third of women's faces is relatively wide. Note that the male lower face is both relatively and absolutely wider than that of the female face.

The inclination of the forehead is more vertical in women than it is men (Fig. 4.2). More often in men, frontal sinus development creates a prominence in the central lower forehead that is absent or vestigial in women. In summary, when compared with men's faces, the upper third of women's faces is relatively flat, vertical, and wide. These values and relations should be kept in mind when reconstructing cranial defects or addressing aesthetic concerns in the frontal area.

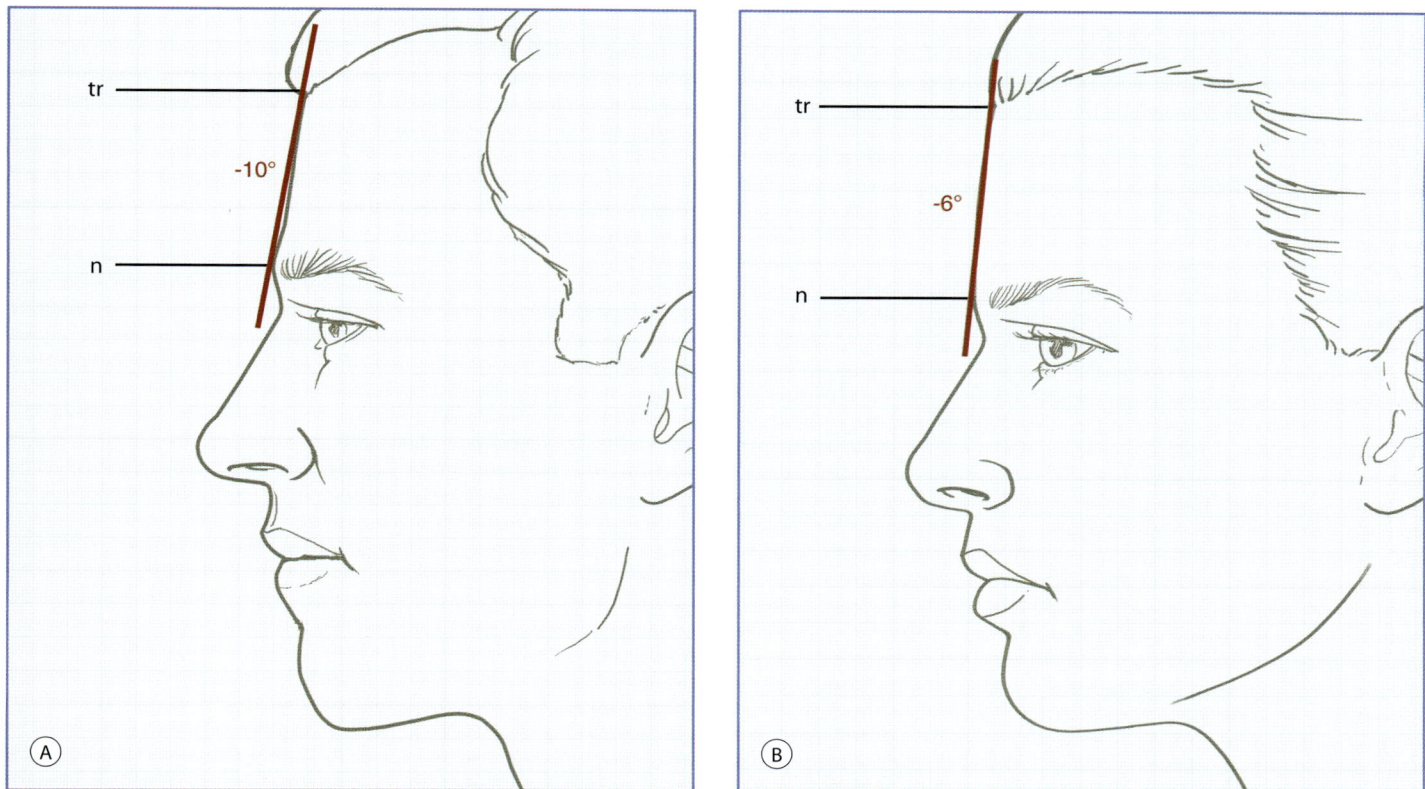

Figure 4.2 Lateral view of (**A**) male and (**B**) female faces demonstrating normal values in degrees for inclination of the forehead in North American white adult men (ages 19–25) (n = 109) and young adult women (n = 200).[1] The inclination of the forehead is more vertical in women than it is men. More often in men, frontal sinus development creates a prominence in the central lower forehead that is absent or vestigial in women. n, nasion; tr, trichion.

The relationship of the orbital rims to the globe is a primary determinant of the appearance of the upper one-third of the face (Fig. 4.3). On average, the surface of the soft tissues overlying the supraorbital rim lies 10 mm anterior to the cornea, while projecting 13 mm beyond the infraorbital rim. When the orbital rims have a greater projection beyond the anterior surface of the cornea, the eyes appear deep-set. When the orbital rims project less, the eyes appear prominent. Certain craniosynostoses result in underdevelopment of the frontal bone and midface, with marked projection of the globe beyond the orbital rims. When this disproportion is severe enough to cause symptoms due to corneal exposure or to be disfiguring, osteotomies are performed to allow skeletal advancement and improvement of globe–rim relationships. When globe–rim disproportions are less severe, they are usually left untreated. Alloplastic augmentation of the orbital rims can be used to improve globe–rim relationships in patients with microform variants of congenital deformities or in 'normal' patients with prominent eyes.[2–5]

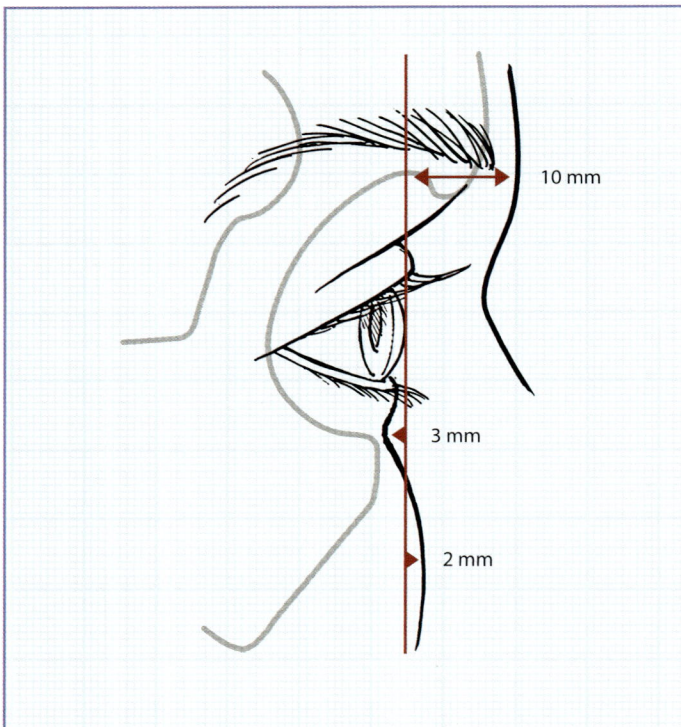

Figure 4.3 Sagittal relations of the anterior surface of the cornea to the soft tissues overlying the supraorbital and infraorbital rims. On average, in the young adult, the supraorbital rim projects 10 mm beyond, the infraorbital rim lies 3 mm behind, and the cheek prominence projects 2 mm beyond the anterior surface of the cornea.[1–3]

SURGICAL ANATOMY

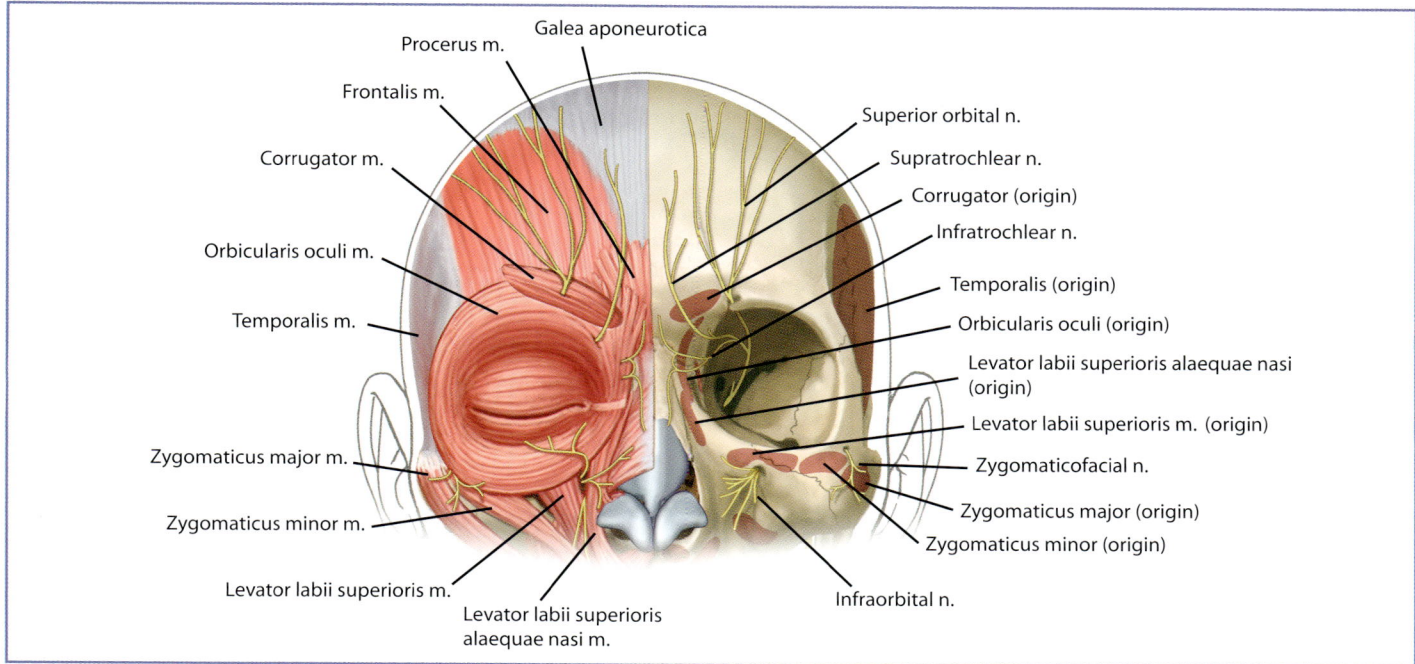

Procerus m.
Galea aponeurotica
Frontalis m.
Corrugator m.
Orbicularis oculi m.
Temporalis m.
Zygomaticus major m.
Zygomaticus minor m.
Levator labii superioris m.
Levator labii superioris alaequae nasi m.
Superior orbital n.
Supratrochlear n.
Corrugator (origin)
Infratrochlear n.
Temporalis (origin)
Orbicularis oculi (origin)
Levator labii superioris alaequae nasi (origin)
Levator labii superioris m. (origin)
Zygomaticofacial n.
Zygomaticus major (origin)
Zygomaticus minor (origin)
Infraorbital n.

Figure 4.4 Anatomy of the frontal area.

Skeleton

The cranium has three distinct layers in the adult: the hard internal and external laminae, and the cancellous middle layer or diploe. The adult bony vault has an average thickness of about 7 mm but varies considerably across areas and individuals.[6] Skull thickness lessens considerably in the elderly. The thickest area is usually the occipital, and the thinnest is the temporal.

The calvaria are covered with periosteum on both the outer and inner surfaces. On the inner surface, it fuses with the dura to become the dura's outer layer. Unlike other areas of the skeleton, and perhaps because of the lack of functional stresses on the skull, the periosteum of the skull seems to have little osteogenic potential in the adult. Therefore the loss or removal of the calvaria requires its replacement if its location is important from a protective or aesthetic standpoint.

The frontal and temporal bones are responsible for the appearance of the upper third of the face. They lie anterior to the coronal suture. The cranial bones posterior to the coronal suture are less aesthetically sensitive and are not further discussed.

The frontal bone consists of vertical and horizontal portions. The larger, vertical portion corresponds to the forehead, while the smaller, orbital or horizontal portion forms the anterior portions of the roofs of the orbital and nasal cavities. The vertical portion of the frontal bone is convex and usually reveals some remnant of the metopic suture. On either side of the midline and about 3 cm above the supraorbital margin are the frontal eminences, which are rounded elevations reflecting the embryologic origin of the frontal bone from two pieces previously separated by the metopic suture.

Just beneath the frontal eminences, and separated from them by a shallow groove, are the superciliary arches. These arches are prominent medially. They are joined to one another by the glabella, which is a smooth elevation in the midline. These elevations are in large part due to the size of the frontal sinuses. They are larger in men than in women.

The supraorbital margin is just inferior to each superciliary arch. It forms the upper boundary of the orbit. Its lateral aspect is well defined and prominent to protect the eye. Medially, it is rounded and merges with the nasal sidewall before it articulates with the nasal bone, the frontal process of the maxilla, and the lacrimal bone. The supraorbital foramen, which transmits the supraorbital nerve and vessels, is located at the junction of the medial and intermediate thirds of the supraorbital margin. The supraorbital margin ends laterally in its zygomatic process, which articulates with the zygoma at the zygomaticofrontal suture. The temporal line runs superiorly from the zygomatic process. It splits into superior and inferior temporal lines.

Muscles

Muscles located in the forehead area relate to the scalp, the nose, the eyelids, and the lower jaw (Fig. 4.4).

The epicranius, which is a broad muscular and tendinous layer, covers the top and the sides of the skull from the occipital bone to the eyebrow. It is composed of the frontalis muscle anteriorly, the occipitalis muscle posteriorly, and an intervening galea aponeurotica. Its posterior counterpart, the occipitalis, arises by short tendinous fibers from the nuchal line of the occipital bone and from the mastoid part of the temporal bone. Its fibers ascend toward the vertex and end in the galea aponeurotica. The frontalis muscle is quadrilateral in shape and covers most of the frontal bone. It has no bony attachments. Its medial fibers are continuous with those of the procerus, its intermediate fibers blend with the corrugator and the orbicularis oculi. Laterally, its fibers also blend with the orbicularis oculi. Its fibers pass upward to join the galea just below the coronal suture. The medial margins of the muscle's two sides meet in the midline for a variable distance above the root of the nose. The frontalis muscle, acting alone, raises the eyebrows. When it works in concert with the occipitalis, the frontalis draws the scalp back to raise the eyebrows and wrinkle the forehead. These muscles are supplied by the facial nerve.

The orbicularis oculi is divided into orbital and palpebral portions. The orbicularis oculi originates from the nasal process of the frontal bone, the frontal process of the maxilla, and the anterior surface of the medial canthal tendon. The fibers are directed laterally to surround the entire circumference of the orbit. The palpebral portion is thin. The orbital portion is thicker. The upper fibers of this portion blend with the frontalis and the corrugator. It often covers the origins of the elevators of the lips and nose. Laterally, it covers the anterior portion of the temporalis fascia. It is supplied by zygomatic and temporal branches of the facial nerve. The orbicularis oculi is the sphincter muscle of the eye.

The corrugator supercilii is a small, narrow, pyramidal muscle that arises from the medial end of the superciliary arch and inserts into the deep surface of the skin in the area of the medial brow. Its fibers originate beneath and pass through those of the frontalis and orbicularis oculi. The corrugator draws the eyebrow downward and medialward. It produces vertical wrinkles in the forehead. It is supplied by zygomatic and temporal branches of the facial nerve.

The procerus arises from the lower part of the nasal bones and inserts into the skin over the lower part of the forehead between the eyebrows. Its fibers intermingle with those of the frontalis. The procerus draws down the medial angle of the eyebrows and produces transverse wrinkles over the bridge of the nose. It is supplied by buccal branches of the facial nerve.

The temporalis is a broad muscle that arises from the whole of the temporal fossa and from the deep surface of the temporal fascia. Its fibers converge as they descend and pass behind the zygomatic arch to insert into the anterior surface of the coronoid and anterior border of the mandibular ramus. This muscle closes the jaws. It is supplied by anterior and posterior deep temporal nerves from the mandibular division of the trigeminal nerve.

CRANIOPLASTY FOR FULL-THICKNESS DEFECTS

Indications

The most frequent indication for cranioplasty is the full-thickness skull defect resulting from the infectious loss of a bone flap after elective craniotomy. In my experience, a frequent cause of craniotomy graft (referred to as a bone flap by most neurosurgeons) loss results not from contamination at surgery but rather from wound closure breakdown. This is precipitated by the common practice of making the osteotomy directly under the scalp incision. The resulting dead space directly beneath the suture line makes the soft tissue closure tenuous. The situation is further aggravated when plates and screws used to stabilize the replaced bone are positioned directly beneath the suture line. Minimal trauma can result in hardware and bone graft exposure with secondary infection (Fig. 4.5). This can be avoided by planning the scalp incision so as to create scalp flaps large enough to allow the craniotomy to be made well within the flap boundaries. This avoids overlying scalp incision and bone incisions, as well as the possibility of fixation hardware being placed directly under the soft tissue closure.

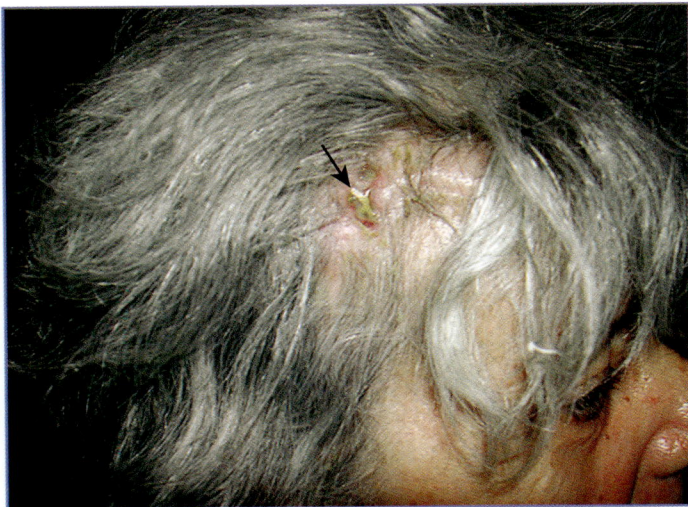

Figure 4.5 Exposed fixation hardware used to immobilize craniotomy graft after elective craniotomy. The craniotomy incision had been made directly beneath the scalp incision. The fixation hardware (arrow) was positioned directly beneath the scalp closure. Treatment required removal of the hardware and bone graft. A cranioplasty was performed 6 months later.

The goals of cranioplasty are to provide protection for the brain and to restore the premorbid contour. In addition, speech problems and hemiparesis may improve by cranial reconstruction if the defect is large enough to allow the scalp to exert direct pressure on the brain.[7-10] Skull defects of greater than 2–3 cm should be considered for repair. However, this decision varies with location. Even small defects in the frontal area can be disturbing to the patient and therefore can be considered for repair. Small defects of the temporal and occipital areas, which are covered by thick muscle, are usually not reconstructed.

Timing of surgery

Cranioplasty is performed when acute infection and risk factors for recurrent infection are eliminated. This assumes the removal of all devitalized tissues and any foreign bodies at the time of craniotomy graft debridement. It requires the treatment of any frontal or ethmoidal sinus inflammatory disease. It also requires that any potential communications between the sinuses and the planned cranioplasty graft be eliminated. Large communications between the sinuses and the anterior cranial fossa, which may be the case after massive trauma requiring frontal sinus cranialization or after tumor removal, require placement of a vascularized barrier for effective isolation. A galea frontalis flap, if available and adequate, or a free tissue transfer may be required. Finally, the adequacy of the soft tissues to provide secure closure at the time of elective cranioplasty must be ensured. This may require a preliminary scalp expansion or flap reconstruction before or at the time of cranioplasty.

A significant reduction in incidence of infection has been shown when 1 year is allowed to elapse between the initial injury or infection and the subsequent reconstruction.[11-13] In my experience, a 6-month infection-free period has been sufficient to ensure that infection has been adequately treated.

Technique

At surgery, the patient is positioned so that a panoramic view of the skull and, if appropriate, the upper face can be draped into the field. This position allows the surgeon to mimic the contralateral anatomy and to avoid unnatural transitions. Preinjury photographs may be helpful. A skull model should be available to aid in the design of complex curvatures and landmarks.

Old scars are usually incised for exposure, and the scalp flap is removed carefully from the underlying dura. Any dural tears are repaired.

Unless prefabricated implants are used, the exposed bone edge is saucerized by removal of the outer table with rongeurs or a high-speed burr. The resultant inner table ledge provides a ledge for implant placement and stabilization.

Materials

Both autogenous bone and alloplastic materials are used to reconstruct the skull. Craniofacial surgeons usually advocate the use of bone for cranioplasty, while the vast majority of neurosurgeons use polymethylmethacrylate (PMMA). In reviewing their experience of 42 posttraumatic reconstructions of frontal defects in which both bone and acrylic were used, Manson et al. found that the material employed was not as important as the timing of reconstruction and the treatment of sinus disease.[11] In the past, I had used bone when there had been recurrent infection or when overlying soft tissues were compromised (e.g. after radiation therapy). Presently, I use alloplastic materials for almost all cranioplasty.

Bone

Bone is championed by many craniofacial surgeons because it becomes revascularized to varying extents by the host, and is therefore less susceptible to infection and late complications. It has the disadvantages of requiring a donor site, being technically demanding and time-consuming to perform, and exhibiting variable resorption and therefore being prone to irregular contour. When bone is used for cranioplasty, resorption of between 25 and 40% has been demonstrated.[11]

Bone donor sites include ribs and calvaria. Split ribs are useful when large defects are to be reconstructed and calvarial bone is in short supply. Split ribs are usually fitted into a shelf made in the adjacent intact skull. In the past, an interlocking chain-link technique[14] was used for stabilization; now, most craniofacial surgeons use a combination of plates and screws to make a stable construct (Fig. 4.6).

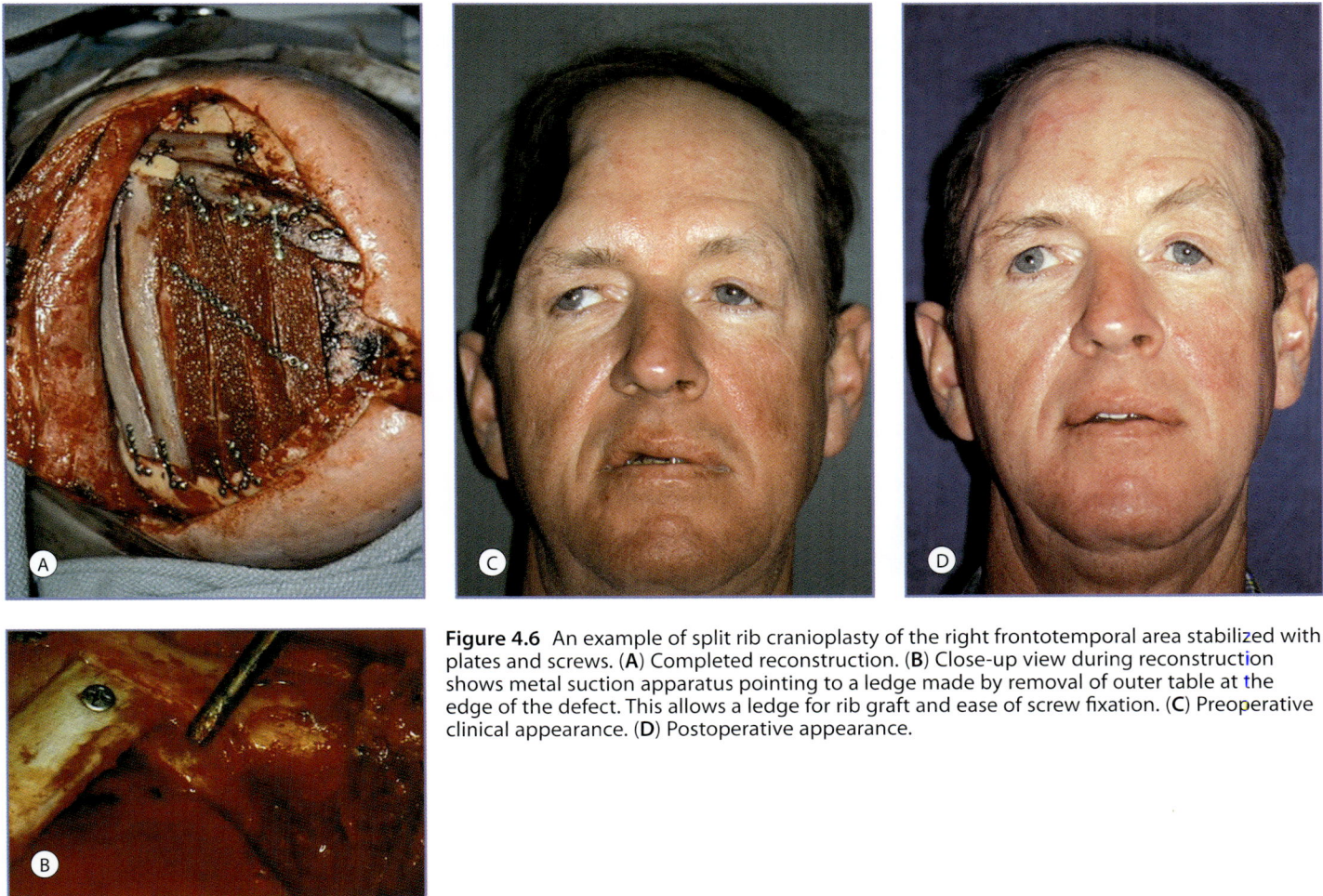

Figure 4.6 An example of split rib cranioplasty of the right frontotemporal area stabilized with plates and screws. (**A**) Completed reconstruction. (**B**) Close-up view during reconstruction shows metal suction apparatus pointing to a ledge made by removal of outer table at the edge of the defect. This allows a ledge for rib graft and ease of screw fixation. (**C**) Preoperative clinical appearance. (**D**) Postoperative appearance.

Calvarial bone has the advantage of being a painless donor site in the surgical field. The calvarial bone is harvested in two ways. The outer table may be harvested from the intact skull, or the inner table may be harvested after craniotomy. Because there is great variability in the thickness of the skull at any given point, and because there is no clinically useful correlation between skull thickness and age, sex, or weight,[6] a coronal computed tomographic image in the area to be harvested is obtained to look for the presence of a diploic space before cranial bone graft harvest is attempted. Although it is shown to be safe in the hands of trained, experienced surgeons, cranial bone graft harvest can have significant complications, including bleeding and dural tear with cerebrospinal fluid leak and meningitis. The parietal area usually serves as the donor site, because this area is usually accessible and the donor site contour deformity is hidden by the patient's hair. This technique is most often used to harvest bone that will reconstruct the internal orbit, reconstruct the nose, or augment an area of the midface skeleton.

The other technique of harvesting cranial bone is to perform a craniotomy with harvest of a full-thickness piece of skull of appropriate size and curvature. The inner table is split from the outer table (Fig. 4.7).

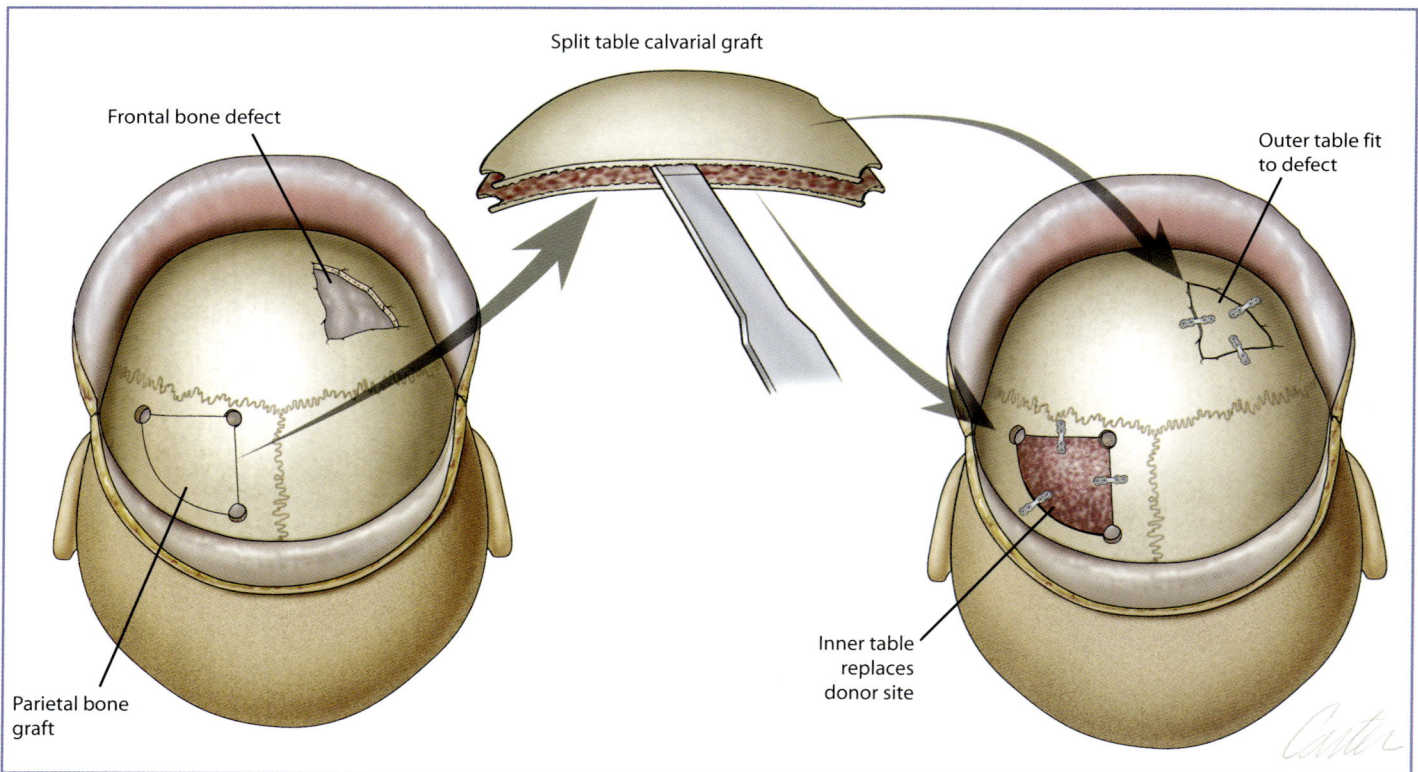

Figure 4.7 Inner table harvest after craniotomy. The outer table is returned to the donor site.

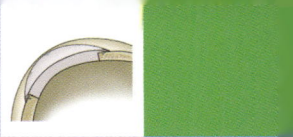

A simple way to do this is with the aid of the Midas Rex drill (Midas Rex Pneumatic Tools, Fort Worth, Texas) and the C-1 bit (Fig. 4.8). This thin bit is placed in the diploe between the two skull cortices. The outer cortex can be replaced, and the inner cortex is used for reconstruction of the defect. Most often, microplates and screws are used to stabilize these reconstructions.

The most current and comprehensive description of the use of autogenous bone has been published as a supplement to volume 116 of the journal *Plastic and Reconstructive Surgery*.[15]

Polymethylmethacrylate (PMMA)

The most commonly used material for skull reconstruction is PMMA. PMMA reconstruction is technically less demanding than reconstruction with autogenous bone and avoids bone donor site morbidity. The aesthetic results are far superior to those obtained with bone. PMMA is radiolucent and therefore does not affect postoperative imaging. It is unaffected by temperature and is strong. When used for full-thickness defects, it can fill intracranial dead space— a problem with bone cranioplasty. Unlike cranioplasty performed with bone, selective overcorrection of the skeletal defect can compensate for overlying soft tissue deficiencies, resulting in a smooth skin surface contour. Eppley found that both porous and non-porous compositions of PMMA presently used for cranioplasty had impact resistance sufficient to offer protection similar to that of native bone.[16] Because it is encapsulated by the host rather than incorporated by surrounding soft tissues, PMMA is believed by some to be more susceptible to infection and late complications.

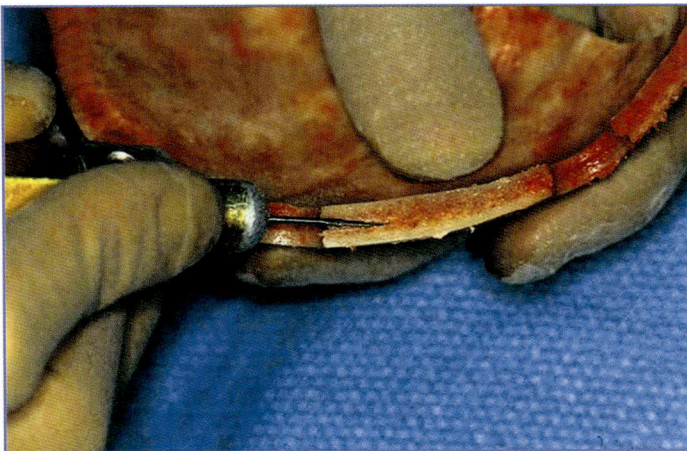

Figure 4.8 Bone flap being split with Midas Rex drill and C-1 bit.

Cranioplasty kits are available that contain a single dose of 30 g of powdered polymer and 17 mL of liquid monomer. The elements are mixed with a spatula in a bowl. The mixing should be conducted under ventilation so that the person mixing is not overcome by fumes. Mixing takes about 30 seconds. The bowl is then covered to avoid evaporation of the monomer. Doughing time varies with the temperature and is about 5 min at 22°C (72°F).

Two techniques are used to shape the implant. One method places the doughy mixture in a plastic sleeve provided in the cranioplasty kit. The sleeve containing the still pliable implant mixture is placed on to the skull defect and molded by digital compression (Fig. 4.9). The molding process occurs under continuous irrigation to avoid thermal damage to the dura and brain. A molding time of 6–8 min is usual. The exothermic polymerization process is allowed to take place away from the surgical field.

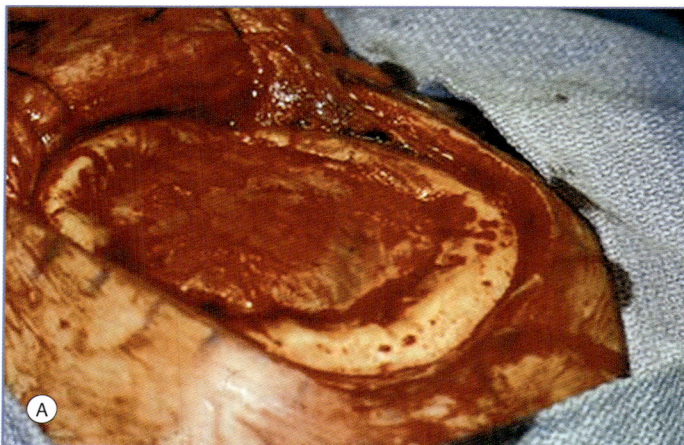

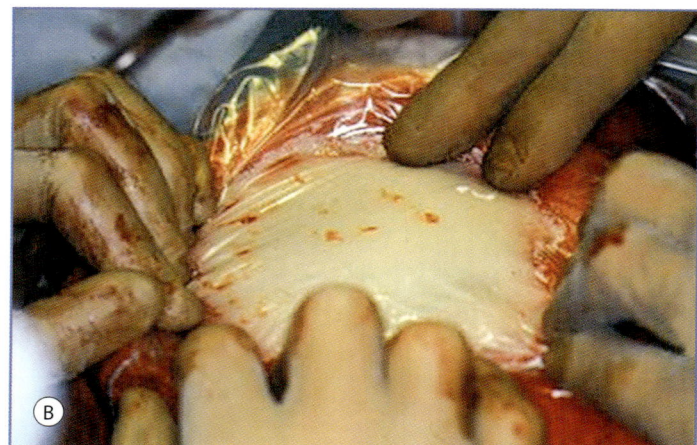

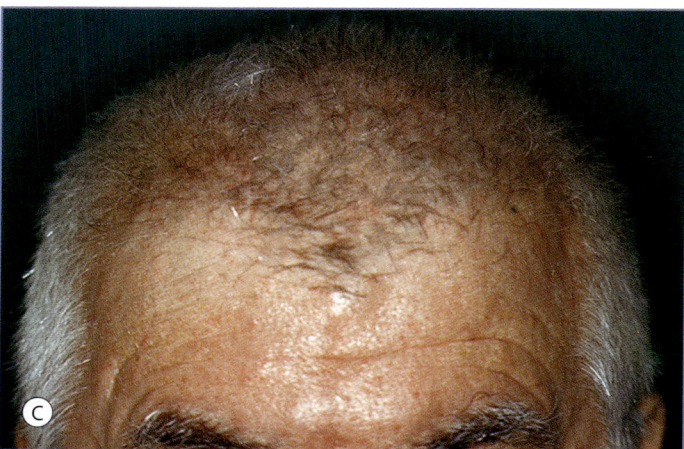

Figure 4.9 Acrylic cranioplasty by plastic sleeve molding technique. (**A**) Intraoperative view of right frontoparietal defect. (**B**) Molding of methylmethacrylate to defect. (**C**) Postoperative result. (From Yaremchuk and Rubin 2000,[17] with permission.)

The other technique for PMMA cranioplasty requires first placing a wire mesh into the skull defect. PMMA is then cured directly on the mesh (Fig. 4.10). This technique allows more risk for burn damage to the dura during the exothermic reaction, which, unlike the sleeve technique, takes place in the surgical field. Irrigation of the implant during the exothermic reaction can avoid heat injury to the dura. Manson et al. showed that the temperature rises less than 3°C when the implant is continuously irrigated.[11]

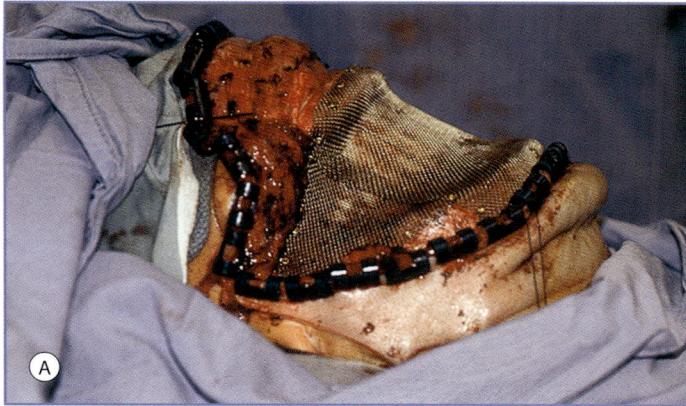

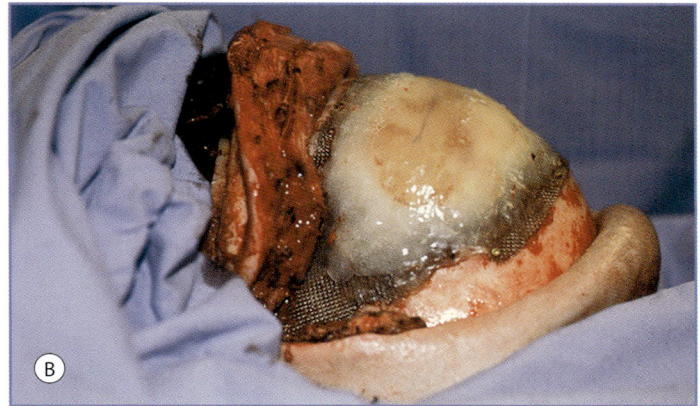

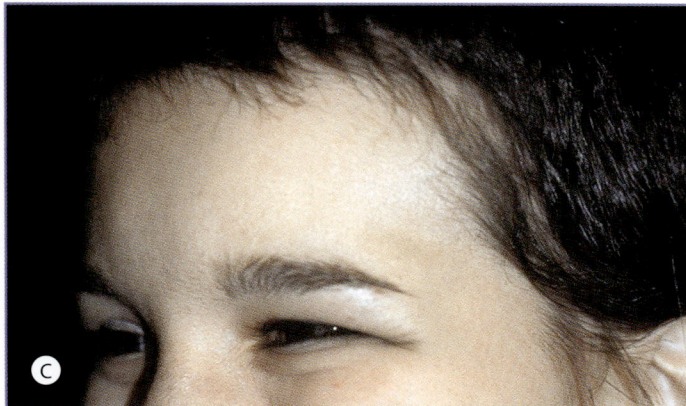

Figure 4.10 Acrylic cranioplasty by mesh onlay technique. (A) Intraoperative view of titanium mesh spanning defect. (B) Polymethylmethacrylate spread over metallic template. (C) Postoperative result.

Stelnicki and Ousterhout developed an in situ model to quantify the effects of saline irrigation on acrylic curing temperature with varying implant thickness.[18] They concluded that in situ polymerization of acrylic implants with saline irrigation is safe if the implant is 6 mm or less in thickness.

Complex curvatures, particularly in the supraorbital area, are formed by adding material to an initial construct. Final adjustments can be made with a contouring burr on a high-speed drill. The implants may be fixed with wires or, more simply and rapidly, with microscrews. The screws are used to fix the position of the implant in one of two ways. In both techniques, the implant must overlie intact skull. Screws may be driven through the acrylic and into underlying bone before it is completely hardened. Another technique, particularly useful in augmenting contour depressions, is first to place the screw in the area to be augmented, leaving the head and two or three threads above the bone surface. The acrylic is then poured over the screw so that it is incorporated in the construct (Fig. 4.11).

The implant may be perforated to allow the dura to be tented up to it. This method lessens the potential for epidural collection. Perforations in the implant also allow drainage and soft tissue ingrowth, which also aids in implant fixation.

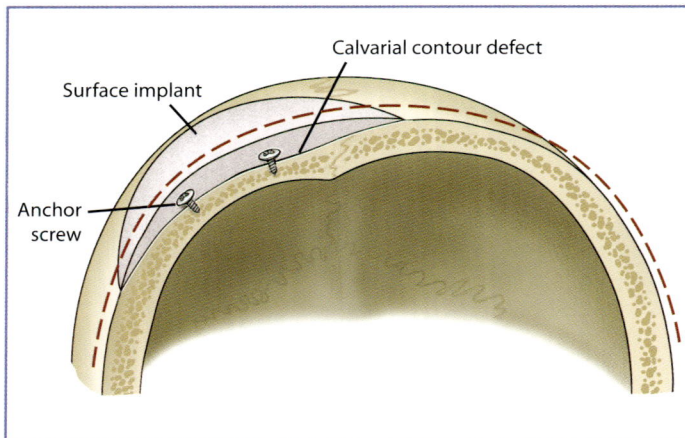

Figure 4.11 Screw stabilization of acrylic onlays. A titanium screw purchases the outer table of the skull in the area of defect. The screw head is left above the skull surface. Acrylic is spread over the screw head to incorporate the construct and to prevent movement of the implant.

Porous polyethylene

Porous polyethylene can be used for the reconstruction of skull defects (Medpor, Porex Surgical, Newnan, Georgia) (Fig. 4.12).

This material has good strength, is contourable, and can be stabilized with plates and screws. Its porosity allows for some soft tissue ingrowth. Various-sized as well as custom implants are available.

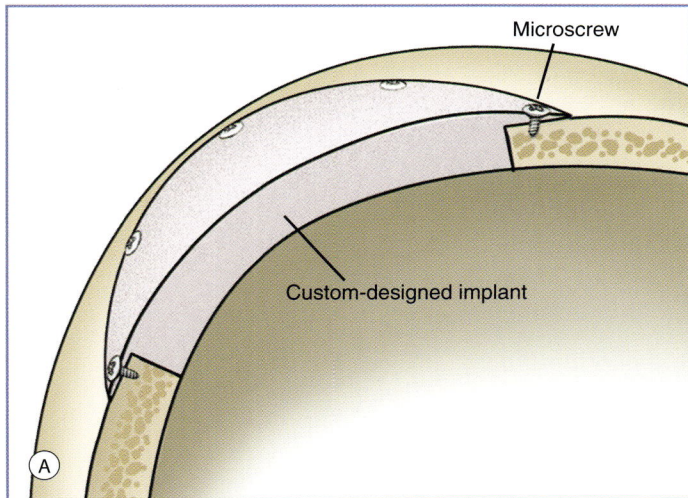

Figure 4.12 Custom porous polyethylene implants are fashioned with a small thin flange that overlies the intact skull. This allows fixation by placing low-profile microscrews through the flange and then into the underlying intact skull. This lessens the likelihood of the implant or fixation hardware eroding through the overlying scalp. (**A**) Illustration of technique. (**B**) Clinical photograph.

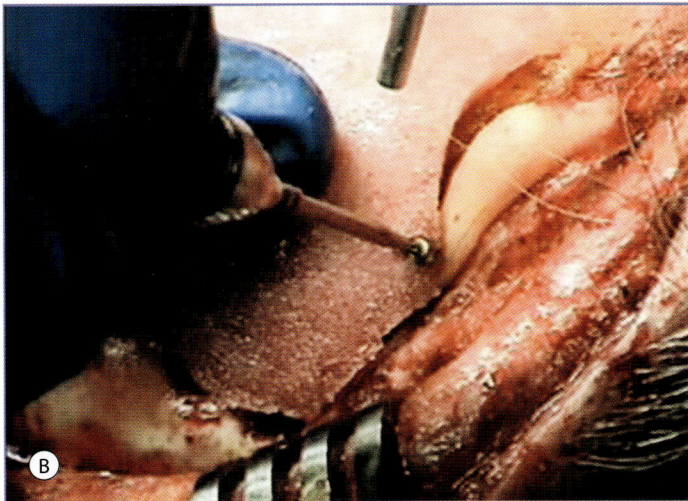

Hydroxyapatite

Hydroxyapatite is a ceramic biomaterial composed of calcium phosphate. It can be manufactured synthetically or formed by chemically converting the naturally porous calcium carbonate skeleton of marine coral. Hydroxyapatite cement has been shown to be osteoconductive, but only minimal direct bone or vascular ingrowth occurs because of the implant's extremely small pore size.[19–22] Any bone ingrowth that occurs is a direct turnover of hydroxyapatite to bone at the periphery of the implant. Implant volume is thought to remain stable because the implant remains largely avascular.

Three forms of hydroxyapatite have been used for facial skeletal reconstruction. Block hydroxyapatite has been used as relatively small interposition grafts.[23] It is extremely brittle, making it difficult to contour. Granular hydroxyapatite has been used as an onlay for orbitocranial defects. The problems with this material included slow cement consolidation and unpredictable volume restoration.[24] A powdered form of hydroxyapatite became available in 1996. When it is mixed with water, the powder becomes a paste that is easily applied to regular surfaces. The paste sets in approximately 20 min. Because of its low flexural resistance, it is recommended for use as an onlay material to improve contour. It has been used with metallic mesh to reconstruct defects. In this application, Moreira-Gonzalez and Zins reported a major complication rate of 42.8%, with some complications occurring as late as 4 years postoperatively. The main problems observed at reoperation were fragmentation of the hydroxyapatite cement, exudation, and severe soft tissue inflammatory reaction.[25] Others have cautioned about the use of this material for vault reconstruction.[26]

Computer-aided design and computer-aided manufacture

Computed tomography imaging of skull defects provides digitized information that can be transferred to design software. Data describing the contour along the edge of the defect and the surface characteristics of the normal cranium surrounding the defect can be used to design a custom-fit implant. The electronic data describing the newly designed prosthesis are then used by a computer-controlled manufacturing system to create a wax model, which is then cast, or to directly mill raw material into the finished implant.[27,28] An alternative method is for anatomically precise stereolithographic biomodels (i.e. exact physical replicas) of the cranium to be constructed. Subsequently, each stereolithographic biomodel is used as a template for the construction of a preliminary implant, which is then inspected by the surgeon physically or online; the surgeon then either approves the implant or requests further modifications. If approved, the final implant is then prepared and packaged sterilely.

Prefabricated implants of various materials, including PMMA–polyhydroxylethylmethacrylate (hard tissue replacement, HTR),[29] porous polyethylene (paper submitted for publication), and PMMA,[30] are available. The use of custom-prefabricated implants can reduce operative time significantly.

When skull defects are large (greater than 6 cm in diameter) or when they involve complex curvatures such as the supraorbital rim, I prefer to reconstruct them with custom porous polyethylene implants prefabricated using computed tomography data. Use of these implants has decreased operative time by at least 50%, thereby more than justifying their fabrication cost (Figs 4.13–4.15).

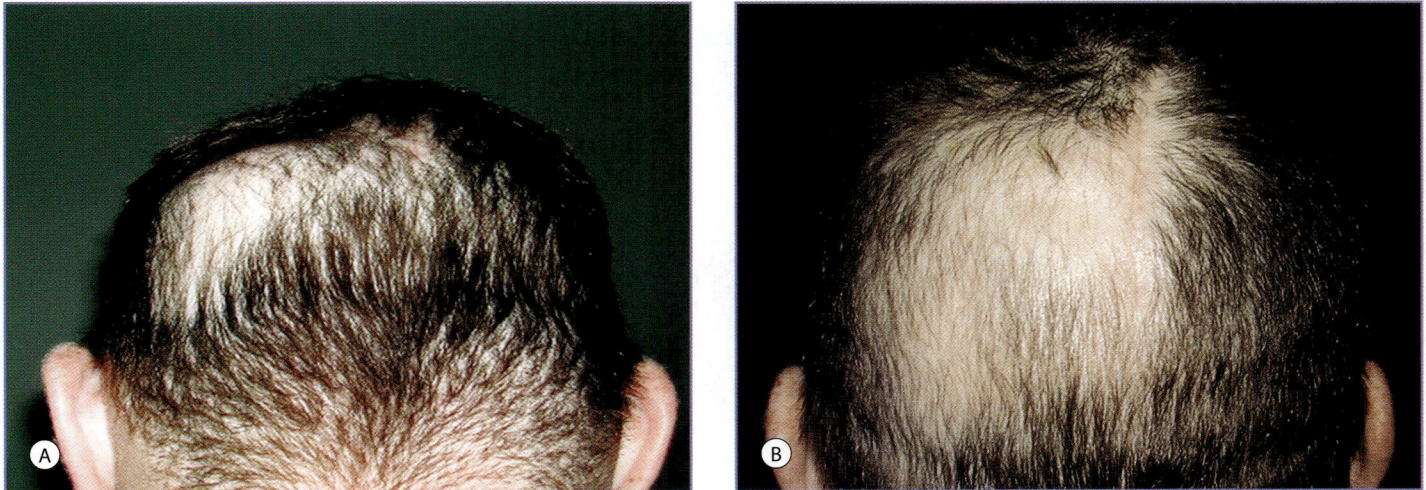

Figure 4.13 An 18-year-old high school student underwent craniotomy to resect a malignant neoplasm. The craniotomy graft was lost to infection. The operative site was subsequently irradiated. After radiation therapy, the patient received a 6-month course of chemotherapy. After this treatment, a three-dimensional computed tomography scan was performed and the data used to manufacture a porous polyethylene implant specific for the defect. Surgery was performed by incising the neurosurgical access incisions. It was necessary to score the galea to expand the scalp and allow wound closure. The implant was fixed to the intact adjacent skull with titanium screws. (A) Preoperative and (B) 1-year postoperative appearance.

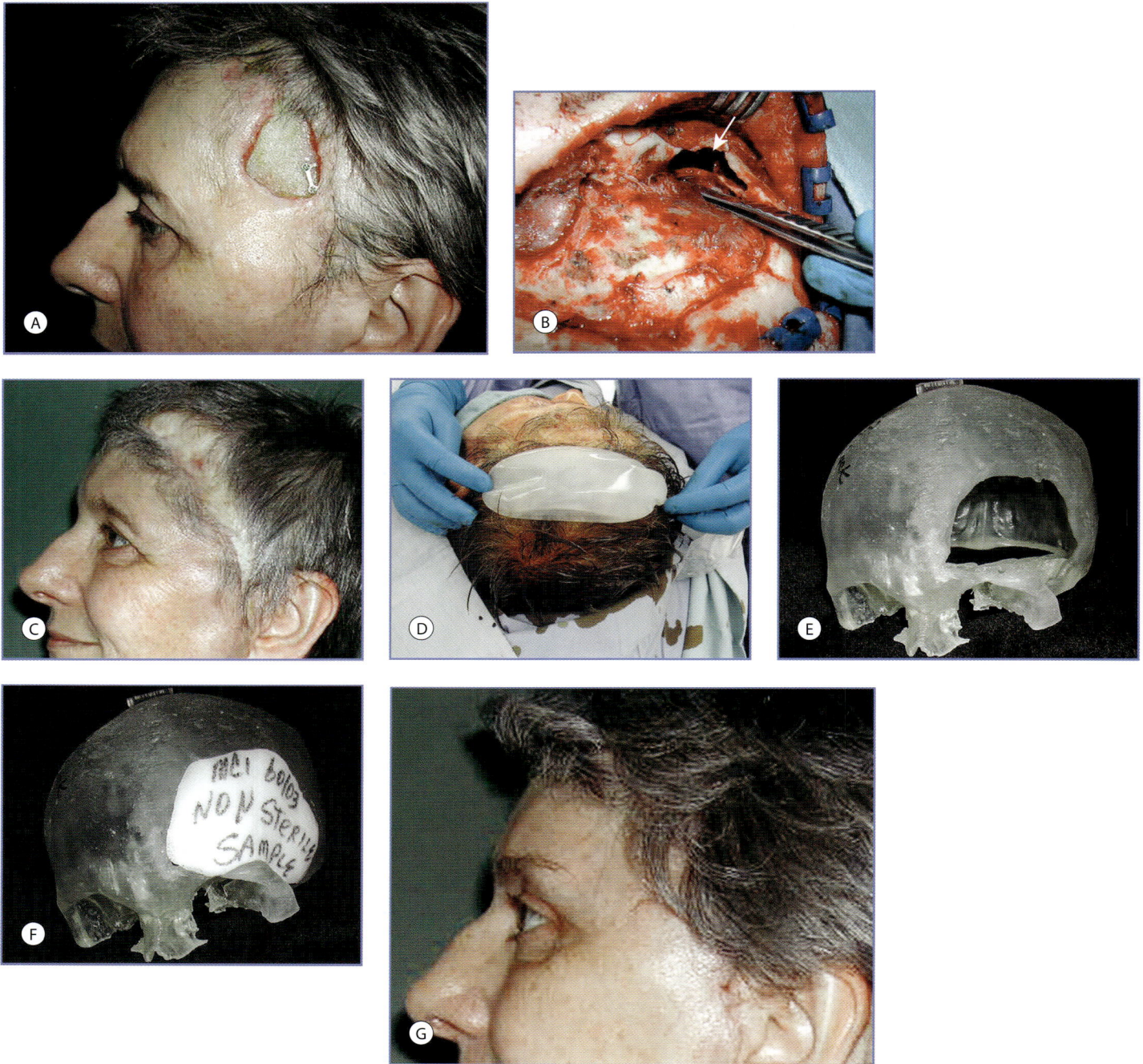

Figure 4.14 A 60-year-old woman presented with an exposed cranial implant. By history, an asymptomatic aneurysm was treated through a left-sided frontotemporal craniotomy. The craniotomy graft was lost to infection. A hydroxyapatite cement and mesh cranioplasty was performed and was subsequently removed due to infection. Six months later, a custom hard tissue replacement implant was fabricated by using three-dimensional computed tomography (CT) data. This became exposed. A CT scan was obtained that showed communication between the frontal sinus and the implant. At surgery, the implant was removed and a rectus abdominis myocutaneous free flap was used to obliterate dead space in the wound, separate the frontal sinus from the anticipated cranioplasty implant, and provide a closed soft tissue wound. Six months later, a tissue expander was placed in the hair-bearing scalp. When the scalp was sufficiently expanded to provide hair-bearing scalp adequate to replace that lost to infection, the expander was removed, and a custom porous polyethylene implant was placed and covered with the expanded, hair-bearing scalp. (**A**) Patient with exposed implant. (**B**) Intraoperative view at time of implant removal. Arrow points to communication with frontal sinus. (**C**) Appearance after rectus abdominis myocutaneous free flap wound closure. (**D**) Tissue expander used to expand hair-bearing scalp. (**E**) Skull model obtained from three-dimensional CT scan data shows cranial defect. (**F**) Skull model and custom implant. (**G**) Appearance after custom implant cranioplasty.

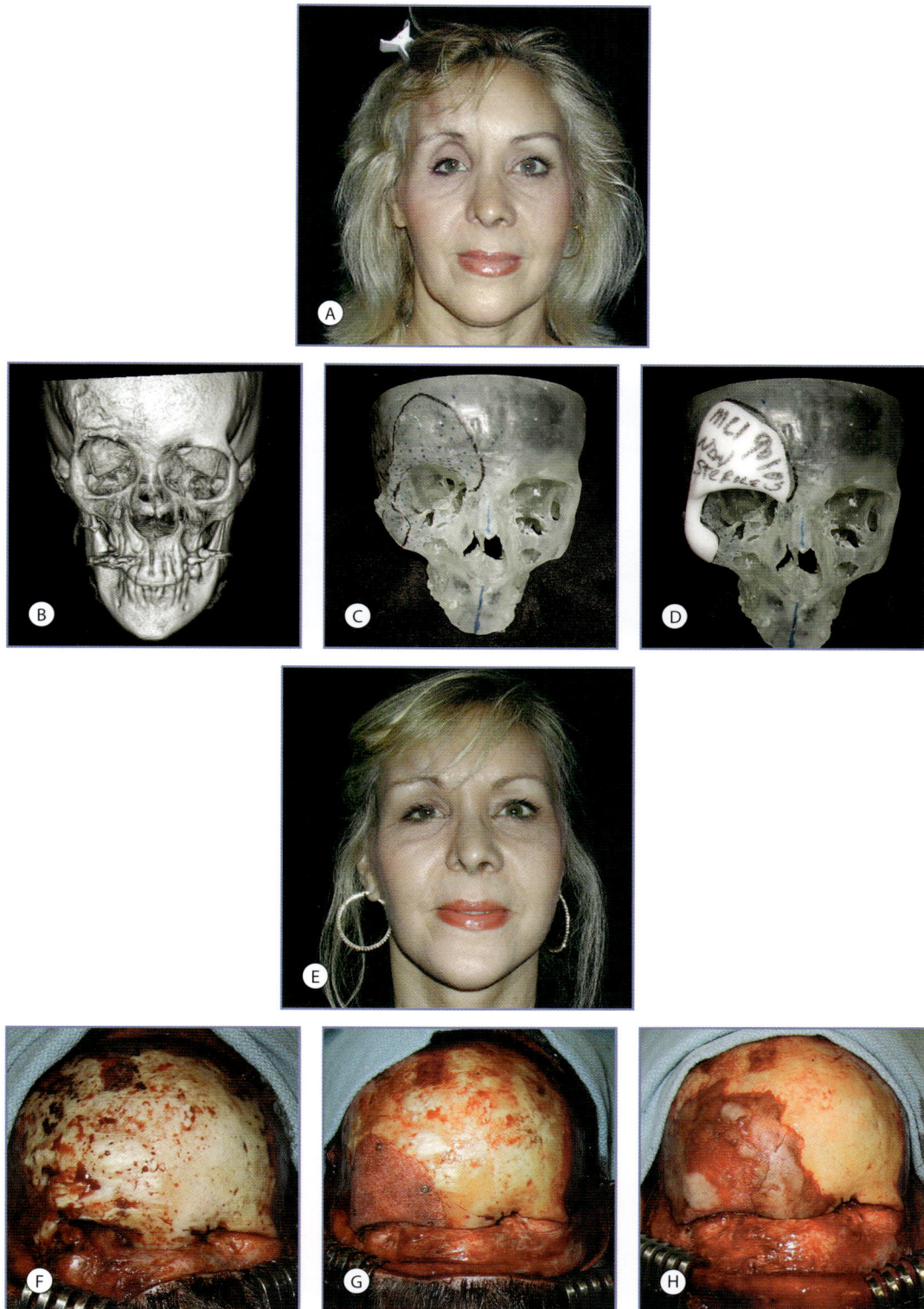

Figure 4.15 A woman with Romberg disease underwent onlay rib frontal cranioplasty at age 21. The grafts resorbed. At age 46, she underwent frontoorbital reconstruction with a custom porous polyethylene implant. Her enophthalmos was corrected by implant augmentation of her internal orbit. (**A**) Preoperative appearance. (**B**) Preoperative three-dimensional computed tomography (CT) shows skeletal deficiency. (**C**) Skull model obtained from three-dimensional CT data. (**D**) Skull model with custom implant. (**E**) Postoperative appearance. (**F**) Intraoperative view. There is no remnant of previously placed onlay bone grafts. (**G**) Intraoperative view shows custom implant in place. (**H**) Intraoperative view shows polymethylmethacrylate used to feather implant native skull transition beneath extremely thin forehead skin.

CRANIOPLASTY FOR CONTOUR DEFORMITIES

Indications

Onlay cranioplasty is most often performed to refine the results of cranioplasties previously performed to reconstruct full-thickness defects or to correct surface irregularities resulting after posttraumatic reconstructions. Onlay cranioplasties may also be performed for purely aesthetic reasons. When this is the case, a change in globe–rim relations is the most frequent indication.

Skeletal surface irregularities

Polymethylmethacrylate is the most frequently used material for onlay reconstructions of surface irregularities. It is immobilized by its insinuation into surface irregularities or by the screw immobilization technique demonstrated in Figure 4.11. Most often, the bicoronal flap is replaced before the PMMA is hardened, and the surface is molded through the overlying scalp. This allows the PMMA to replace both hard and soft tissue deficits, with a resultant smooth skin surface contour (Figs 4.15 and 4.16).

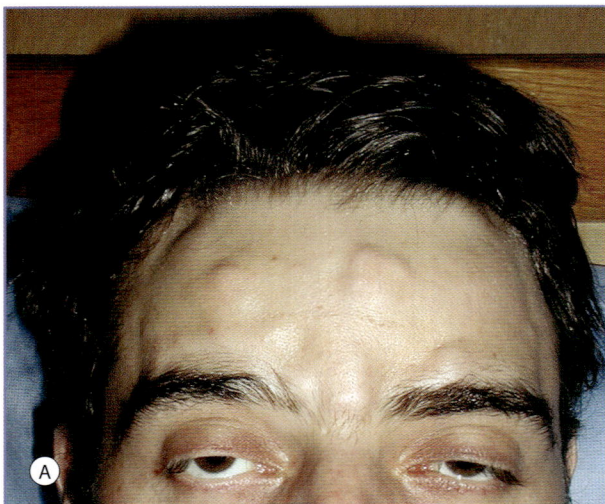

Figure 4.16 A 27-year-old man presented for correction of frontal contour irregularities 1 year after being treated for frontal bone fractures and intracranial injuries. Using coronal incision access, the fixation hardware was removed and the frontal area resurfaced with polymethylmethacrylate (PMMA). (**A**) Preoperative frontal view shows frontal contour irregularities. (**B**) Intraoperative view shows prominent plates and screws and the adjacent resorbed bone replaced at the time of fracture repair. (**C**) Intraoperative view after reconstruction with PMMA.

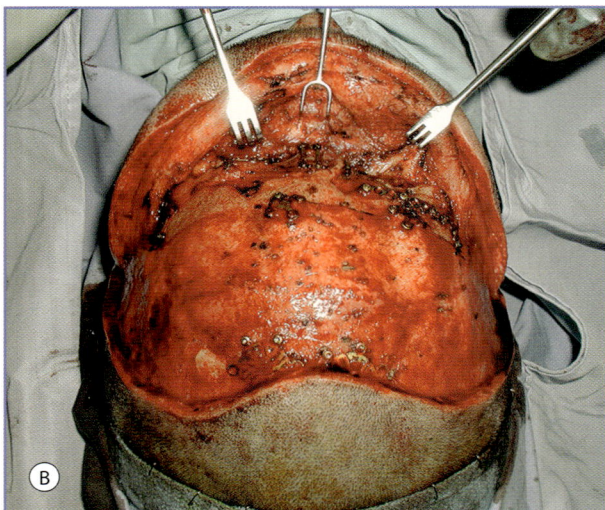

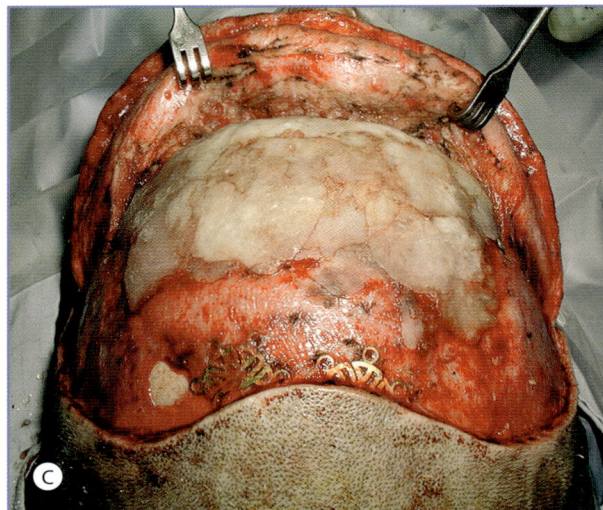

When the frontal area is augmented for aesthetic concerns, a combination of implants and PMMA is employed. Implants can help ensure a uniform thickness, defined projection, or symmetric complex curvature. PMMA is used to create smooth transitions between the implants and the native skull (Fig. 4.17).

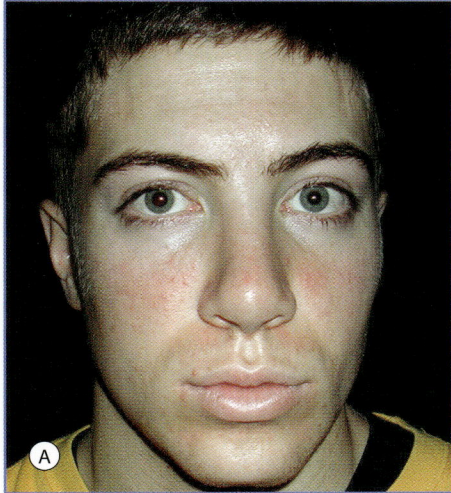

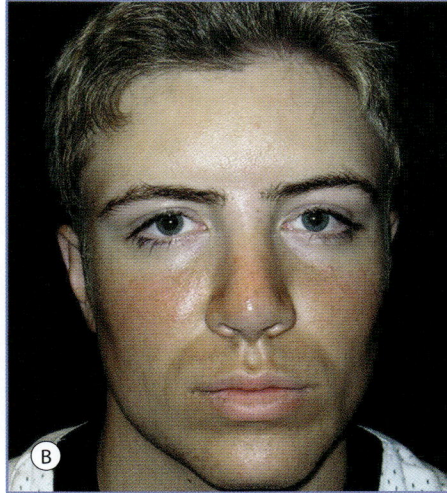

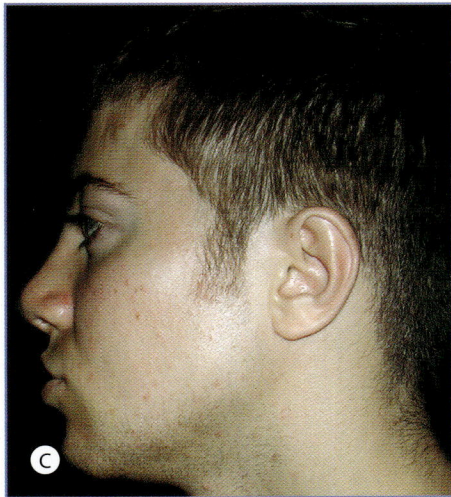

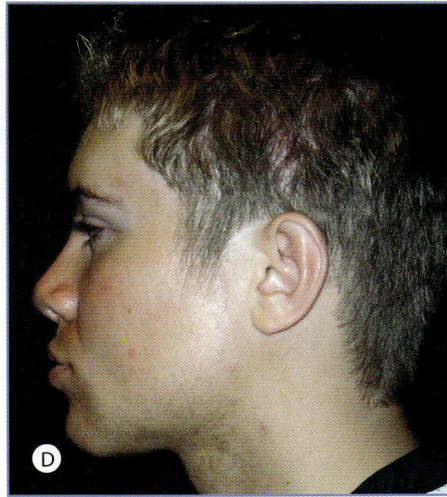

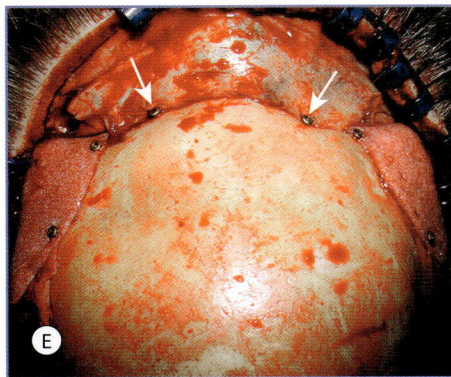

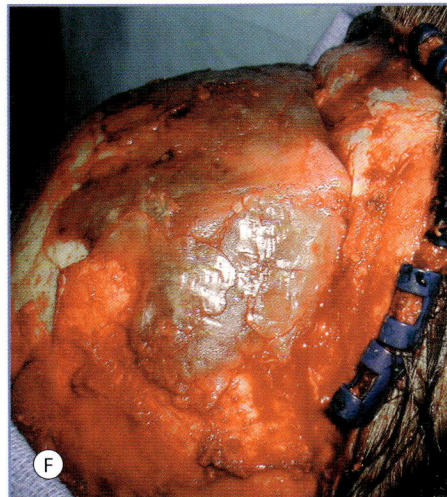

Figure 4.17 A 25-year-old man underwent augmentation of his supraorbital rims to make his eyes appear less prominent. Titanium screws were placed so that the screw heads projected 5 mm beyond the supraorbital rim. Porous polyethylene implants were positioned laterally. Polymethylmethacrylate (PMMA) was used to cover the rim screws and the porous polyethylene implants. Lateral canthopexies were also performed. (**A**) Preoperative and (**B**) postoperative frontal appearance. (**C**) Preoperative and (**D**) postoperative lateral appearance. (**E**) Intraoperative view from coronal approach. Arrows point to screws at supraorbital rim used to ensure measured projection of supraorbital rim PMMA only. (**F**) Intraoperative lateral view.

Temporal depressions

Disinsertion and reattachment of the temporal muscle leads to its atrophy. The subsequent loss of volume of this muscle may result in a visible depression in the temporal area. Alloplastic materials can be used to augment the volume of the temporal muscle and thereby restore contour. Alloplastic materials can be placed behind the muscle or between the muscle and the overlying soft tissues. Thin (1.5 mm) sheets of porous polyethylene are placed beneath the edges of the zygomatic arch and lateral orbital rim, or PMMA is fashioned over titanium screws placed at the lateral orbital rim. Porous polyethylene implants are available in shapes specifically designed for this application. They are modified as appropriate during the surgery (Fig. 4.18).

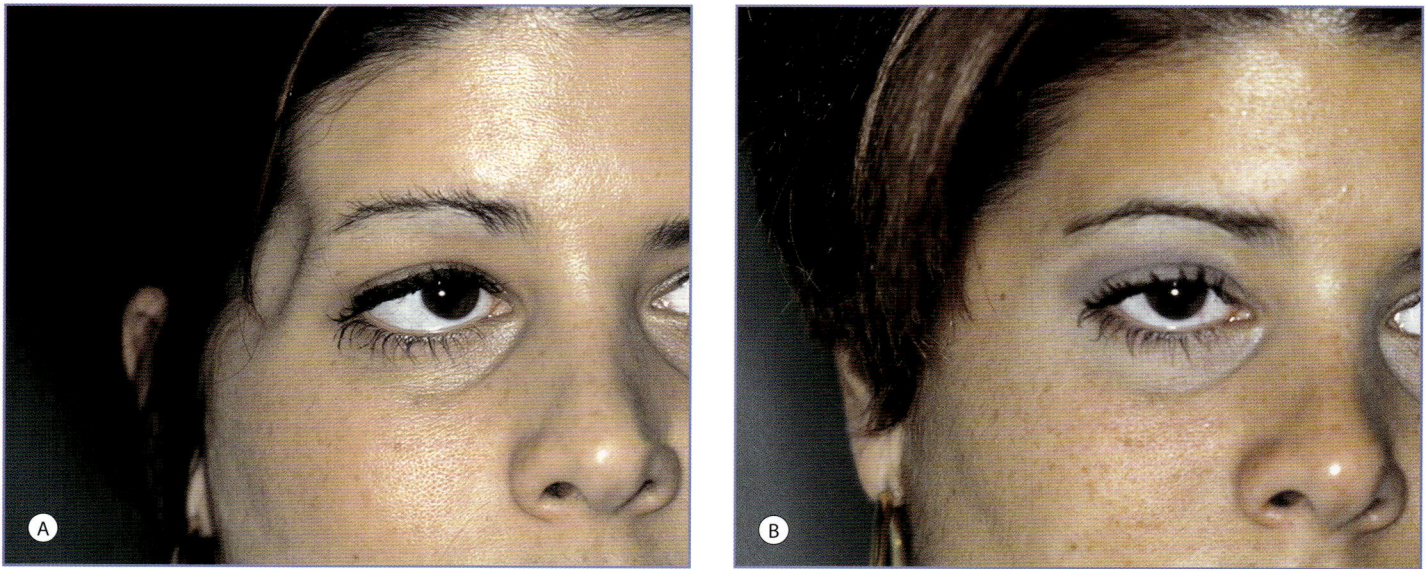

Figure 4.18 A 28-year-old woman developed temporal depression after craniotomy. The preoperative contour was restored with polymethylmethacrylate augmentation. (**A**) Preoperative and (**B**) postoperative appearance.

REFERENCES

1. Farkas LG, Hreczko TA, Katic MJ. Appendix A. Craniofacial norms in North American Caucasians from birth (one year) to adulthood. In: Farkas LG, ed. Anthropometry of the head and face. 2nd edn. New York: Raven Press; 1994.
2. Whitaker LA, Morales L, Farkas LG. Aesthetic surgery of the supraorbital ridge and forehead structures. Plast Reconstr Surg 1986; 78(1):23–32.
3. Bartlett SP, Wornom I, Whitaker LA. Evaluation of facial skeletal aesthetics and planning. Clin Plast Surg 1991; 18(1):1–9.
4. Pessa JE, Desvigne LD, Lambros VS, et al. Changes in ocular globe-to-orbital rim position with age: implication for aesthetic blepharoplasty of the lower eyelids. Aesthetic Plast Surg 1999; 23(5):337–342.
5. Marchac D. Relationship of the orbits to the upper eyelids. Clin Plast Surg 1981; 8(4):717–724.
6. Pensler J, McCarthy JG. The calvarial donor site: an anatomic study in cadavers. Plast Reconstr Surg 1985; 75(5):648–651.
7. Grantham EG, Landis HP. Cranioplasty and posttraumatic syndrome. J Neurosurg 1948; 5:19.
8. Carmichael FA. The reduction of hernia cerebri by tantalum cranioplasty. A preliminary report. J Neurosurg 1945; 2:379.
9. Tabaddor K, LaMorgese J. Complication of a large cranial defect. Case report. J Neurosurg 1976; 44(4):506–508.
10. Stula D. The problem of 'sinking skin-flap syndrome' in cranioplasty. J Craniomaxillofac Surg 1982; 10:142.
11. Manson PN, Crawley WA, Hoopes JE. Frontal cranioplasty: risk factors and choice of cranial vault reconstructive material. Plast Reconstr Surg 1986; 77(6):888–904.
12. Hammon WM, Kempe LG. Methyl methacrylate cranioplasty: 13 years' experience with 417 patients. Acta Neurochir 1971; 25(1):69–77.
13. Rish BL, Dillon JD, Meirowsky AM, et al. Cranioplasty: a review of 1030 cases of penetrating head injury. Neurosurgery 1979; 4(5):381–385.
14. Munro IR, Guyuron B. Split rib cranioplasty. Ann Plast Surg 1981; 7(5):341–346.
15. October supplement. Plast Reconstr Surg 2005; 116.
16. Eppley BL. Biomechanical testing of alloplastic PMMA cranioplasty materials. J Craniofac Surg 2005; 16(1):140–143.
17. Yaremchuk MJ, Rubin JP. Surgical repair of major defects of the scalp and skull. In: Schmidek HH, ed. Operative neurosurgical techniques. 4th edn. Philadelphia: Saunders; 2000.
18. Stelnicki EJ, Ousterhout DK. Prevention of thermal tissue injury induced by the application of polymethylmethacrylate to the calvarium. J Craniofac Surg 1996; 7(3):192–195.
19. Constantino PD, Friedman CD, Jones K, et al. Experimental hydroxyapatite cement cranioplasty. Plast Reconstr Surg 1992; 90(2):174–185.
20. Burstein FD, Cohen SR, Hudgins R, et al. The use of hydroxyapatite cement in secondary craniofacial reconstruction. Plast Reconstr Surg 1999; 104(5):1270–1275.
21. Constantino PD, Friedman CD, Jones K, et al. Hydroxyapatite cement: I. Basic chemistry and histologic properties. Arch Otolaryngol Head Neck Surg 1991; 117(4):379–384.
22. Constantino PD, Friedman CD, Jones K, et al. Hydroxyapatite cement: II. Obliteration and reconstruction of the cat frontal sinus. Arch Otolaryngol Head Neck Surg 1991; 117:22.
23. Rosen HM. Porous, block hydroxyapatite as an interpositional bone graft substitute in orthognathic surgery. Plast Reconstr Surg 1989; 83(6):985–990.
24. Burstein FD, Cohen SR, Hudgins R, et al. The use of porous granular hydroxyapatite in secondary orbitocranial reconstruction. Plast Reconstr Surg 1997; 100(4):869–874.
25. Moreira-Gonzalez A, Zins J. The use of hydroxyapatite bone cement in the repair of large full thickness cranial defects: a caution. Presented at the American Association 84th Annual Meeting, Scottsdale, Arizona, 2005.
26. Matic D, Phillips JH. A contraindication for the use of hydroxyapatite cement in the pediatric population. Plast Reconstr Surg 2002; 110(1):1–5.
27. Wehmoller MW, Eufinge H, Kruse D, et al. CAD by processing of computed tomography data and CAM of individually designed prostheses. Int J Oral Maxillofac Surg 1995; 24:90–97.
28. Eufinger H, Wehmoller MW, Machtens E, et al. Reconstruction of craniofacial bone defects with individual alloplastic implants based on CAD/CAM manipulated CT data. J Craniomaxillofac Surg 1995; 23:175–181.
29. Eppley BL, Kilgore M, Coleman JJ. Cranial reconstruction with computer generated hard-tissue replacement patient-matched implants: indications, surgical techniques, and long term follow up. Plast Reconstr Surg 2002; 109:864–871.
30. Taub PJ, Rudkin GH, Clearihue WJ, et al. Prefabricated alloplastic implants for cranial defects. Plast Reconstr Surg 2003; 111:1232–1240.

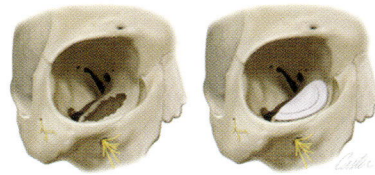

Chapter 5

Internal orbit

ENOPHTHALMOS

The size and shape of the orbit determine the position of the eye. Enophthalmos is the recession of the ocular globe within the bony orbit. Two to three millimeters of enophthalmos is clinically detectable, and more than 5 mm is disfiguring. The principal mechanism in its development is the displacement of a relatively constant volume of orbital soft tissue into an enlarged bony orbit. Posttraumatic fat atrophy and scar contracture are real, but less important, factors in causing a mismatch of soft tissue and orbital volume.[1-3] Enophthalmos may result from fractures involving only the orbital floor or medial orbital wall. These are termed *pure blowout* fractures. More often, enophthalmos is part of an orbital deformity whereby not only the internal orbit is disrupted, but also the adjacent facial skeleton. The internal orbit disruption is referred to as an *impure blowout* fracture in these situations.

Because enophthalmos most often presents with an inadequately treated orbital fracture where the orbital floor is disrupted, the condition is characteristically accompanied by inferior displacement of the globe. Recession of the globe changes the drape of the upper lid on the globe, tending to deepen the superior tarsal fold and cause a lowering or pseudoptosis of the upper lid (Fig. 5.1).

Because posttraumatic enophthalmos is primarily due to alterations in the configuration of the bony internal orbit rather than to changes in the amount or character of its soft tissue contents, the treatment strategy for restoring eye position is the anatomical reconstruction of the internal orbit. This is best accomplished by defining the location and extent of injury preoperatively with computed tomography (CT) scans, widely exposing the injured area, retrieving displaced orbital soft tissues, and reconstructing the invariably comminuted fractured skeleton.[1-3]

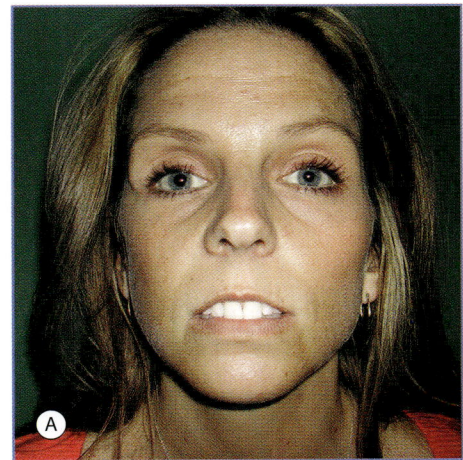

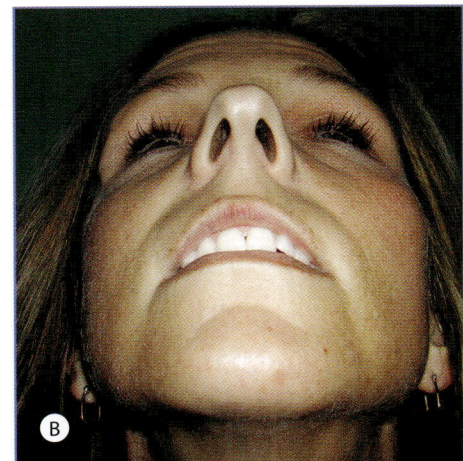

Figure 5.1 A 30-year-old woman with posttraumatic enophthalmos. Note inward displacement of the globe, deepening of the supratarsal sulcus, and pseudoptosis of the upper lid. (**A**) Frontal and (**B**) worm's eye views.

ORBITAL ANATOMY

The internal orbit may be conceptualized as a modified pyramid with an apex, a base, and four walls. The optic foramen, which transmits the optic nerve and the ophthalmic artery, forms the apex of the pyramid. It is located at the farthest superior medial portion of the internal orbit. The base of the pyramid is formed by the orbital rims. The roof, floor, medial wall, and lateral wall constitute the pyramid's walls.

While the entire lateral wall consists of thick bone created by the articulation of the greater wing of the sphenoid and the orbital process of the zygoma, the floor, medial wall, and roof vary in their thickness. They can be divided into concentric thirds based on bone thickness. The anterior third of the internal orbit consists of increasingly thicker bone as it merges with the orbital rim. The posterior third also consists of thick bone, with relatively flat walls. The middle third consists of thin bone and allows this portion of the orbit to act as a crush zone, thereby protecting the optic nerve and globe by absorbing impact forces.

The floor medial to the infraorbital canal and the inferior portion of the medial wall is typically involved in the blowout fracture. This area has a convex shape that produces a constriction behind the globe. Loss of this convexity transforms the internal orbit shape from pyramidal to spherical, increasing orbital volume and tending toward enophthalmos (Figs 5.2 and 5.3).

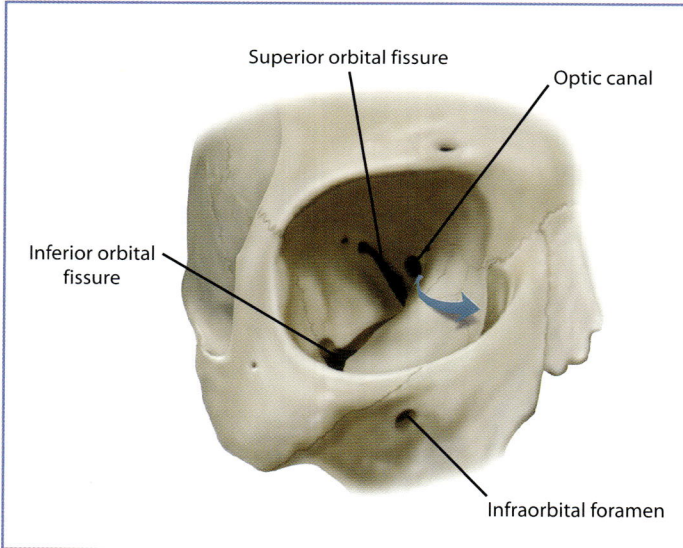

Figure 5.2 The orbit with its constituent bones and communications. Note the convex shape of the inferomedial aspect of the internal orbit.

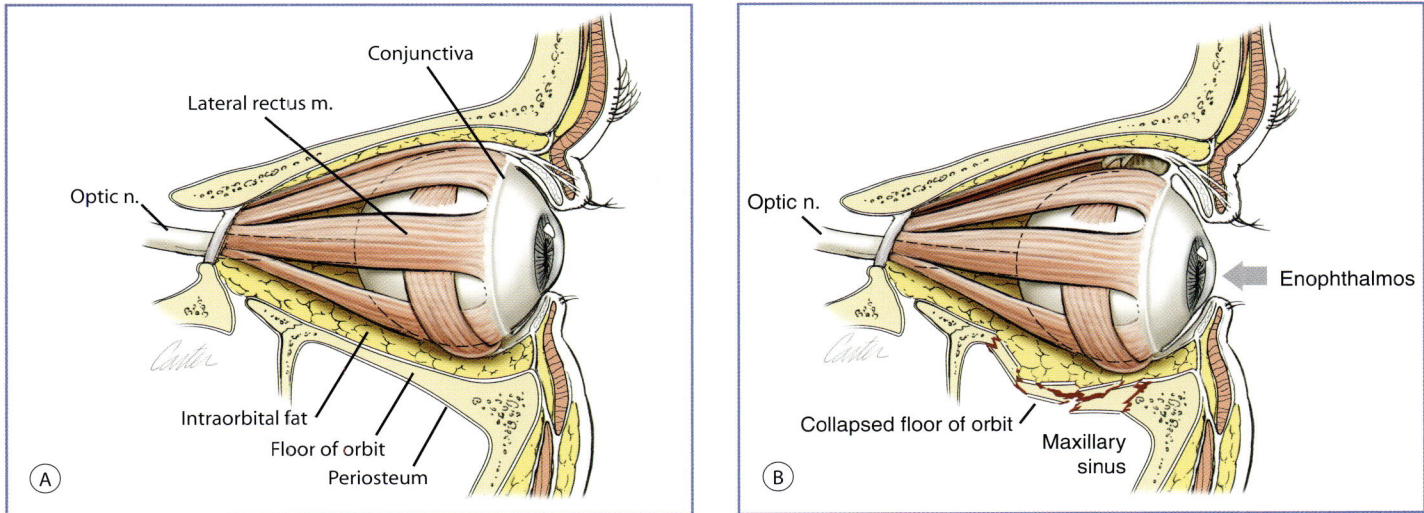

Figure 5.3 Sagittal section of orbit. (**A**) Normal. (**B**) Disrupted orbital floor. Loss of convexity of floor increases orbital volume and tends toward enophthalmos.

Certain injuries, usually involving the lateral orbital wall or roof, may result in inward displacement of larger fracture segments. These *blow-in* fractures decrease orbital volume, resulting in globe proptosis.

There are nine openings within each orbit. Most important are the optic foramen and the superior and inferior orbital fissures. The optic foramen, located at the apex, transmits the optic nerve. The superior orbital fissure, located between the roof and the lateral wall, near the apex, transmits the oculomotor, the trochlear, and the ophthalmic division of the trigeminal and the abducent nerves. The inferior orbital fissure separates the lateral wall from the floor. Through this fissure, the orbit communicates with the temporal, infratemporal, and pterygopalatine fossae. It transmits the maxillary nerve, its zygomatic branch, and the ascending branches from its sphenopalatine branch. It also transmits the infraorbital vessels and the vein that connects the inferior ophthalmic vein with the pterygoid venous plexus. The supraorbital foramen, infraorbital canal, anterior and posterior ethmoidal foramina, and zygomatic foramen transmit their respective neurovascular structures. There is also a canal for the nasolacrimal duct.

81

PREOPERATIVE EVALUATION

Physical examination

The clinical diagnosis of significant internal orbital disruption is based on globe malposition. In the uninjured state, the cornea extends approximately 16–17 mm *anterior* to the lateral orbital rim. Immediately after injury, however, globe position may appear normal or proptotic owing to soft tissue swelling. A difference in globe position is most easily determined by viewing the position in the worm's eye position. On frontal view, a deepening of the supratarsal sulcus and a lowering of the upper lid margin (pseudoptosis) reflect an increase in orbital volume and subsequent recession of the globe. When the lateral orbital rim is intact (isolated floor or medial wall blowout fractures), the severity of enophthalmos can be determined with a Hertel exophthalmometer, which measures the difference between the anterior corneal surface and the lateral orbital rim.

Radiologic imaging

Computed tomography imaging is necessary to determine the presence and extent of injury. Plain x-rays will confirm the presence of fractures but will not define the injury or the status of the soft tissues. The ideal preoperative evaluation consists of thin-slice axial and coronal CT sections using both bone and soft tissue windows. (Software packages allow reconstruction of sagittal sections.) By adding together the consecutive CT slices where a defect appears, one can determine the size of a floor or wall injury. Defects greater than 25% of the orbital floor will result in clinically measurable enophthalmos. Those involving more than half of the floor will result in obvious enophthalmos. Diplopia may result from eye muscle contusion or muscle entrapment. This can be differentiated on physical examination by forced duction test and often by high-resolution CT scan.

OPERATIVE TECHNIQUE

Timing

In the acute phase, CT findings coupled with forced duction testing provide the best guide to the need for surgery. As noted above, a CT scan can define the amount of floor disruption and therefore predict the likelihood of enophthalmos. It can also define the relation of the extraocular muscles to the fracture segments.

If surgery is thought appropriate, it should be performed soon after injury, when dissection is more straightforward and the soft tissue scarring and contracture are less problematic. Late and secondary reconstructions are less successful than appropriate reconstruction performed in the acute phase. When indications for acute management are unclear, exploration is performed if enophthalmos greater than 2 mm develops at any time within the first 6 weeks following injury.[4,5]

PEARL

The size of orbital floor defects can be quantified by adding coronal and sagittal CT scan sections.

Exposure

Proper repositioning of the globe requires exposure and anatomical reconstruction of the internal orbit. I prefer a transconjunctival retroseptal incision, often with a lateral canthotomy extension, to approach the orbital floor and lower medial and lateral walls. The coronal flap is used to approach the upper medial and lateral walls as well as the orbital roof. I avoid techniques such as skin and skin–muscle flaps, which delaminate and relaminate the lower lid. Postoperative scarring can only lower the lid margin.[6] Extensive subperiosteal dissection of the lateral orbit will detach the lateral canthus. It should be repositioned at closure.

Mobilization and retrieval of orbital contents

A small conical space and fragile contents make surgery in the internal orbit challenging using loupe magnification, the soft tissue contents of the orbit are freed from the injured skeleton by subperiosteal dissection. Care is taken to avoid damaging the lacrimal sac and structures in the inferior orbital fissure. Ideally, intact bony edges are identified for orientation and to provide stable constructs on which to position grafts or implants. This dissection can be exceedingly difficult in extensive injuries, particularly when surgery has been delayed and prolapsed orbital soft tissues have healed to damaged mucosa in the maxillary or ethmoid sinuses, or to the temporalis muscle in the temporal fossa. The orbital contents must be separated from these structures and replaced in the orbit.

An inferior orbitotomy increases internal orbit access and thereby simplifies soft tissue mobilization.[7] This maneuver is frequently used for secondary or late reconstructions (Fig. 5.4).

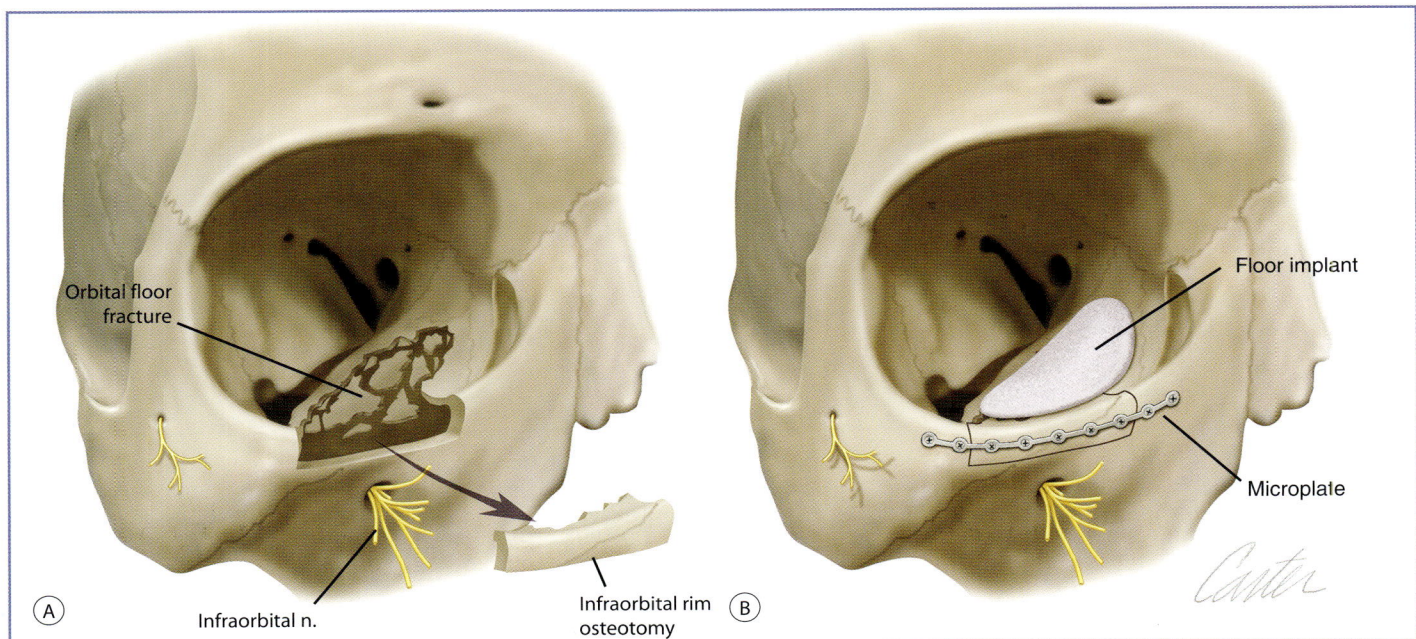

Figure 5.4 Inferior orbitotomy simplifies retrieval of prolapsed orbital contents from the maxillary sinus and identification of intact bony landmarks. Anatomical replacement of the osteotomized rim segment is simplified by adapting a microplate to the rim, drilling holes, and temporarily fixing the intact rim prior to making the osteotomy. (**A**) Location of orbitotomy. (**B**) Replacement of rim segment and reconstruction of defect.

Once the prolapsed contents of the orbit are retrieved, temporarily interposing a piece of silicone sheeting between the soft tissues and the area to be reconstructed is helpful (Fig. 5.5). This maneuver prevents the soft tissues falling back into the sinus, thereby lessening their subsequent handling and allowing easier control during placement of the implant or graft. Once reconstruction is complete, the silicone sheet is removed.[8]

Internal orbit reconstruction

The internal orbit is reconstructed to restore its preinjury anatomy with the anticipation that proper globe position will result. This requires definition of the injured area, which is best accomplished by identifying intact bone and hence the limits of the defect. This process is complicated by the location and extent of the injury. The bony landmark that is usually most difficult to identify is the posterior ledge of the remaining intact orbital floor. When the orbital floor disruption extends far posterior and intact bone cannot be visualized, it can be located by placing the end of an elevator against the posterior wall of the maxillary sinus and elevating it until it meets resistance; this indicates contact with the intact posterior remnant of the orbital floor. This structure is usually 35–40 mm from the infraorbital rim (Fig. 5.6).

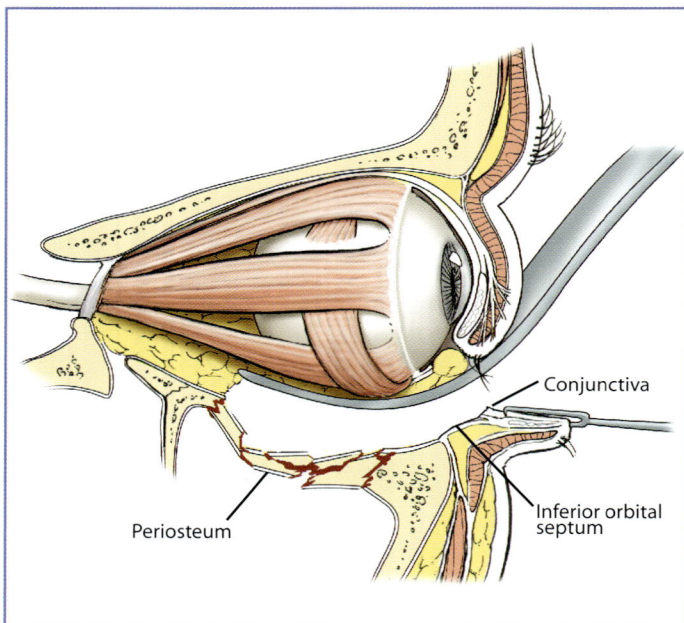

Figure 5.5 A retractor is lifting the orbital contents which have been retrieved from the maxillary antrum. A thick piece of silicone sheeting is often placed beneath the retrieved orbital contents to prevent the soft tissues from prolapsing into the maxillary antrum when the retractor is repositioned.

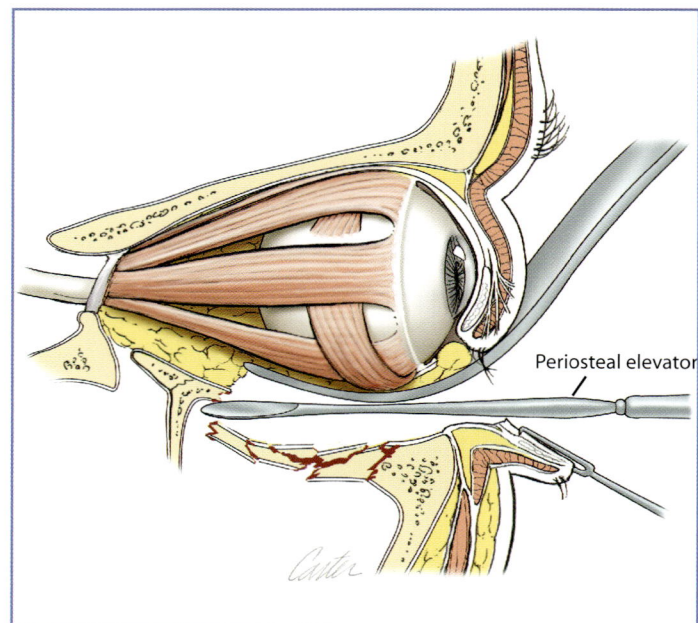

Figure 5.6 Identification of the intact posterior ledge can be simplified by placing an elevator against the posterior wall of the maxillary antrum, and elevating it until it meets the restriction of the intact posterior ledge. The presence of an intact ledge must be confirmed preoperatively by computed tomography scans to avoid putting the optic nerve at risk. An implant placed on this ledge provides a posterior landmark for orientation and a stable construct for implant placement.

When reconstructing injuries to one orbital wall, the surgeon first defines the defect by identifying intact bone edges and then spans the defect with an implant or autogenous graft (Fig. 5.7). The size of the defect and the normal configuration of the injured area will dictate the dimensions, thickness, and number of grafts. For example, a small floor defect is usually reconstructed with a single thin graft, thereby replicating the relatively flat shape of the orbital floor. A similarly dimensioned inferomedially located defect usually requires a thick graft, or stacked grafts, to recreate the convex shape of the orbit in this area. Failure to replicate this convexity effectively increases the volume of the orbit from normal and tends toward enophthalmos. Similarly, placement of an overly thick graft to reconstruct the floor would also create an internal orbit shape different from normal. In this case, the abnormal convexity beneath the globe would elevate it, resulting in an ocular dystopia. For injuries involving only the floor, I routinely use an alloplastic implant. Most often, it is a sheet of porous polyethylene or metallic mesh. To ensure stability of the construct, I routinely immobilize the implant with a screw.

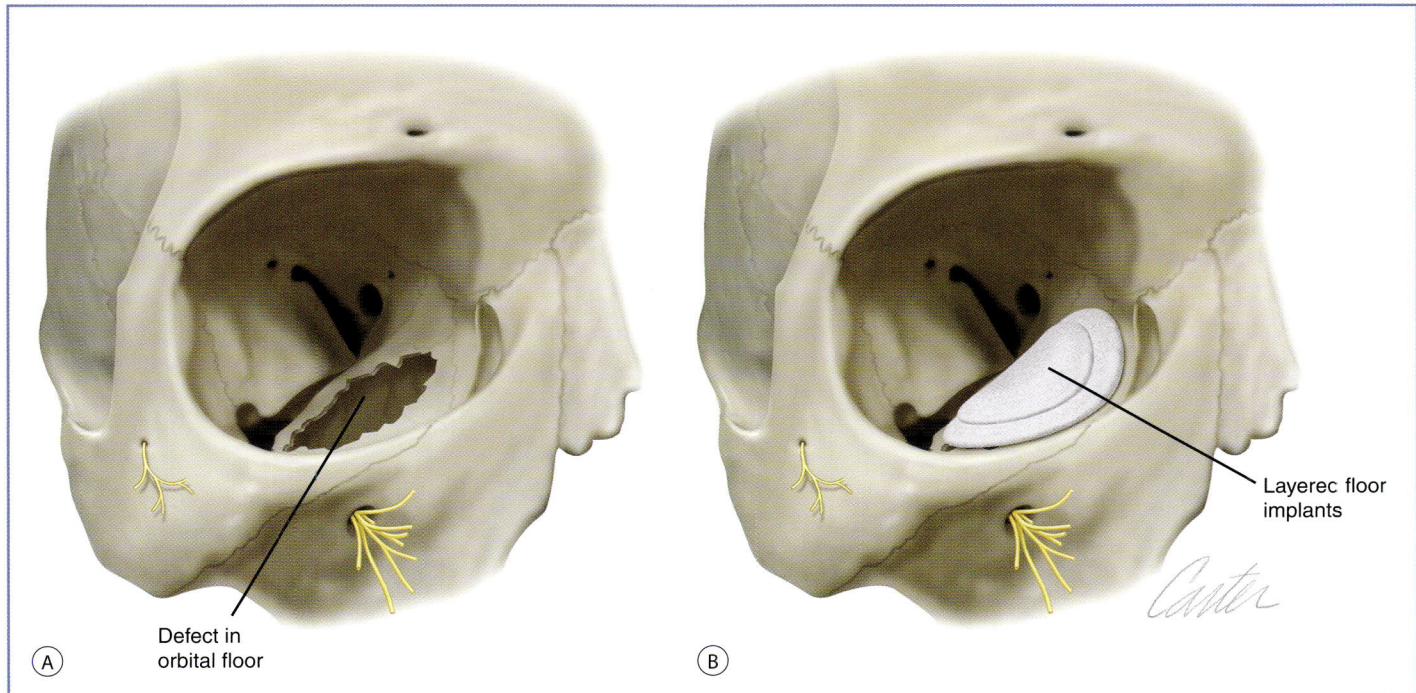

Defect in orbital floor

(A)

Layerec floor implants

(B)

Figure 5.7 Orbital floor reconstructed with graft spanning the defect. Stable adjacent ledges make bone graft or implant positioning relatively straightforward. (**A**) Orbital floor with defect and (**B**) reconstructed.

Multiple wall injuries are sequentially reconstructed using titanium mesh. The mesh may be a platform for autogenous bone or other implants (Fig. 5.8).

When injuries are devastating and mucosalization of an alloplastic implant is thought unlikely, I prefer to reconstruct the internal orbit with autogenous bone, usually rib.

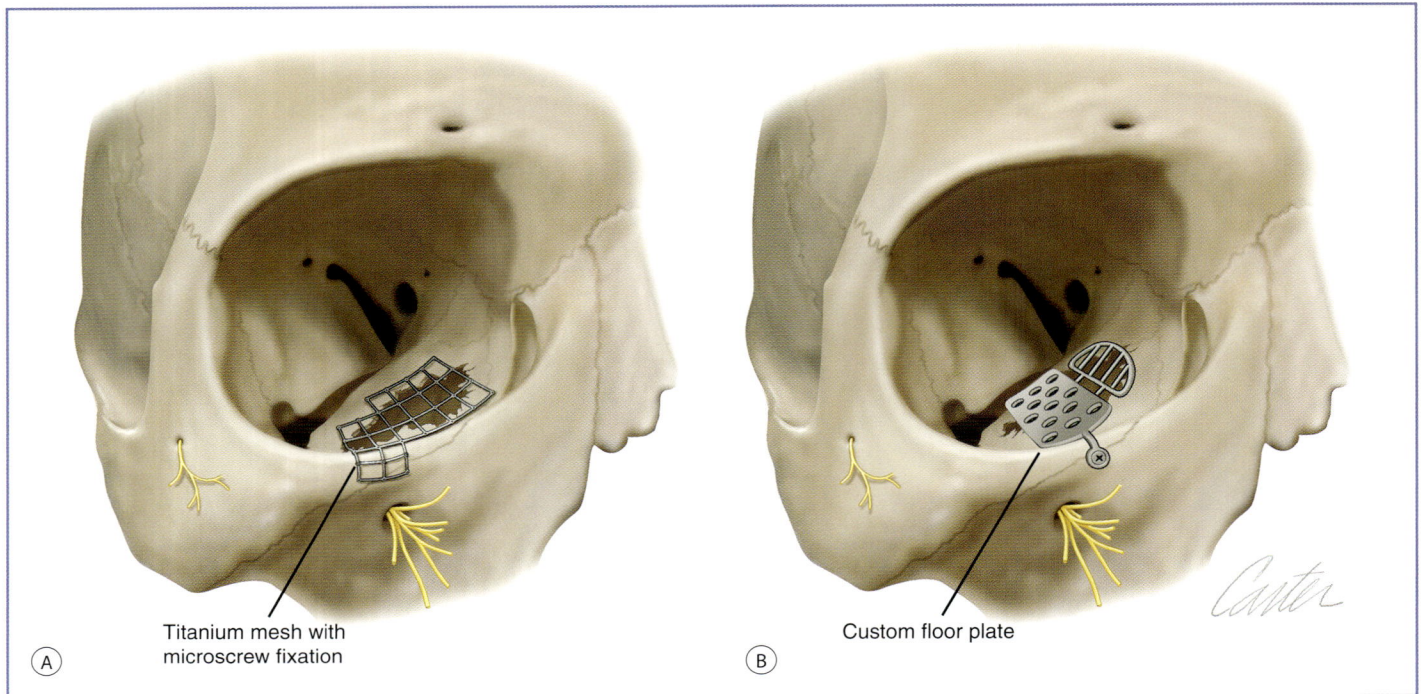

Titanium mesh with microscrew fixation

(A)

Custom floor plate

(B)

Figure 5.8 Methods of spanning large orbital defects. (**A**) Titanium mesh can be molded to the appropriate contour and fixed to the orbital rim. (**B**) Custom-made floor plate that provides a stable construct in which to place a graft.

Implant materials

Materials available for reconstruction include bone, cartilage, smooth and porous plastics, and metal.

Reconstruction with autogenous bone has the conceptual advantage that it will, in time, become revascularized and incorporated into the skeleton, thereby resisting migration, extrusion, and infection. Revascularization, however, may also predispose the graft to resorb, with a concomitant change in internal orbit architecture and hence volume and globe position. Clinical experience has shown that calvarial grafts tend to resorb less than grafts taken from other donor sites. Cranial bone grafts have more dense cortical bone than ilium or rib, which tend to be predominantly cancellous. Experimental evidence suggests that the volume persistence of calvarial grafts may result from the fact that cortical bone is less susceptible to revascularization than cancellous bone, and hence less susceptible to osteoclastic activity (see Ch. 2).[9] Calvarial bone can be difficult to shape and control during internal orbit reconstruction.

To avoid changes in graft shape and volume, as well as to avoid the morbidity and operative time associated with autogenous graft harvest, alloplastic implants have long been used for orbital floor reconstruction. These include polytetrafluoroethylene, silicone, dense and porous polyethylene, resorbable materials, metal plates, and polymethylmethacrylate. High rates of extrusion have been documented for the rigid, smooth-surfaced implants made of silicone (3.1%) and nylon (12%). There are also many reports of late complications, especially with silicone, polytetrafluoroethylene, and nylon plates. These have been noted to occur as late as 21 years after placement, and include infection, extrusion, migration with hematoma formation, and lower eyelid deformity.[10] Clinical experience obtained from treating these complications suggests that these problems are related to capsule formation around smooth-surfaced implants, with the concomitant tendency toward implant migration.

Porous polyethylene is the author's preferred non-metallic orbital implant. This implant has a pore size that allows vascular ingrowth and some incorporation into the recipient site.[11] In a personal experience with over 200 patients since 1987, there has been no known instance of infection or graft extrusion using this material. Clinical experience suggests that the soft tissue ingrowth into the material limits the tendency for migration seen with smooth-surfaced implants. Others have presented anecdotal data suggesting that this soft tissue ingrowth has the potential to include adjacent ocular motility muscles, with the possibility of ocular motility disorder. To avoid this potential problem, polyethylene implants are now available with a smooth surface on one side and a porous surface on the other. The smooth surface is intended to face the orbital soft tissue contents and the porous side to face the sinuses. The smooth surface is intended to prevent soft tissue ingrowth and possible motility problems, while the porous side allows soft tissue ingrowth with concomitant immobilization and mucosalization.

Injuries involving two or more walls of the orbit are problematic. Rigid fixation techniques allow these complex injuries to be subdivided into a series of smaller, more manageable areas for reconstruction. Titanium metal implants are attached to the orbital rim and are used to span large defects.[12–14] This support function can be accomplished with a number of implant designs (Fig. 5.8). The implant alone may be used to restore the internal orbital contour or may serve as a platform on which to place grafts or implants. Laminated implants of titanium metal and polyethylene are available. A titanium mesh infrastructure is sandwiched between a sheet of smooth polyethylene on one side, and a sheet of porous polyethylene on the other. The metal facilitates implant conformability and screw fixation. The smooth laminate is intended to interface with the soft tissue contents, preventing their prolapse into the metallic mesh. The porous laminate is intended to interface with the mucosal surface.

CLINICAL EXAMPLES

Clinical examples of patients treated with the techniques described are presented in Figures 5.9–5.13.

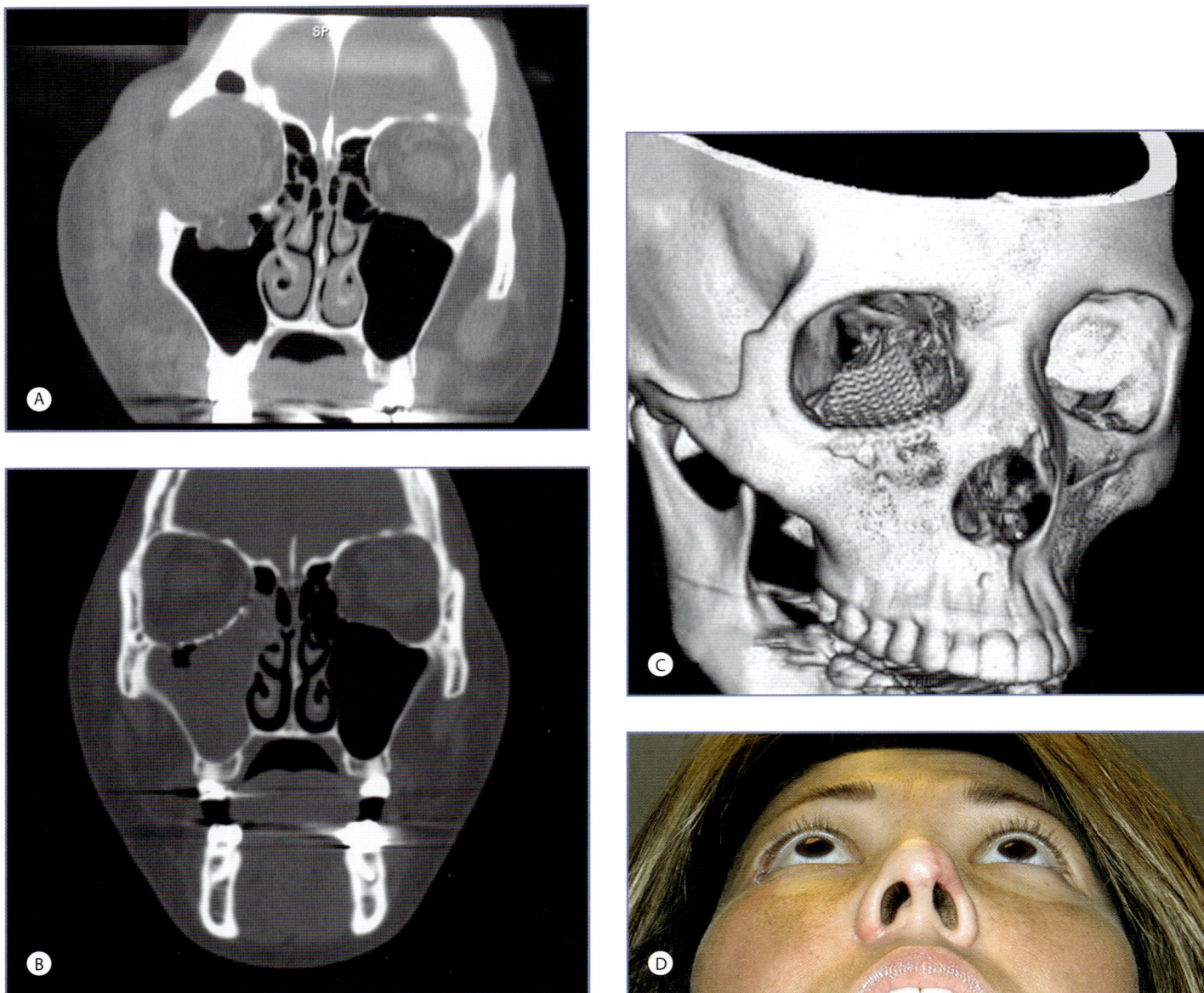

Figure 5.9 Computed tomography (CT) scans of a 23-year-old woman who suffered an orbital floor blowout fracture in a motor vehicle accident. (**A**) Preoperative coronal CT shows floor defect. The injury was reconstructed with a titanium mesh plate used to span the floor defect. (**B**) Postoperative coronal CT shows reconstruction. (**C**) Postoperative three-dimensional CT shows reconstruction. The mesh was wrapped around the inferior orbital rim, where it was immobilized with a titanium microscrew. (**D**) Postoperative worm's eye view.

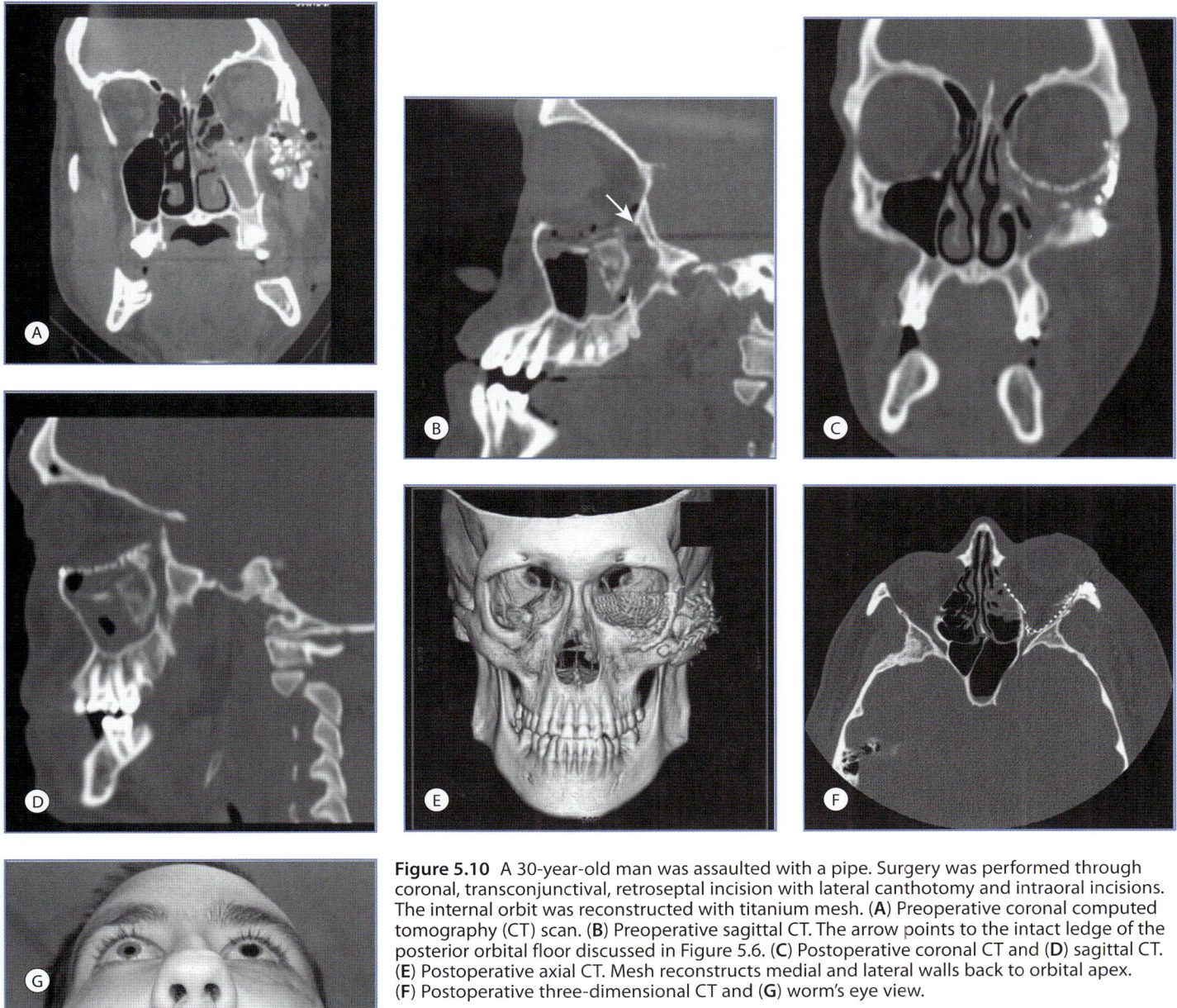

Figure 5.10 A 30-year-old man was assaulted with a pipe. Surgery was performed through coronal, transconjunctival, retroseptal incision with lateral canthotomy and intraoral incisions. The internal orbit was reconstructed with titanium mesh. (**A**) Preoperative coronal computed tomography (CT) scan. (**B**) Preoperative sagittal CT. The arrow points to the intact ledge of the posterior orbital floor discussed in Figure 5.6. (**C**) Postoperative coronal CT and (**D**) sagittal CT. (**E**) Postoperative axial CT. Mesh reconstructs medial and lateral walls back to orbital apex. (**F**) Postoperative three-dimensional CT and (**G**) worm's eye view.

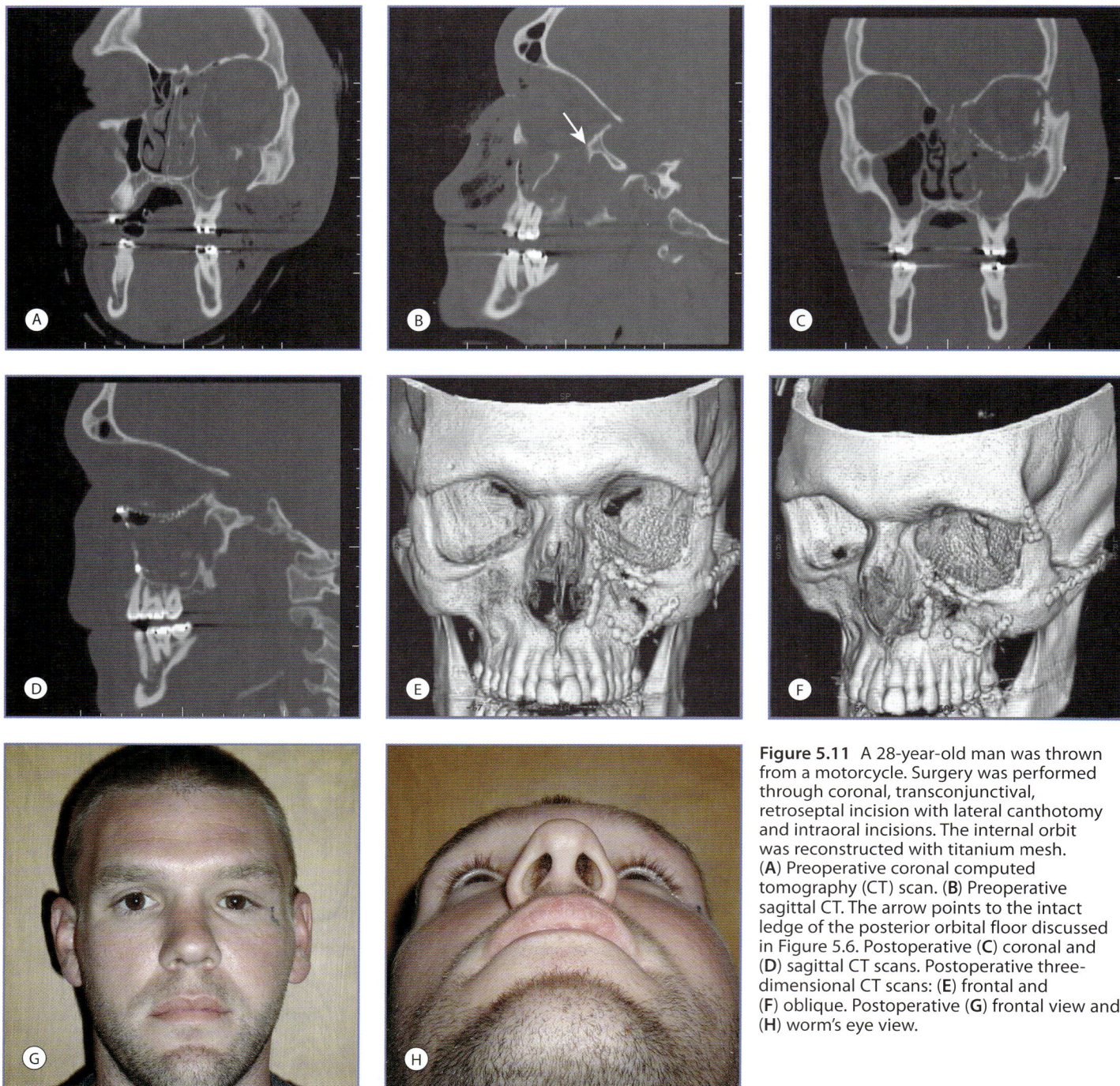

Figure 5.11 A 28-year-old man was thrown from a motorcycle. Surgery was performed through coronal, transconjunctival, retroseptal incision with lateral canthotomy and intraoral incisions. The internal orbit was reconstructed with titanium mesh. (**A**) Preoperative coronal computed tomography (CT) scan. (**B**) Preoperative sagittal CT. The arrow points to the intact ledge of the posterior orbital floor discussed in Figure 5.6. Postoperative (**C**) coronal and (**D**) sagittal CT scans. Postoperative three-dimensional CT scans: (**E**) frontal and (**F**) oblique. Postoperative (**G**) frontal view and (**H**) worm's eye view.

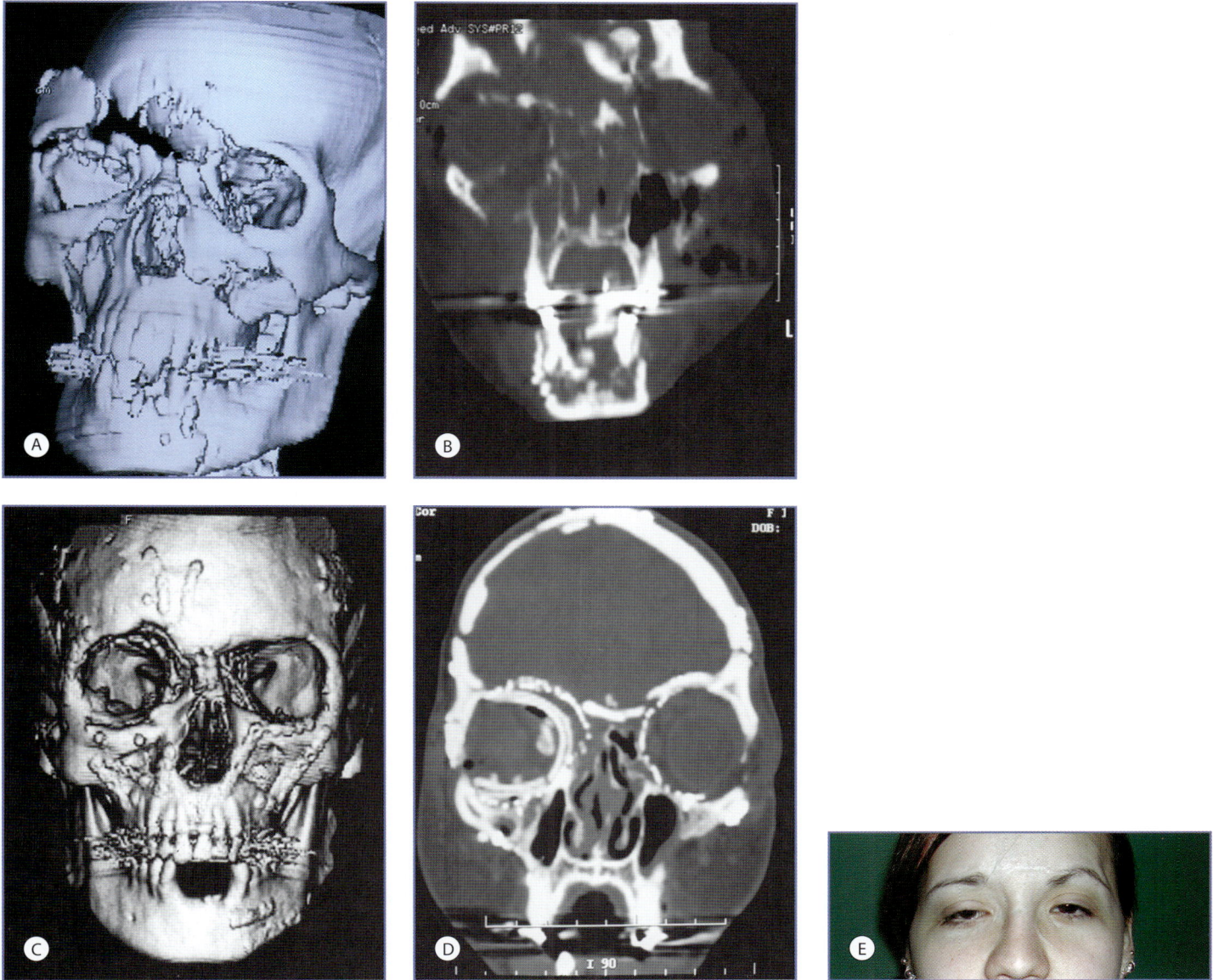

Figure 5.12 A 19-year-old woman suffered panfacial injuries in a motor vehicle accident. A staged reconstruction was performed during her acute hospitalization. The internal orbits were reconstructed with both titanium mesh and split rib grafts. (**A**) Preoperative three-dimensional computed tomography (CT) scan. (**B**) Preoperative coronal CT. (**C**) Postoperative three-dimensional CT. (**D**) Postoperative coronal CT. (**E**) Postoperative appearance.

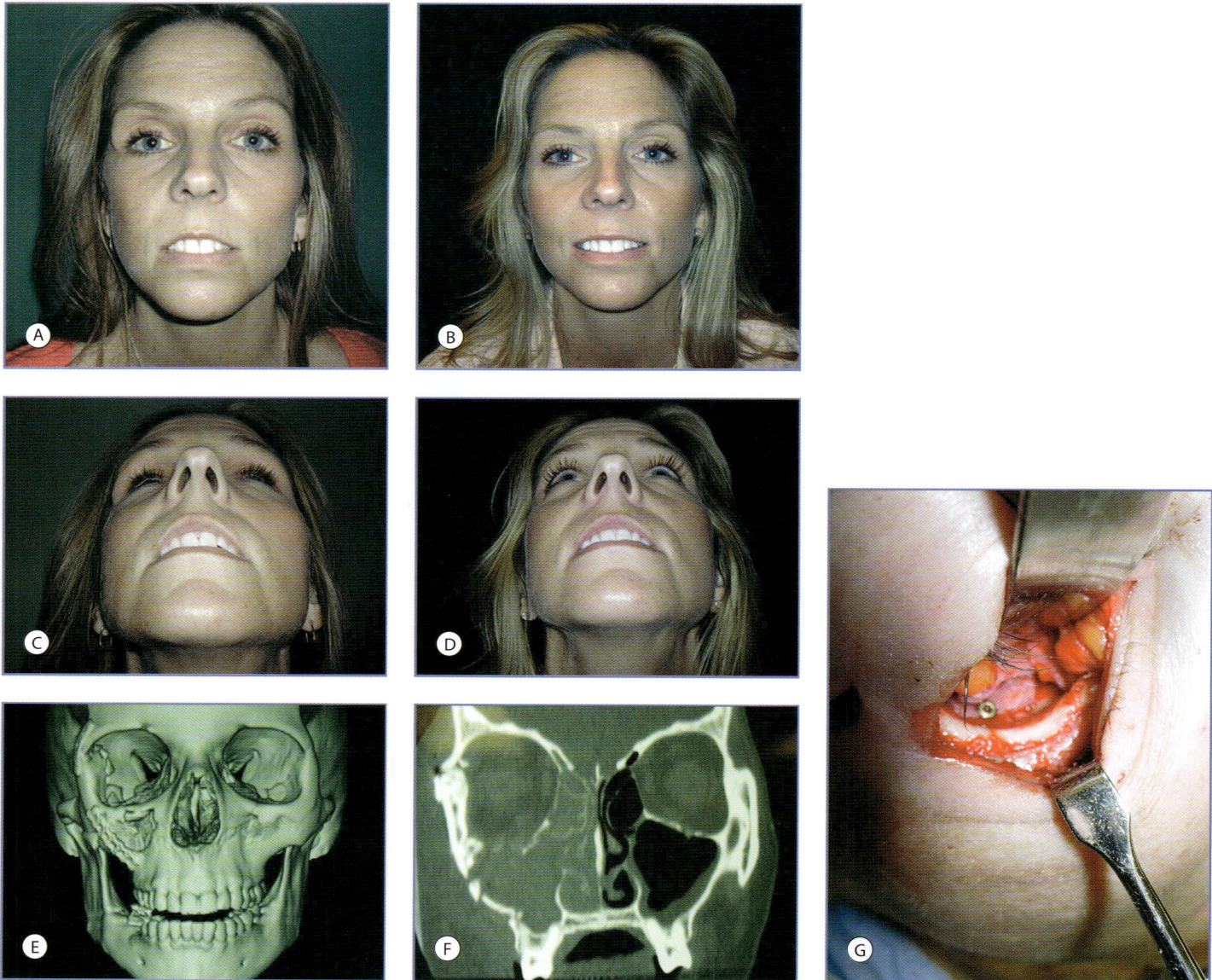

Figure 5.13 A 32-year-old woman was struck by an automobile and suffered multiple injuries including a right orbital fracture. The internal orbit was not reconstructed acutely, and the patient developed enophthalmos as well as a loss of malar prominence. The patient presented for secondary reconstruction 9 months after her initial repair. Surgery was performed through a transconjunctival retroseptal with lateral canthotomy and intraoral incisions. The internal orbit was reconstructed with porous polyethylene immobilized with titanium screws. The lateral and inferior orbital rims were augmented with screw-immobilized porous polyethylene. (**A**) Preoperative and (**B**) postoperative frontal view. (**C**) Preoperative and (**D**) postoperative worm's eye view. (**E**) Preoperative three-dimensional CT shows initial reconstruction. (**F**) Preoperative coronal CT shows enlarged, unrepaired internal orbit. (**G**) Intraoperative view of internal orbit reconstruction with screw-immobilized porous polyethylene implants. The lower lid is being retracted inferiorly. The orbital contents are being retracted superiorly.

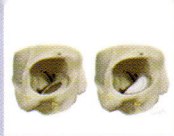

REFERENCES

1. Bite U, Jackson IT, Forbes GS, et al. Orbital measurements in enophthalmos using three dimensional CT imaging. Plast Reconstr Surg 1985; 75:502–511.

2. Manson PN, Clifford CM, Su CT, et al. Mechanisms of global support and post-traumatic enophthalmos. I. The anatomy of the ligament sling and its relation to intramuscular cone orbital fat. Plast Reconstr Surg 1985; 77:193–200.

3. Manson PN, Grivas A, Rosenbaum A, et al. Studies on enophthalmos. II. The measurement of orbital injuries and their treatment by quantitative computed tomography. Plast Reconstr Surg 1985; 77:201–209.

4. Hawes MJ, Dortzbach RK. Surgery on orbital floor fractures (influence of time and repair and fracture size). Ophthalmology 1983; 90:1066–1072.

5. Wilkins RB, Havins WE. Current treatment of blowout fractures. Ophthalmology 1982; 89:464–472.

6. Yaremchuk MJ, Kim WK. Soft tissue alterations with acute, extended open reduction and internal fixation of orbital fractures. J Craniofac Surg 1992; 3:134–140.

7. Tessier P. Inferior orbitotomy. A new approach to the orbital floor. Clin Plast Surg 1982; 9:569–575.

8. Glassman RD, Manson PN, Petty P, et al. Techniques for improved visibility and lid protection in orbital explorations. J Craniofac Surg 1990; 1:69–72.

9. Chen NT, Glowacki J, Bucky LP, et al. The roles of revascularization and resorption on endurance of craniofacial onlay bone grafts in the rabbit. Plast Reconstr Surg 1994; 93:725–782.

10. Rubin JP, Yaremchuk MJ. Complications and toxicities of implantable biomaterials used in facial reconstructive and aesthetic surgery: a comprehensive review of the literature. Plast Reconstr Surg 1997; 100:1336–1353.

11. Romano J, Iliff N, Manson PN. Use of Medpor porous polyethylene implants in 140 patients with facial fractures. J Craniofac Surg 1993; 4:142–150.

12. Glassman RD, Manson PN, Vanderkolk CA, et al. Rigid fixation of internal orbital fractures. Plast Reconstr Surg 1990; 86:1103–1110.

13. Rubin PAD, Shore JW, Yaremchuk MJ. Complex orbital fracture repair using rigid fixation of the internal orbital skeleton. Ophthalmology 1992; 99:553–561.

14. Yaremchuk MJ, Manson PN. Reconstruction of the internal orbit using rigid fixation techniques. In: Yaremchuk MJ, Gruss JS, Manson PN, eds. Rigid fixation of the craniomaxillofacial skeleton. Boston: Butterworth-Heinemann; 1992.

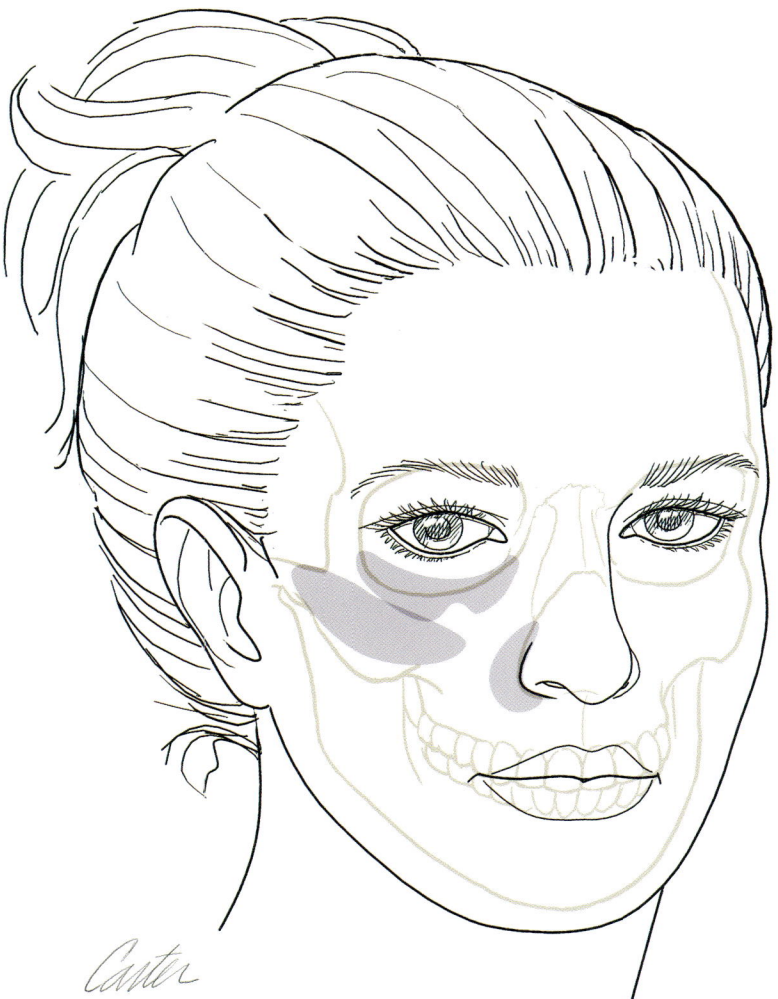

Carter

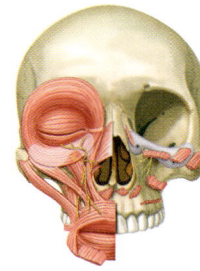

Chapter 6

Infraorbital rim

The upper midface skeleton has direct and indirect influences on the appearance of the face and particularly the eyes. The relationship between the globe and the orbital rims will determine if the eyes appear prominent or deep-set. Because the infraorbital rim and upper midface skeleton support the lower eyelids and the cheek soft tissues, their projection impacts on lid and cheek position. Patients with retrusive skeletons are more likely to undergo premature lower lid and cheek descent with aging. This lack of skeletal support predisposes to lower lid malposition after blepharoplasty, and limits the efficacy and longevity of midface lifting. This chapter demonstrates the impact that infraorbital rim augmentation, either alone or together with other soft tissue manipulations, has on periorbital appearance. It includes techniques not only for augmenting the infraorbital rim with alloplastic implants, but also for resuspending the midface soft tissues, as well as repositioning the lower lid and lateral canthus.

GLOBE–RIM RELATIONS

The relationship of the globe to the orbital rims is a primary determinant of the appearance of the upper third of the face. Normal values—that is, averages calculated from groups of young, healthy adults—have been published, and they are presented in Figure 6.1.[1–4]

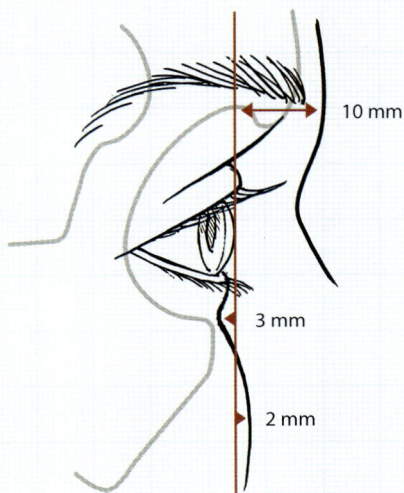

Figure 6.1 Sagittal relations of the anterior surface of the cornea to the soft tissues overlying the supraorbital and infraorbital rims. On average, in the young adult, the supraorbital rim projects 10 mm beyond, the infraorbital rim lies 3 mm behind, and the cheek prominence projects 2 mm beyond the anterior surface of the cornea.[1–4]

On average, the surface of the soft tissues overlying the supraorbital rim lies 10 mm anterior to the cornea, and the surface of the soft tissues overlying the infraorbital rim lies 3 mm behind the anterior surface of the cornea. This implies that the supraorbital rim usually projects 13 mm beyond the infraorbital rim. When the orbital rims have a greater projection beyond the anterior surface of the cornea, the eyes appear deep-set. When the orbital rims project less, the eyes appear prominent. In addition to being predisposed to corneal exposure–related problems, overly prominent eyes are usually considered less attractive. Globe to orbital rim measurements have a wide range and are influenced by ethnicity and sex, and change with aging.

Ethnicity and sex

The considerable variability in globe to orbital rim relations is a result of the wide variations in human facial skeleton morphology. Migliori and Gladstone determined the normal range of globe protrusion for white and black adults.[5] Using the Hertel exophthalmometer, which measures projection of the anterior surface of the cornea beyond the lateral orbital rim, they found that the average for white adults was 10 mm; for black adults, it was 12 mm. In addition to determining a range of normal values, they documented racial and sexual differences in globe projection. When globe projection was measured relative to the lateral orbital rim, men's globes, on average, were 2 mm more prominent than women's, and black men's and women's globes were 2 mm more prominent than those of white men and white women.

Aging

Pessa et al. showed that the globe–orbital rim relationship changes with age.[3] They studied two groups of individuals, young and old, using three-dimensional computed tomography. Their findings are summarized in Figure 6.2.

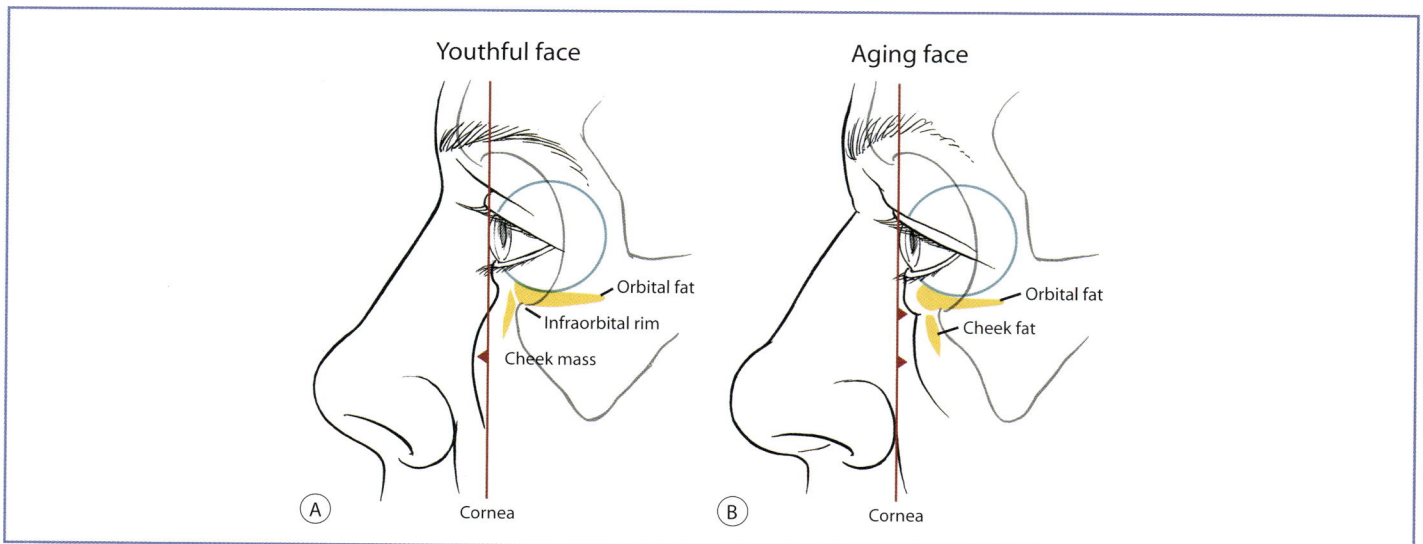

Figure 6.2 Changes in the sagittal position of orbital fat, infraorbital rim, and cheek prominence that occur with aging, as measured by Pessa. (**A**) In the youthful face, the cheek mass lies anterior to the surface of the cornea, and the orbital fat lies slightly anterior to the orbital rim. (**B**) With aging, the cheek mass moves posterior to the surface of the cornea. The infraorbital rim also recedes, and the orbital fat moves slightly anteriorly. These changes in position of the cheek mass and infraorbital rim were statistically significant, but the anterior movement of the orbital fat was not. The red line is dropped vertically from the cornea. (After Pessa et al. 1999,[3] with permission.)

In the youthful face, the cheek fat lies anterior to the cornea and the orbital fat lies slightly anterior to the orbital rim. With aging, the cheek mass tends to lie posterior to the anterior surface of the cornea, the orbital fat moves slightly anterior, and the infraorbital rim has a significant movement posteriorly. Hence retrusion of the infraorbital rim with aging will make the eyes appear more prominent by changing globe–rim relations, and it will significantly impact the appearance of the lower lid bags, particularly in those who tend toward maxillary hypoplasia.

BLEPHAROPLASTY

The relative prominence of the eyes impacts on the position and shape of the lower lid, and therefore it is an important consideration in aesthetic blepharoplasty. Plastic surgeons have long recognized that patients with prominent eyes are predisposed to the lower lid descent that may be exaggerated and symptomatic after conventional blepharoplasty. Eye prominence results from a deficiency in skeletal support, as has been discussed, but may also result from excess of orbital soft tissue volume. Eye prominence correlates with a more inferior position of the lower lid (resulting in scleral show) and a more medial position of the lateral canthus.[6] Descent of the lower lid increases the height of the palpebral fissure while the more medial position of the lateral canthus decreases its width. Hence patients with poorly projecting upper midface skeletons have 'round eyes' as compared with the long, narrow eyes characteristic of young people with a normal periorbital morphology.[4,7,8] Furthermore, in the skeletally deficient, the lack of infraorbital rim projection and cheek prominence often allows their lower lid fat compartments to be visible, giving them 'early bags' (Fig. 6.3).

> **PEARL**
>
> Deficient infraorbital rim projection predisposes to lower lid descent with aging.

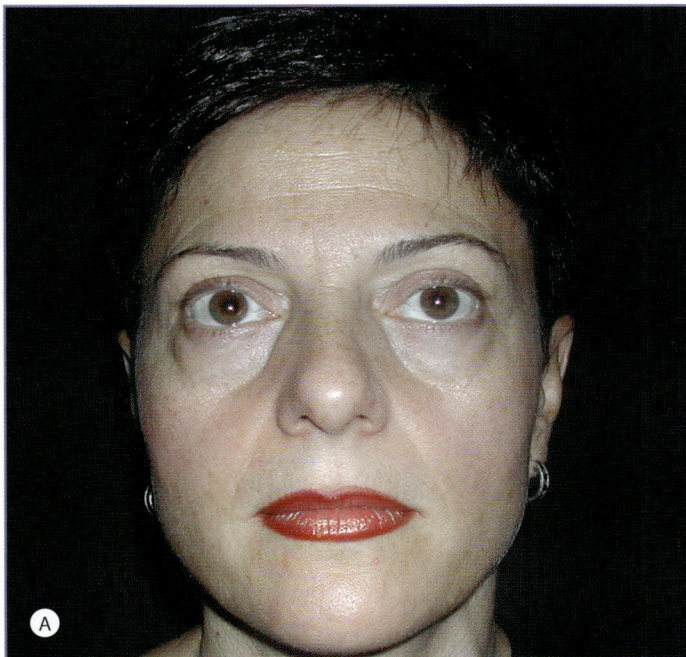

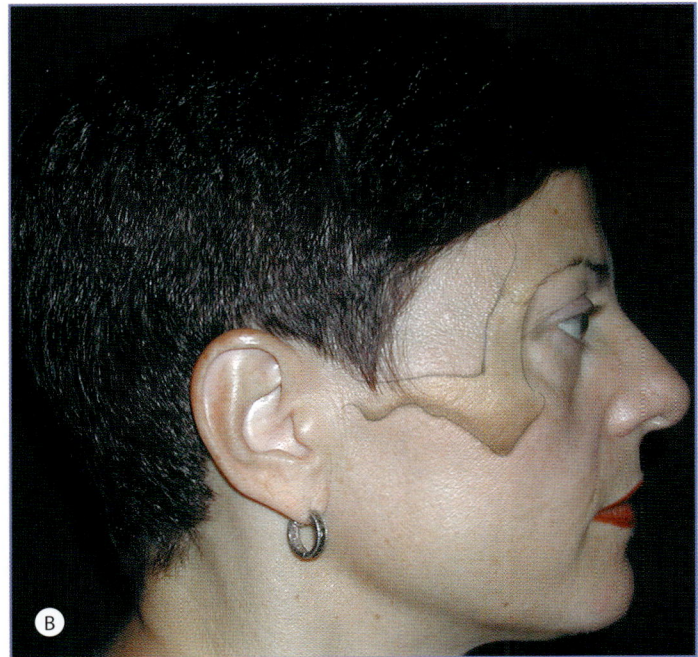

Figure 6.3 (**A**) Frontal and (**B**) lateral views of a woman with midface skeletal morphology (negative vector) predisposing to lower lid and cheek descent, resulting in a 'round eye' appearance with prominent bags. On lateral view (**B**), the artist has drawn in the underlying facial skeleton. (From Yaremchuk 2004,[9] with permission.)

Negative vector

Patients with prominent eyes have long been recognized to develop symptomatic lower lid descent (with exaggeration of their round eyes) after conventional lower blepharoplasty. Rees and LaTrenta studied the influence of periorbital skeletal morphology in predicting the likelihood of symptomatic lower lid malposition after lower blepharoplasty.[10] They found that patients whose eyes were prominent, because of either maxillary hypoplasia or thyroid ophthalmopathy, had a high incidence of lid malposition and dry eye symptoms after blepharoplasty. Patients with prominent eyes were therefore considered 'morphologically prone' to develop symptomatic lid malposition after lower blepharoplasty.

Later, Jelks and Jelks categorized globe–orbital rim relationships and the tendency for the development of lower lid malposition after blepharoplasty (Fig. 6.4).[11] On sagittal view, they placed a line or 'vector' between the most anterior projection of the globe and the malar eminence and lid margin. A *positive* vector relationship exists when the most anterior projection of the globe is posterior to the lid margin and the malar eminence. A *negative* vector relationship exists when the most anterior projection of the globe lies anterior to the lower lid and the malar eminence. They warned that patients whose orbital morphology has a negative vector relationship are prone to lid malposition after lower blepharoplasty.

> **PEARL**
>
> Deficient infraorbital rim projection predisposes to lower lid descent after blepharoplasty.

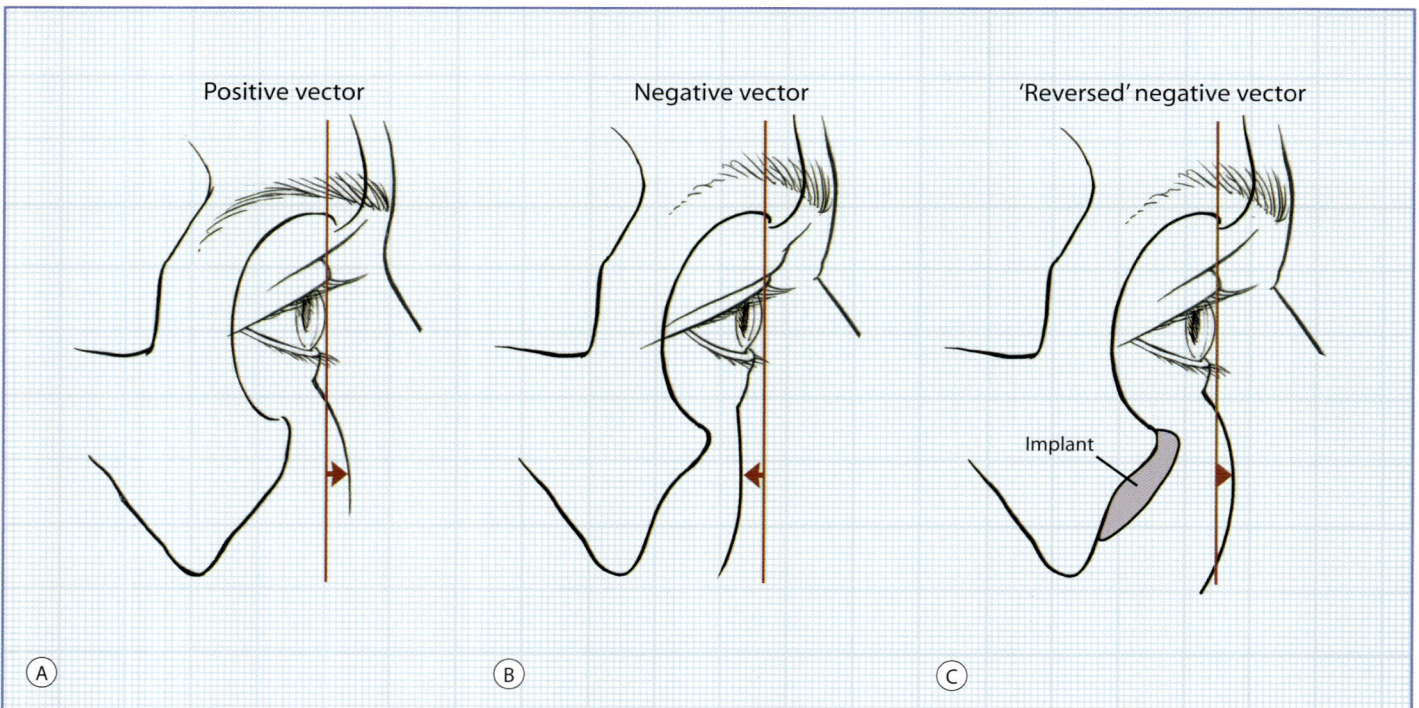

Figure 6.4 Jelks and Jelks categorized globe–orbital rim relationships by placing a line or 'vector' between the most anterior projection of the globe and the malar eminence and lid margin.[11] (**A**) Positive vector relationship. In the youthful face with normal globe-to-skeletal rim relations, the cheek mass supported by the infraorbital rim lies anterior to the surface of the cornea. The position of the cheek prominence beyond the anterior surface of the cornea is termed a *positive vector*. (**B**) Negative vector relationship. In patients with maxillary hypoplasia, the cheek mass lies posterior to the surface of the cornea. The position of the cheek prominence beyond the anterior surface of the cornea is termed a *negative vector*. (**C**) 'Reversed' negative vector relationship. Alloplastic augmentation of the infraorbital rim can reverse the negative vector. (After Yaremchuk 2003,[8] with permission.)

Reversing the negative vector

Augmentation of the infraorbital rim in patients with a retruded infraorbital rim can bring it into a better relationship with the globe, thereby 'reversing the negative vector'.[12]

As will be described, infraorbital rim augmentation is part of the strategy for normalizing the appearance in patients who are morphologically prone. It can be adapted for morphologically prone patients who are first seeking to improve their periorbital appearance, or for those whose lid malposition and round eye appearance have been exaggerated by previous lower blepharoplasty.

PREOPERATIVE EVALUATION

As depicted in Figure 6.1, in young, healthy adults, the average projection of the soft tissues overlying the supraorbital rim beyond the surface of the cornea is about 10 mm, and the projection of the cornea beyond the soft tissues overlying the infraorbital rim is 3 mm. These relations are the approximate goals of augmentation of the supraorbital rims. Documenting the amount of disproportion is useful for preoperative planning and postoperative evaluation, and it can be done with measurements by a Luedde exophthalmometer or with life-sized photographs. A Luedde exophthalmometer placed on the lateral orbital rim and placed perpendicular to the anterior surface of the cornea allows more objective comparison of the anterior projection of the cornea and tissues overlying the infraorbital rim. A disproportion in sagittal globe–rim relations is usually obvious, and correction is made by clinical judgment.

PEARL

Infraorbital rim augmentation can provide support for the resuspended lower lid and cheek in patients with midface skeletal deficiency.

101

SURGICAL ANATOMY (Fig. 6.5)

The infraorbital rim has lateral zygomatic bone and medial maxillary bone contributions. The zygomaticomaxillary suture is situated approximately at the midpupillary line. Approximately 8–10 mm beneath the orbital floor (3–6 mm in severely hypoplastic midfaces) and along the zygomaticomaxillary suture exits the infraorbital nerve. The infraorbital nerve travels beneath the levator superioris and above the levator anguli oris. Its branches supply the skin of the lower lid, the side of the nose, and most of the cheek and upper lip. The zygomaticofacial nerve exits through its small foramen located on the lateral aspect of the zygoma, approximately 8–10 mm beneath the infraorbital rim and in line with the lateral orbital rim. It supplies a small portion of the skin of the upper cheek. Whereas the infraorbital nerve must be protected, the zygomaticofacial nerve is routinely sacrificed during infraorbital rim augmentation, with the ensuing sensory loss rarely noted by the patient.

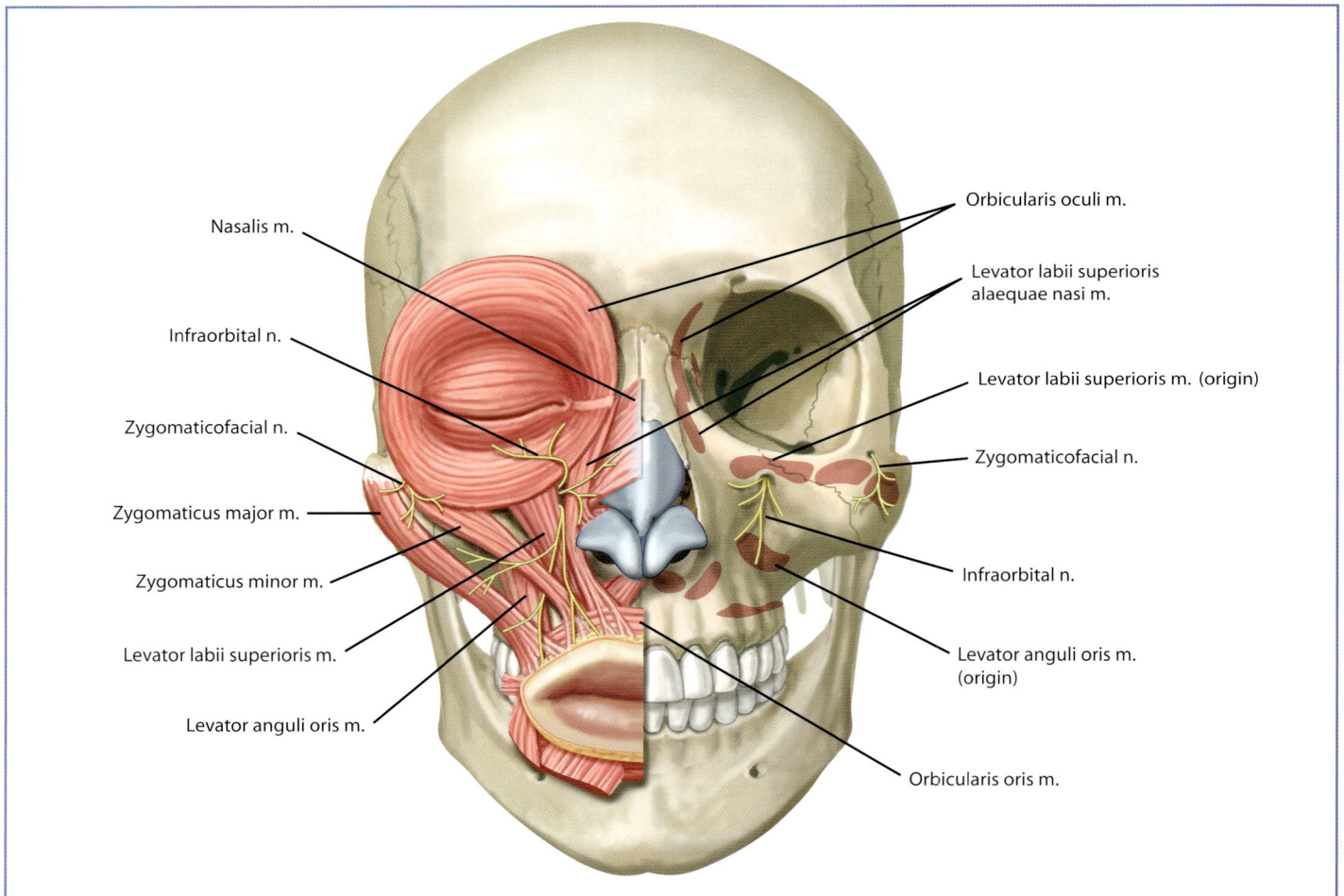

Figure 6.5 Midface skeletal anatomy with muscle origins and nerve foramina.

In exposing the surface of the infraorbital rim area for implant augmentation, the origins of the upper lip elevators are detached from their skeletal origins. The zygomaticus major muscle originates from the lateral surface of the zygoma just medial to the zygomaticotemporal suture, and sometimes intermingles with the orbicularis oculi. It passes obliquely downward and forward to the corner of the mouth, where it inserts into skin and mucosa. The zygomaticus minor lies medial to the zygomaticus major. It originates from the malar surface of the zygoma immediately lateral to the zygomaticomaxillary suture, and passes downward and medially to insert into the lip just medial to the corner of the mouth. The levator labii superioris originates from the lower margin of the orbit just above the infraorbital foramen. It travels downward and medially to insert into the orbicularis oris as well as the skin of the lip. The levator labii superioris alaequae nasi originates from the frontal process of the maxilla lateral to the nose. It inserts into the skin and alar cartilage of the nose and, more significantly, into the skin and musculature of the lip. Branches of the infra-orbital nerve are adherent to the underside of the levator muscles.

The orbicularis oculi originates from the nasal process of the frontal bone, the frontal process of the maxilla, and from the anterior surface of the medial canthal tendon. The fibers are directed laterally to surround the entire circumference of the orbit. The orbicularis oculi's maxillary origins are elevated during the placement of an infraorbital rim implant. The manipulation of this muscle may lead to a transient decrease in lower lid tone.

THE IMPLANT

An implant specifically designed to augment the anterior sagittal projection of the orbital rim is available (it can, of course, be carved from any implant material).[12] This implant can provide up to 5 mm of anterior projection and is trimmed to meet the specific needs of the patient. A small flange allows it to rest on the most anterior aspect of the orbital floor. This flange allows easier positioning of the implant and a possible area for screw fixation to the skeleton (Fig. 6.6).

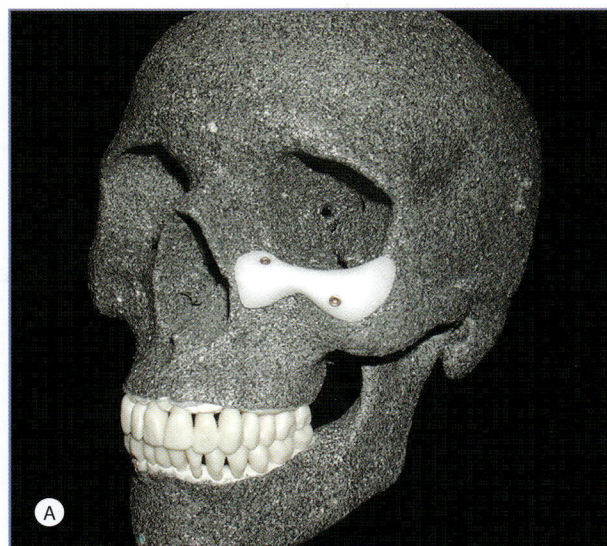

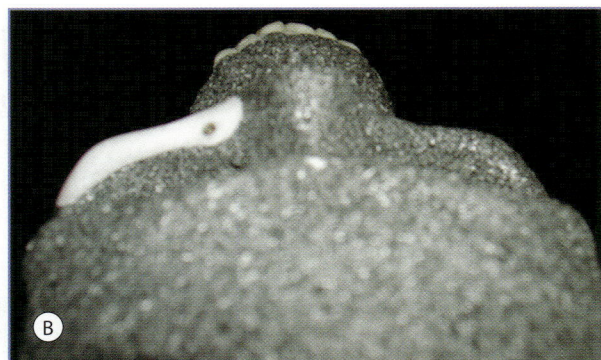

Figure 6.6 Implants designed specifically for infraorbital rim augmentation allow up to 5 mm of anterior projection (Porex Surgical, Newnan, Georgia). They are carved to meet the specific needs of the patient. Screw fixation ensures application of the implant to skeleton, thereby preventing gaps between the implant and the skeleton and aiding a smooth implant–skeleton transition. (A) Oblique and (B) overhead view. Note the rim projection provided by implant.

OPERATIVE TECHNIQUE TO AUGMENT
THE INFRAORBITAL RIM (Figs 6.7 and 6.8)

The infraorbital rim and adjacent anatomy must be exposed sufficiently to ensure ideal implant placement, smooth implant–facial skeleton transition, and screw fixation. Direct rim, subciliary skin, or subciliary skin–muscle flap incisions can provide this exposure. A transconjunctival incision alone is inadequate for implant placement and screw stabilization. A transconjunctival retroseptal incision, if used, requires lengthening with a lateral canthotomy or combination with intraoral and lateral extent of lower blepharoplasty incisions. It is important to identify the infraorbital nerve, which exits from the infraorbital foramen about 1 cm below the margin of the orbit. This may be 3–6 mm in patients with significant maxillary hypoplasia—the usual candidates for this surgery. The orbicularis oculi and the origins of the lip elevators are separated from the underlying skeleton in a subperiosteal plane to expose the infraorbital rim.

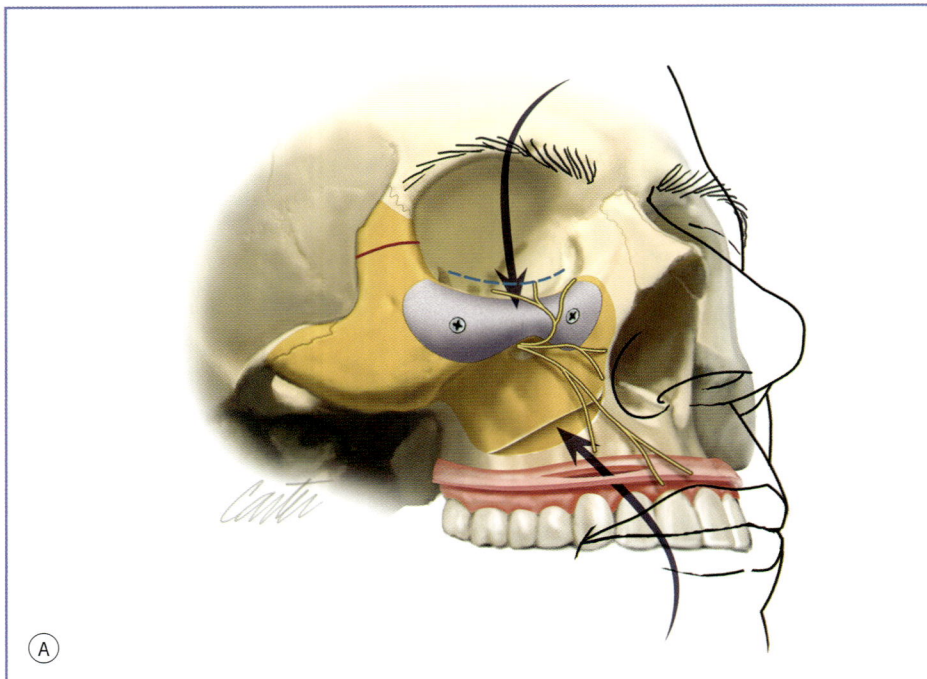

Figure 6.7 (**A**) Overview of the operation to increase projection of infraorbital rim and 'reverse the negative vector' in patients with upper midface skeletal deficiency. I prefer a transconjunctival retroseptal incision (broken line) with the lateral extent of a lower lid blepharoplasty incision (solid line) to expose the infraorbital rim. This approach preserves the integrity of the lateral canthus, and hence the palpebral fissure. Transcutaneous blepharoplasty or transconjunctival with lateral canthotomy incisions are alternative approaches that provide greater exposure but are accompanied by a greater risk of palpebral fissure distortion. An intraoral incision is used to access the lower midface skeleton and to identify and protect the infraorbital nerve. The lower lid and midface soft tissues are freed by subperiosteal dissection. The implant is immobilized with titanium screws. (**B**) Clinical photograph shows screw immobilization of infraorbital rim implant. Two Senn retractors are retracting the lower lid. A malleable retractor is retracting the orbital contents. (**C**) Clinical photograph shows screw immobilization of the inferior lateral aspect of the implant through intraoral access. Retractors are retracting the right upper lip and cheek the arrow points to the infraorbital nerve.

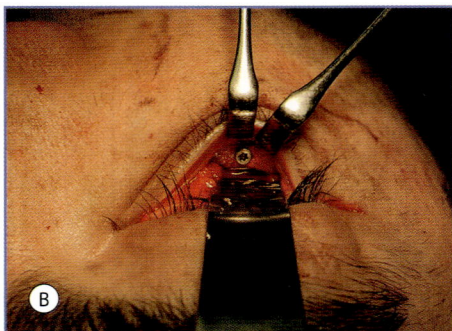

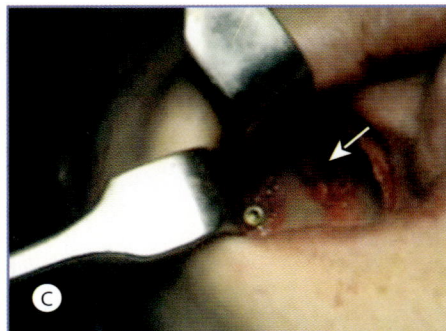

The implant is carved to fit the specific needs of the patient. Segmenting the implant may facilitate placement of the implant through limited skeletal access.

The implant is fixed to the skeleton with titanium screw to allow precise application of the implant to the surface of the skeleton. This ensures the desired augmentation, because gaps between the implants and the skeleton effectively result in unplanned increases in augmentation. Screw fixation also allows the implant to be contoured after it has been positioned on the skeleton, thereby providing an imperceptible transition between the area augmented and the adjacent skeleton.

PEARL

Segmenting the implant may facilitate its placement when using limited access incisions.

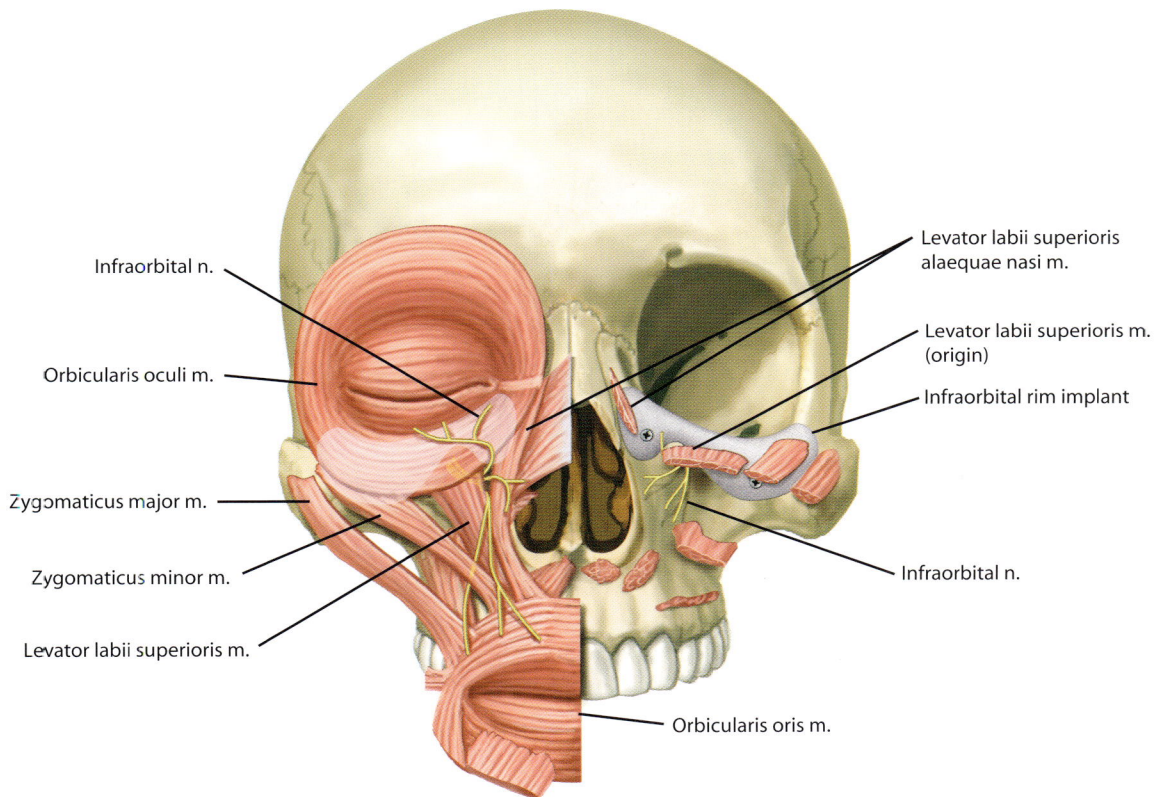

Figure 6.8 Position of infraorbital rim implant relative to underlying skeleton and overlying lip elevators.

Clinical examples

Patients who have undergone infraorbital rim augmentation are shown in Figures 6.9 and 6.10.

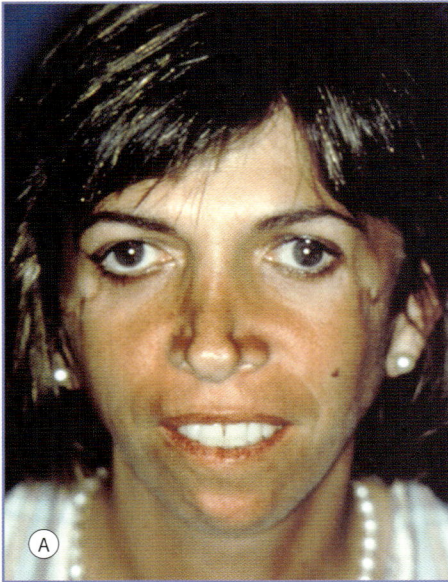

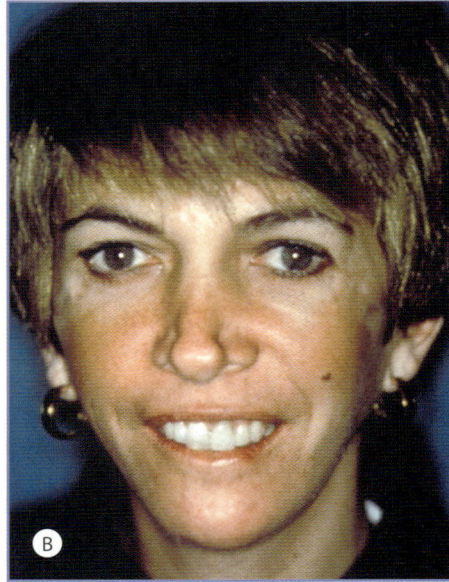

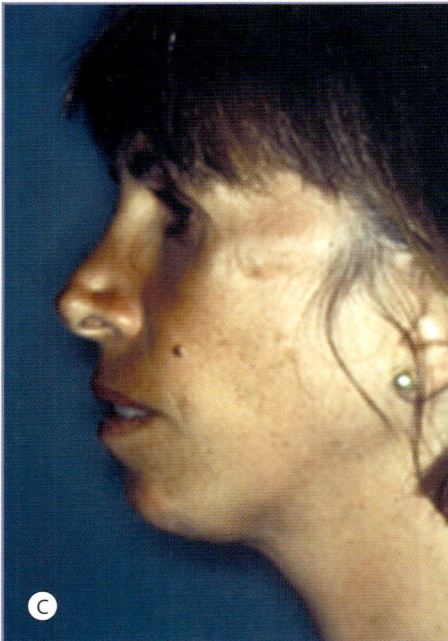

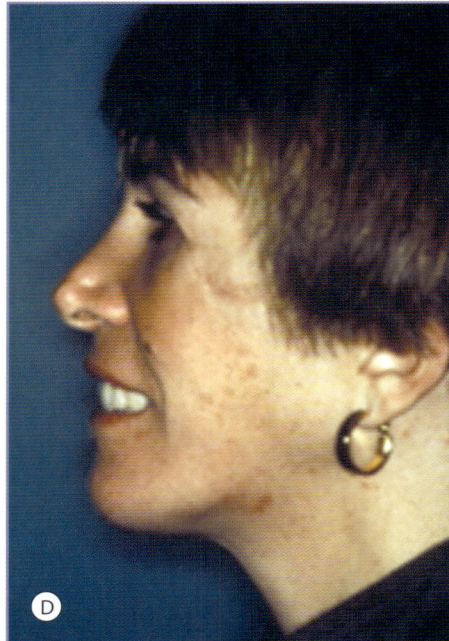

Figure 6.9 A 35-year-old woman presented with malar and lateral orbital deficiency due to Treacher Collins syndrome. Silicone implants placed during her teenaged years had been removed because of infection. Rib grafts used to reconstruct the malar and zygomatic arch had resorbed, leaving fixation wires visible through thin skin. The zygomatic arch, malar area, and coloboma of the lateral infraorbital rim were reconstructed with custom-carved porous polyethylene implants that were fixed with metal screws. Surgery was performed through bicoronal, intraoral, and transconjunctival incisions. In addition, lateral canthopexies and a sliding advancement genioplasty were performed. At 2.5 years postoperatively, an area of implant prominence was treated with imbricating and overlying attenuated soft tissue and contouring the implant prominence. The patient was last seen 6 years postoperatively and was contacted recently. It has been 15 years since the surgery, and she has had no further surgeries, with a stable, satisfactory result. (**A**) Preoperative and (**B**) postoperative frontal views. (**C**) Preoperative and (**D**) postoperative lateral views.

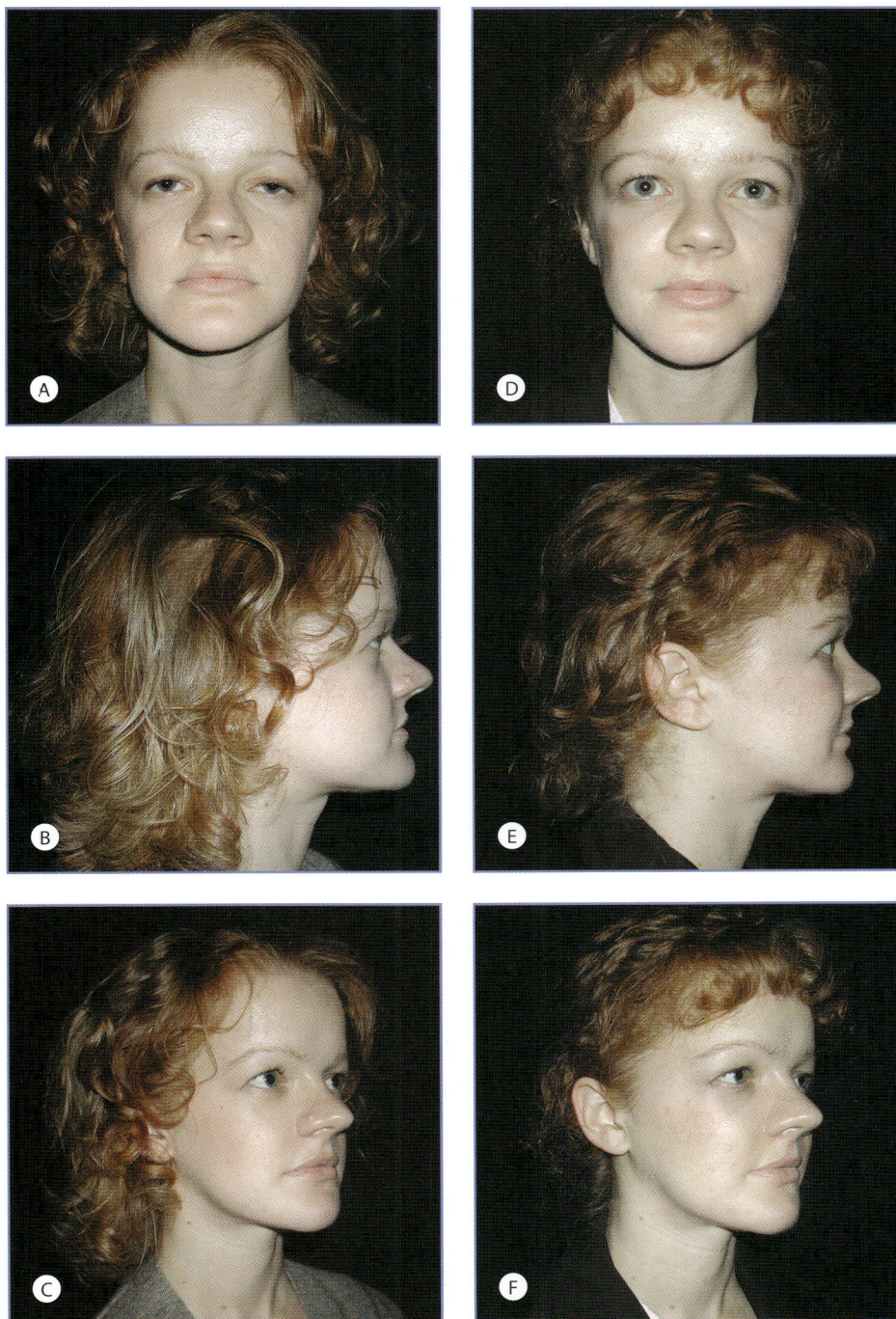

Figure 6.10 A 30-year old woman with craniocleidoclavicular syndrome had undergone LeFort I advancement, sagittal split osteotomy, and sliding advancement genioplasty in the past. Infraorbital rim augmentation was performed through transconjunctival and intraoral incisions. (**A–C**) Preoperative frontal, lateral, and oblique views. (**D–F**) Postoperative frontal, lateral, and oblique views.

INFRAORBITAL RIM AUGMENTATION AND BLEPHAROPLASTY

Patients with hypoplastic orbital rims tend to age prematurely. The deficiency in skeletal support for the lower lid and midface soft tissues results in their early descent, with concomitant rounding of the palpebral fissure and absence of a distinct cheek–lid interface. Patients with this facial skeletal morphology are prone to further lower lid descent, which is often symptomatic, after blepharoplasty.

A treatment for lower lid retraction after blepharoplasty in the morphologically prone has received little attention in the literature. In his textbook, McCord proposed treating postblepharoplasty patients with lower lid retraction and prominent eyes by loosening the lower lid margin with a full-thickness transverse blepharotomy, performing a canthotomy, placing a small spacer graft, and suprapositioning the lateral canthus.[13] This type of procedure was originally used in patients with Graves disease. In a more recent review article, he demonstrated the use of spacer grafts combined with midface lifting (to vertically recruit cheek tissues instead of transverse blepharotomy) and periosteal strip canthoplasty (or fascia grafts).[14] Baylis, Goldberg, and Groth stated that patients with prominent eyes frequently require the use of spacers for the correction of lower eyelid retraction.[15] For patients with marked proptosis, they suggested considering (without documenting) orbital decompression or orbital rim onlay advancement in addition to soft tissue repositioning.

The periorbital appearance of patients with hypoplastic infraorbital rims (morphologically prone, negative vector) can be normalized with a procedure that combines infraorbital rim augmentation, subperiosteal midface elevation and, if necessary, lateral canthopexy.[9] An alloplastic implant increases the sagittal projection of the infraorbital rim, effectively reversing the negative vector. The implant provides support for the cheek and lid tissues. The midface elevation repositions the descended cheek and recruits lower lid tissue. The lateral canthopexy repositions the lateral canthus and provides additional support for the lower lid. This operation can be adapted for morphologically prone patients who are first seeking improvement in their periorbital appearance, or for those whose lid malposition and round eye appearance have been exaggerated by previous lower blepharoplasty. It is adapted from experience treating the posttraumatic,[16-18] Graves ophthalmopathy, and postblepharoplasty lower lid retraction.[8]

Operative technique

This procedure involves three basic maneuvers. Subperiosteal freeing and elevation of the lower lid and midface recruits lid tissues and allows lower lid repositioning. Augmentation of the infraorbital rim with an alloplastic implant effectively changes the facial skeletal morphology, thereby providing support for the lower lid and midface soft tissues. Lateral canthopexy restores palpebral fissure shape and provides additional lower lid support (Fig. 6.11).

Periorbital access

Various combinations of incisions may be used to expose the infraorbital rim while mobilizing adjacent lid and midface soft tissues. My preference is to combine the lateral extent of the lower lid blepharoplasty incision with a transconjunctival retroseptal incision and an upper gingival buccal sulcus incision. If necessary, this transconjunctival incision can be connected with the lateral blepharoplasty transcutaneous incision with a lateral canthotomy. These additional incisions prolong palpebral edema and risk canthal distortion. Approaches that delaminate and relaminate the lower lid, such as lower lid skin only or lower lid skin–muscle flaps, are avoided.

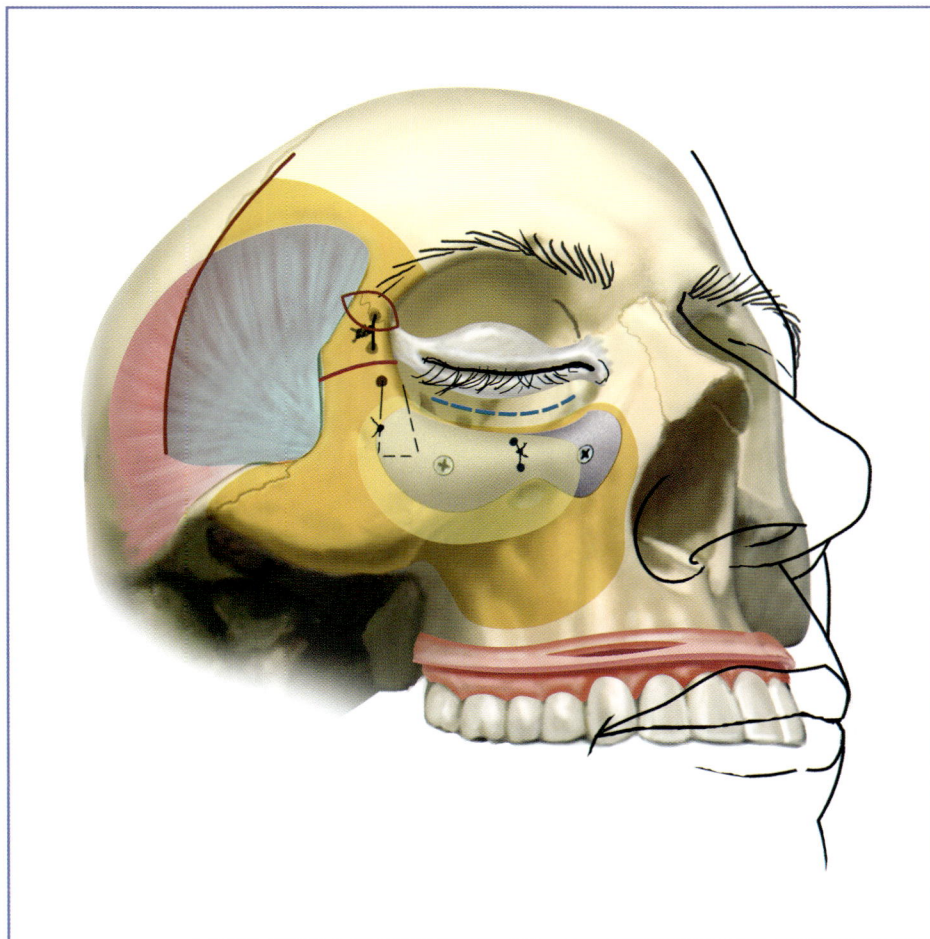

Figure 6.11 Overview of operation to correct 'round eye' appearance in prominent eye patients with midface skeletal deficiency. Cutaneous incisions (solid lines) include temporal and lateral extent of upper and lower lid blepharoplasty incisions. An intraoral incision (broken line) is used to access the midface skeleton. The lower lid, midface and temporal soft tissues are freed by subperiosteal dissection. An implant augments the projection of the infraorbital rim area and is immobilized with screws. The midface soft tissues are resuspended using sutures tied to drill holes placed in the infraorbital rim. The lateral canthopexy is performed by purchasing the lateral canthus with figure-of-eight sutures of 30-gauge wire, which is passed from within the orbit through drill holes placed in the lateral orbital rim and tied over the resultant bridge of bone.

Midface and lower lid mobilization

Through a temporal (or bicoronal) incision, the lateral orbital soft tissues are mobilized. The superficial layer of the deep temporal fascia is incised at the level of the zygomatic frontal suture to expose the superficial temporal fat pad.[19] This dissection is carried inferiorly until it reaches the zygomatic arch and lateral orbital rim previously exposed through the lateral blepharoplasty incision. Using the intraoral incision, the midface soft tissues are separated from the underlying skeleton and masseter muscle. This allows en bloc elevation of the malar midface soft tissues and lower lid.[8]

Implant placement

Infraorbital rim implants (Porex Surgical, Newnan, Georgia) are custom carved to meet the specific needs of the patient.[12] Approximately 3–5 mm of augmentation at the infraorbital rim has been employed. All implants are fixed to the skeleton with titanium screws (Synthes Corp., Paoli, Pennsylvania).

Midface elevation and fixation

Sutures are used to elevate and secure the malar midface and lid soft tissues. Through the intraoral incision, two figure-of-eight sutures of 3-0 polyglycolic acid are used to purchase the midface soft tissues. These sutures incorporate the incised periosteum, origins of the released lip elevators, and cheek subcutaneous tissue. A suture placed at the midpupil level is passed through the lower lid incision and secured to the rim implant. Another suture is placed in the lateral aspect of the malar fat pad (placed approximately 3 cm beneath the lateral canthus) and is tied to a drill hole placed in the lateral orbital rim. The elevated suborbicularis oculi fat and adjacent musculature now rest on the augmented skeleton and help to support the freed and elevated lid margin (Figs 6.12 and 6.13).

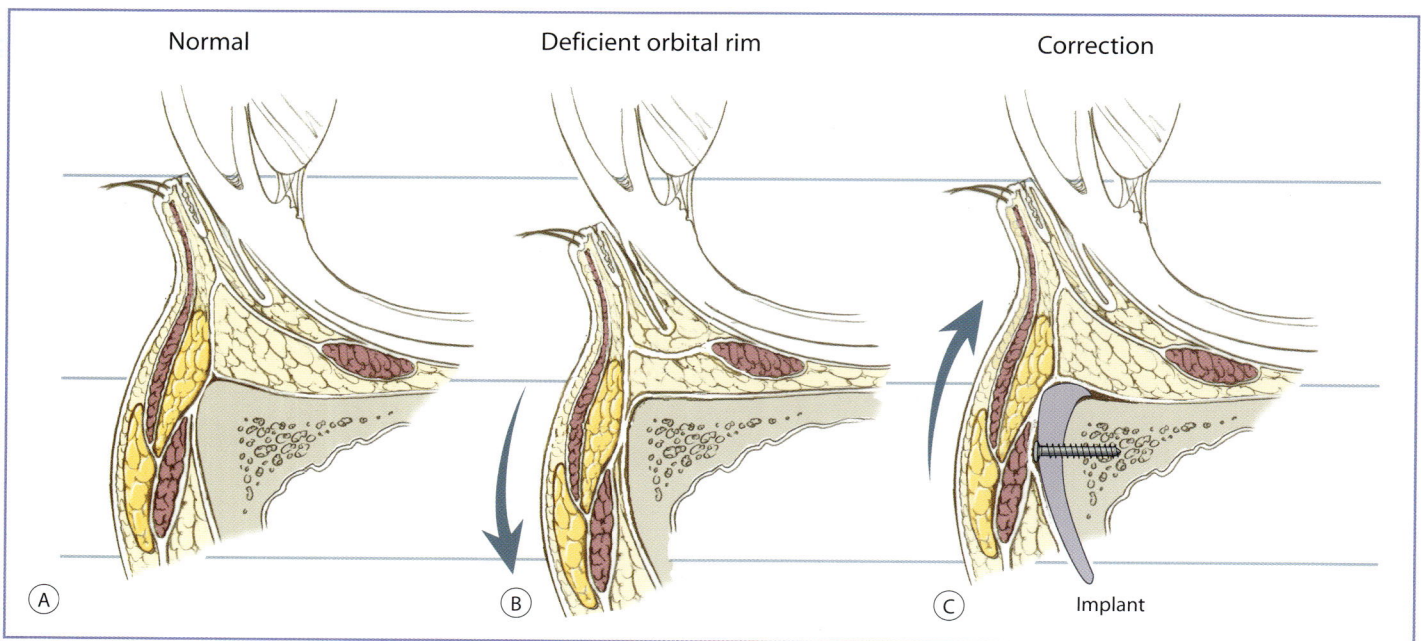

Normal   Deficient orbital rim   Correction

A   B   C   Implant

Figure 6.12 Sagittal sections of lower lid, globe, and orbital rim taken at midpupil in a normal subject (**A**), a 'morphologically prone' patient with lid descent after previous blepharoplasty (**B**), and a morphologically prone patient with lid descent who has undergone infraorbital rim implant augmentation and midface elevation (**C**).

This technique of midface elevation is adapted from Phillips, Gruss, Wells, and Challet's method of subperiosteal midface soft tissue repositioning used after extensive facial skeletal degloving performed to access and treat the fractured midface.[18] This author also uses it to restore a youthful cheek–lid interface during rejuvenative aesthetic surgery,[7] and together with lateral canthopexy[8] to reposition the inferiorly displaced lower lid occurring after blepharoplasty in patients with normal skeletal anatomy.

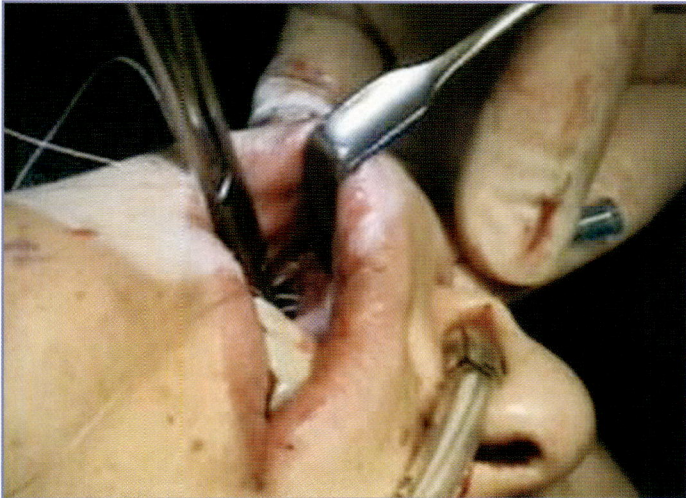

Figure 6.13 Clinical photograph shows suture elevation of cheek mass during subperiosteal midface lift. Through an intraoral approach, the cheek soft tissue mass is being purchased with a figure-of-eight suture. A needle has been placed percutaneously at a point 3 cm beneath the lateral canthus.

Lateral canthopexy

A lateral canthopexy is performed to narrow the palpebral fissure and to provide additional support for the elevated lower lid margin. Through the lateral extent of the lower blepharoplasty incision, both limbs of the lateral canthus are purchased with a figure-of-eight 30- or 32-gauge titanium wire suture. In the postblepharoplasty patient, if scarring limits the upward mobility of the lateral canthus, the lateral third of the middle lamellae is incised with needle tip electrocautery.

Through coronal access, or if the temporal incision is used the lateral extent of an upper lid blepharoplasty incision, two drill holes are placed in the lateral orbital rim just at and 2 mm below the zygomaticofrontal suture. Each end of the wire is then passed from within the orbit through the drill holes to the lateral orbital rim. The wires are then twisted to one another over the bridge of bone between the two holes (Fig. 6.14).[20,21]

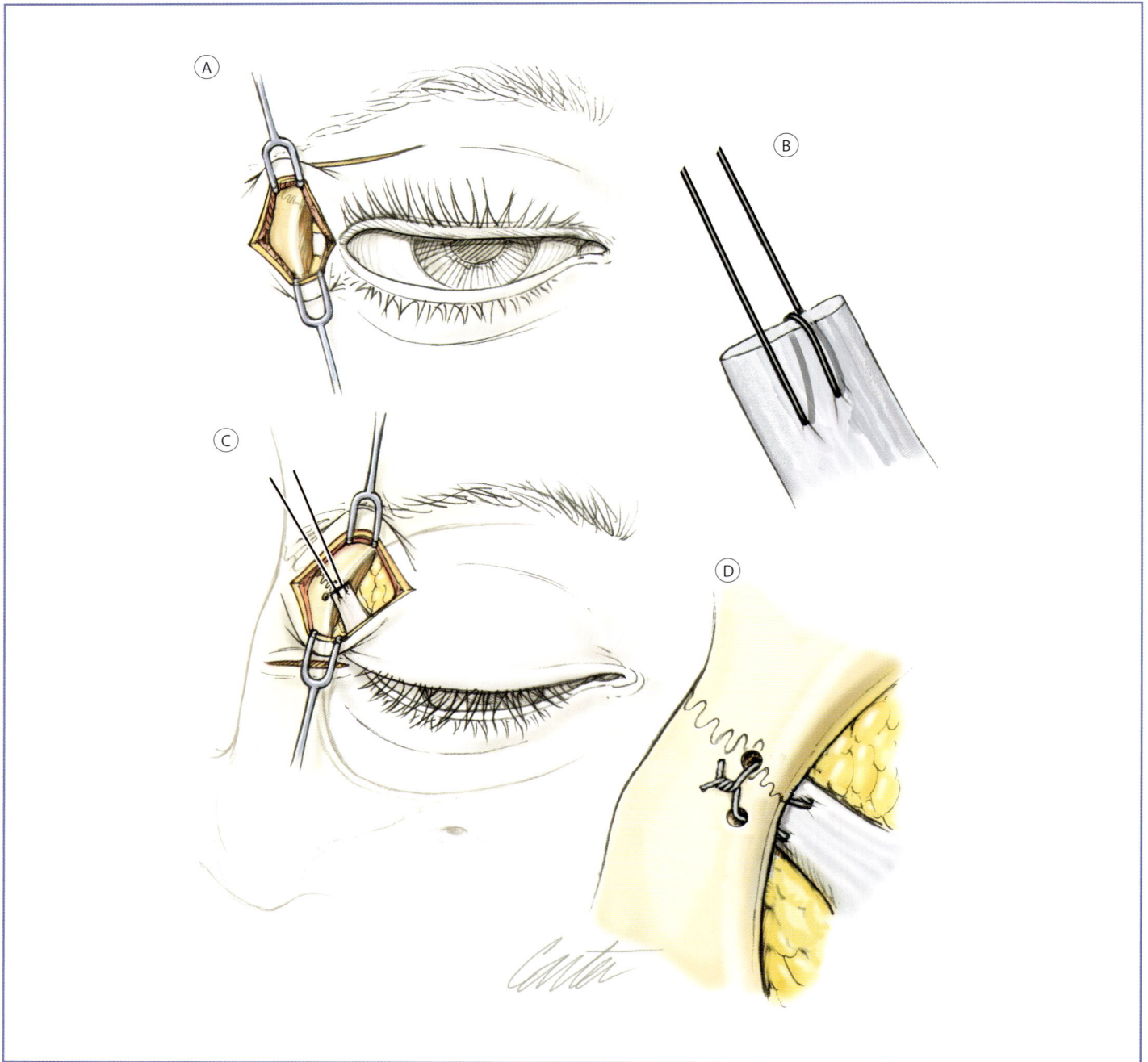

Figure 6.14 Technique of lateral canthopexy. (**A**) Through the lateral extent of the lower lid blepharoplasty incision, the lateral canthus is identified and freed from Whitnall's tubercle by subperiosteal dissection. (**B**) The lateral canthus is purchased by a figure-of-eight, 30-gauge titanium wire suture. (**C**) The ends of the suture are passed along the lateral orbit from the lower lid to the upper lid (or coronal) incision. To ensure adequate vertical mobility of the lateral canthus and lateral lid margin, it may be necessary to incise the lateral third of the scarred and contracted lid lamellae. (**D**) Each end of the wire suture is passed from within the orbit through drill holes made in the lateral orbital rim that were placed at the zygomaticofrontal suture and 2–3 mm below it. The ends of the wire suture are twisted to one another over the bridge of bone. Passing the wire from inside to outside, the orbit applies the lid to the globe (see Fig. 6.15).

Drill hole placement determines the lateral canthal position, which should be 2–3 mm above the medial canthal plane. The lateral canthus is not supraplaced. The amount of wire twisting will determine the amount of canthal elevation. The strand of twisted wire ends is left approximately 0.5 cm long. This length allows the end to be placed into one of the drill holes or into the orbit to avoid its postoperative visibility or palpability. If the height of the lateral canthus needs readjustment postoperatively, the stump can be retrieved and twisted more to raise the canthus, or untwisted to lower it.

The bridge of bone canthopexy is preferred for both practical and conceptual reasons. Drill holes placed in the lateral orbital rim can be placed after precise measurement, allowing for predictable and symmetric lateral canthus positioning. The bridge of bone provides a secure fixation point. The passing of the canthopexy wires from inside the orbit to outside applies the lid to the globe. This maneuver avoids the lid–globe dysjunction in the lateral commissure, which is common when canthopexy sutures are tied to the outer surface of the lateral orbit (Fig. 6.15).

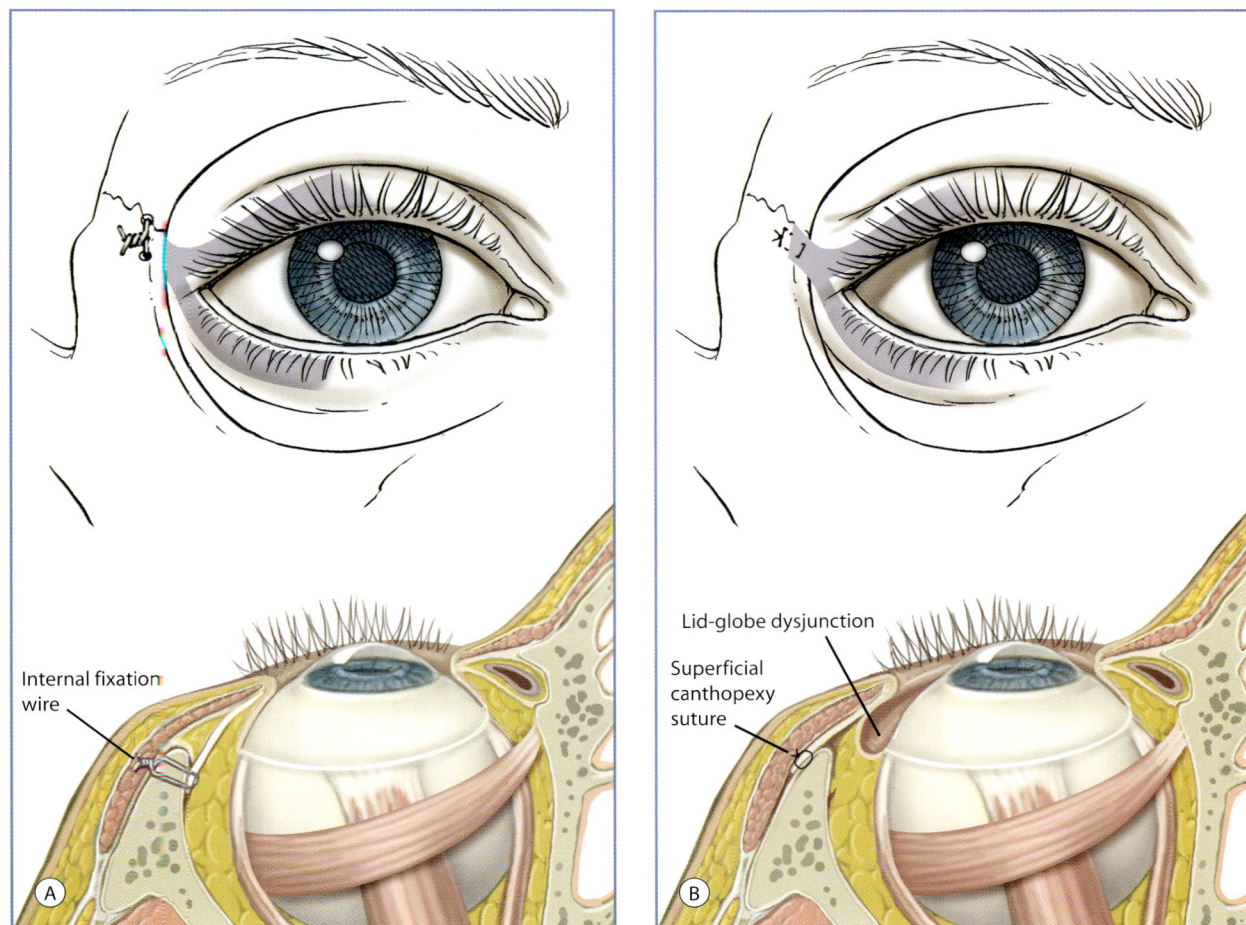

Internal fixation wire

Lid-globe dysjunction

Superficial canthopexy suture

A **B**

Figure 6.15 The position of the lateral canthus relative to the lateral orbital rim determines the relation of the lower lid to the surface of the globe. (**A**) The lateral canthopexy stitch is passed through the inner surface of the lateral orbital wall and tied on its outside surface. (**B**) The lateral canthopexy stitch is attached to the periosteum of the anterior surface of the lateral orbital rim. Note the gap between the surface of the globe and the lateral aspect of the lower lid.

Lateral canthopexy, because it does not violate the lid margin, maintains or has the potential to restore palpebral fissure shape, including the lateral canthal angle. Canthoplasty procedures, by design, alter the shape of the palpebral fissure, because they disassemble and reassemble the lateral canthus while shortening the lower lid margin (Fig. 6.16).

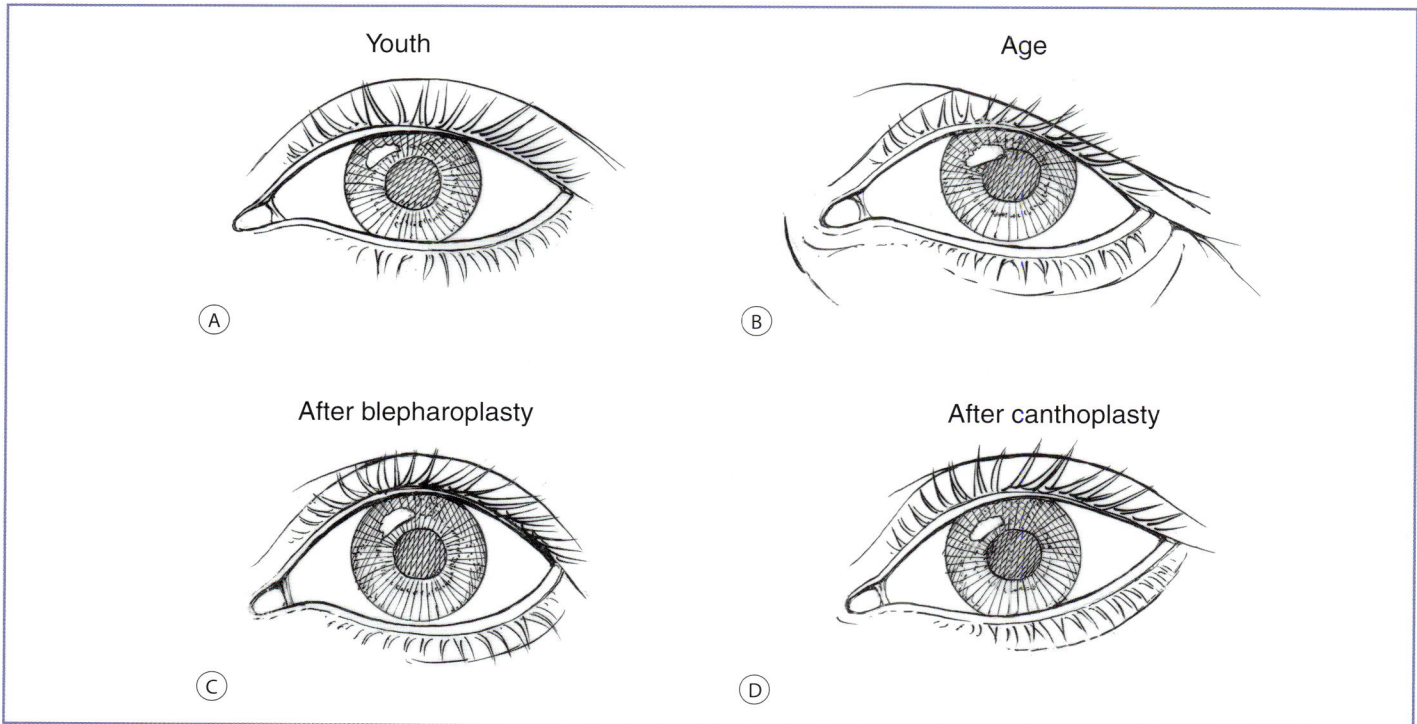

Youth

Age

(A)

(B)

After blepharoplasty

After canthoplasty

(C)

(D)

Figure 6.16 The shape of the palpebral fissure is a primary determinant of periorbital appearance. (**A**) In young adults with normal skeletal morphology, the palpebral fissure is long and narrow. (**B**) With aging, descent of the lower lid and medial migration of the lateral canthus round the shape of the palpebral fissure. (**C**) Standard blepharoplasty techniques that remove lower lid skin (and often muscle) tend to lower the lower lid margin, further rounding the palpebral fissure. (**D**) Canthoplasty procedures, by design, alter the shape of the palpebral fissure, because they disassemble and reassemble the lateral canthus while shortening the lower lid margin. Lateral canthopexy, because it does not violate the lid margin, maintains or has the potential to restore palpebral fissure shape, including the lateral canthal angle.

Temporal soft tissue elevation

The temporal soft tissues are elevated and redistributed to avoid the 'Madam Butterfly' look.[22] When a coronal incision is used to perform the lateral canthopexy, a lateral brow lift will avoid any upper lid bunching after lateral canthal elevation. When the latter extent of an upper lid blepharoplasty incision is used, a small ellipse of skin and underlying orbicularis oculi muscle is removed at the time of closure.

A suction drain is placed through a stab wound incision in the temporal scalp and placed beneath the composite lid–midface flap. A temporary tarsorrhaphy stitch is placed to limit postoperative chemosis. Compressive dressings are not used, because they direct fluid toward the more distensible lid soft tissues.

PEARL

A temporary tarsorrhaphy stitch will help control postoperative chemosis.

Clinical examples

Examples of patients who have undergone infraorbital rim augmentation and midface elevation are presented in Figures 6.17 and 6.18. Examples of patients who have undergone infraorbital rim augmentation, midface elevation, and lateral canthopexy are presented in Figures 6.19–6.21.

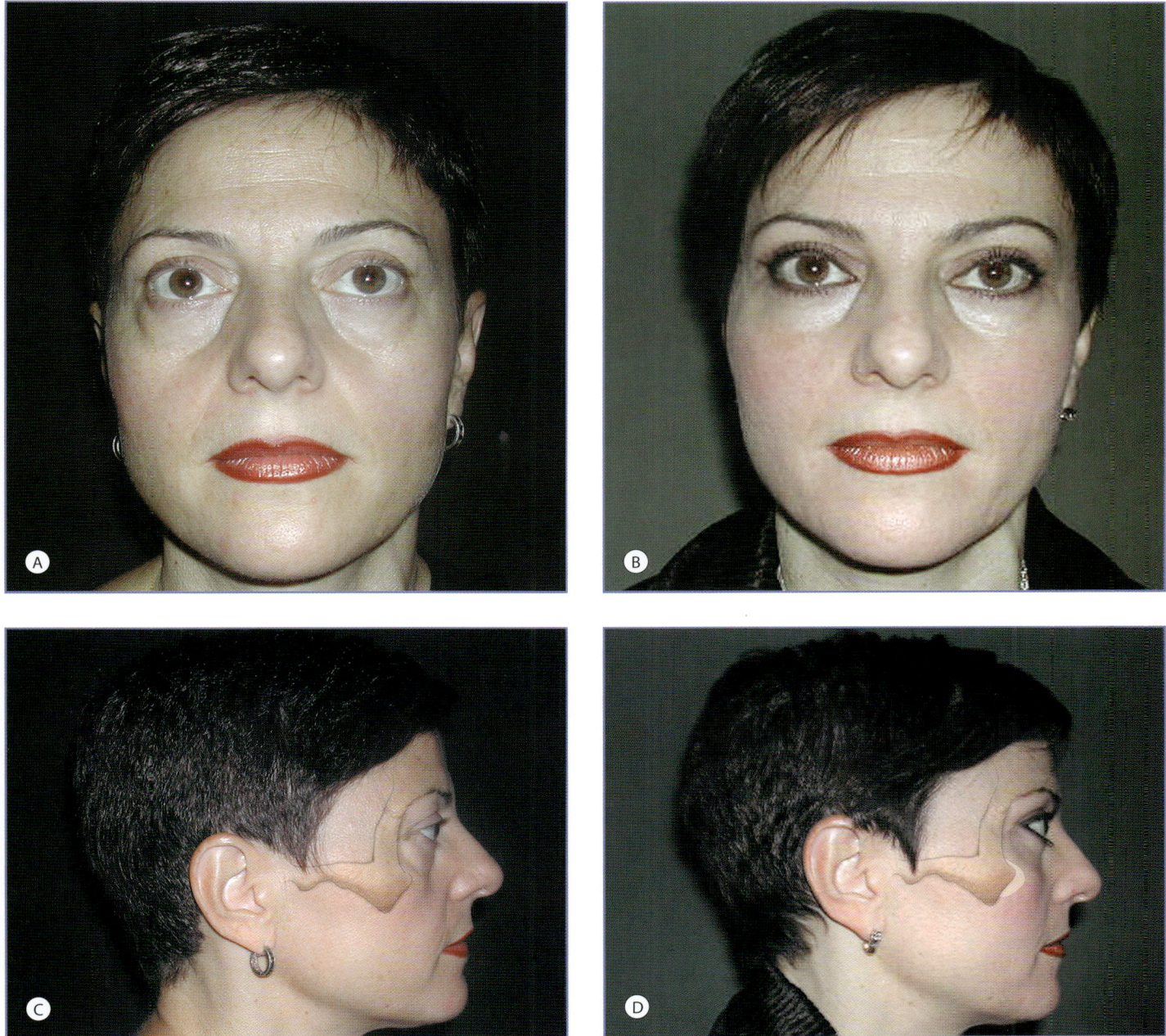

Figure 6.17 The 49-year-old woman shown in Figure 6.3 underwent infraorbital rim augmentation and midface lift. No fat was removed from the lower lids. (**A**) Preoperative frontal view. (**B**) One-year postoperative frontal view. Note that the infraorbital implant did not extend sufficiently medial to correct tear-through deformity. Note also that without direct manipulation of lower lid fat, the 'early bags' are ameliorated but not eliminated. (**C**) Preoperative lateral view with artist's rendition of underlying facial skeleton. (**D**) One-year postoperative lateral view with artist's rendition of augmented facial skeleton. (From Yaremchuk 2004,[9] with permission.)

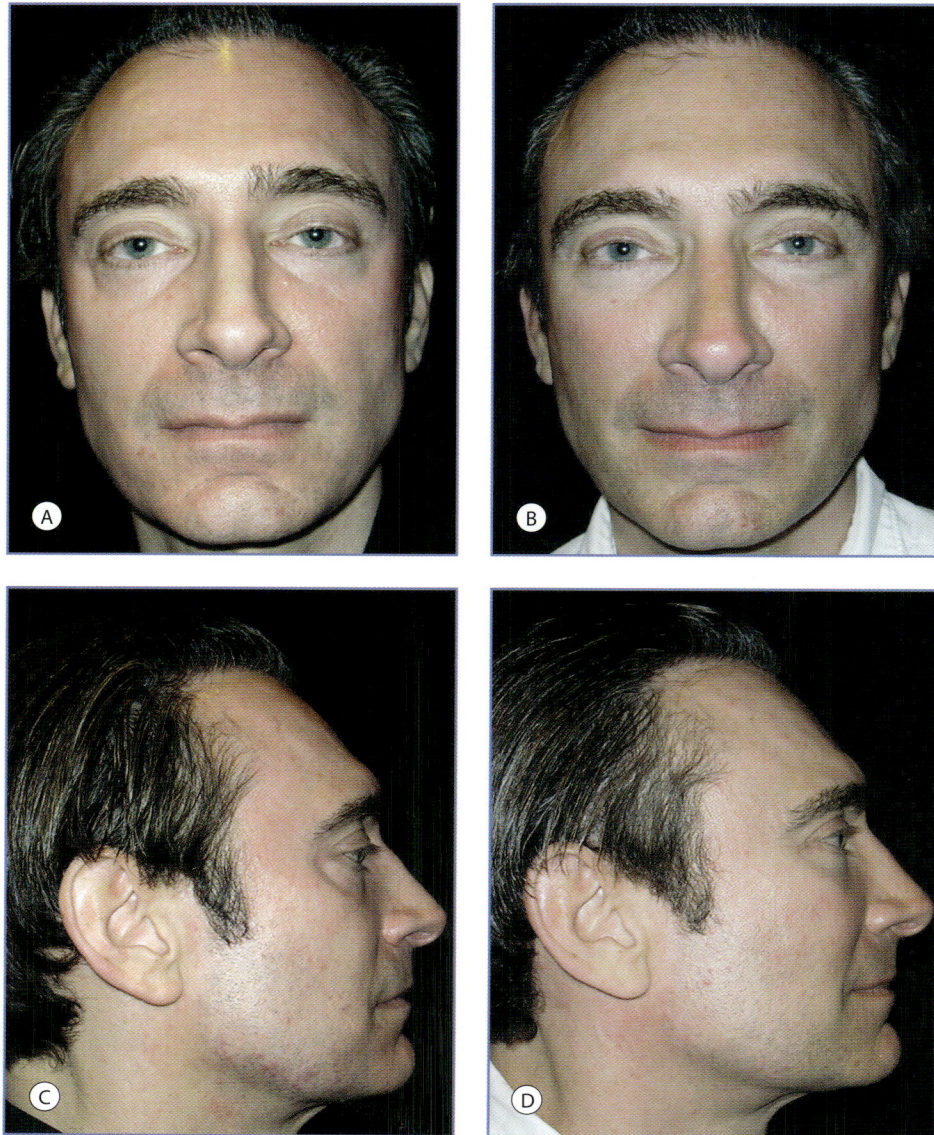

Figure 6.18 A 50-year-old man underwent infraorbital rim augmentation and blepharoplasty. (**A**) Preoperative and (**B**) postoperative frontal views. (**C**) Preoperative and (**D**) postoperative lateral views.

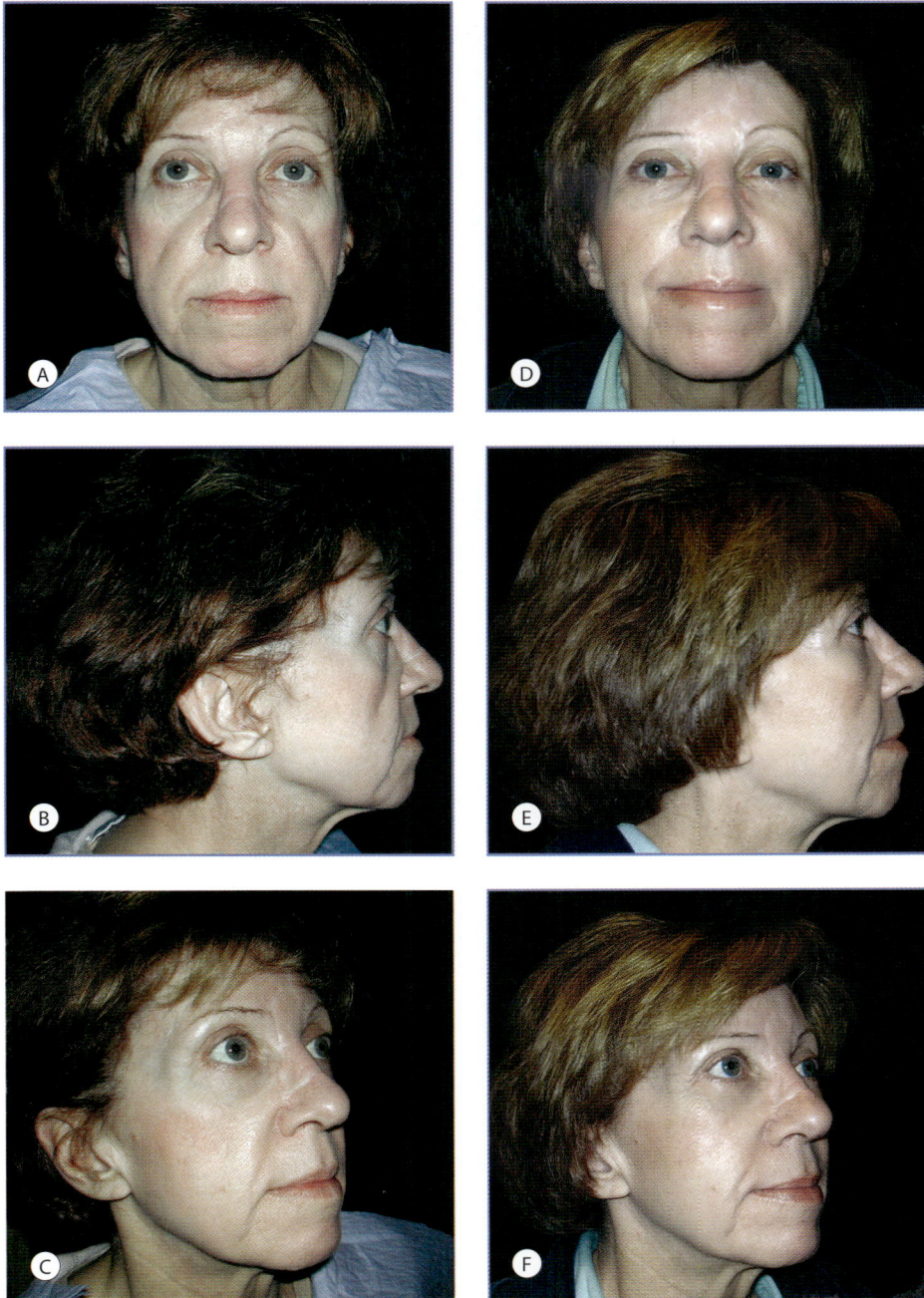

Figure 6.19 This 58-year-old woman underwent infraorbital rim augmentation, midface lift, and lateral canthopexy. Two millimeters of skin and a small amount of fat were removed from the lower lid. (**A–C**) Preoperative frontal, lateral, and oblique views. (**D–F**) Postoperative frontal, lateral and oblique views. Left brow distortion is a result of a forehead flap procedure used for skin cancer related nasal reconstruction performed by another surgeon in the remote past.

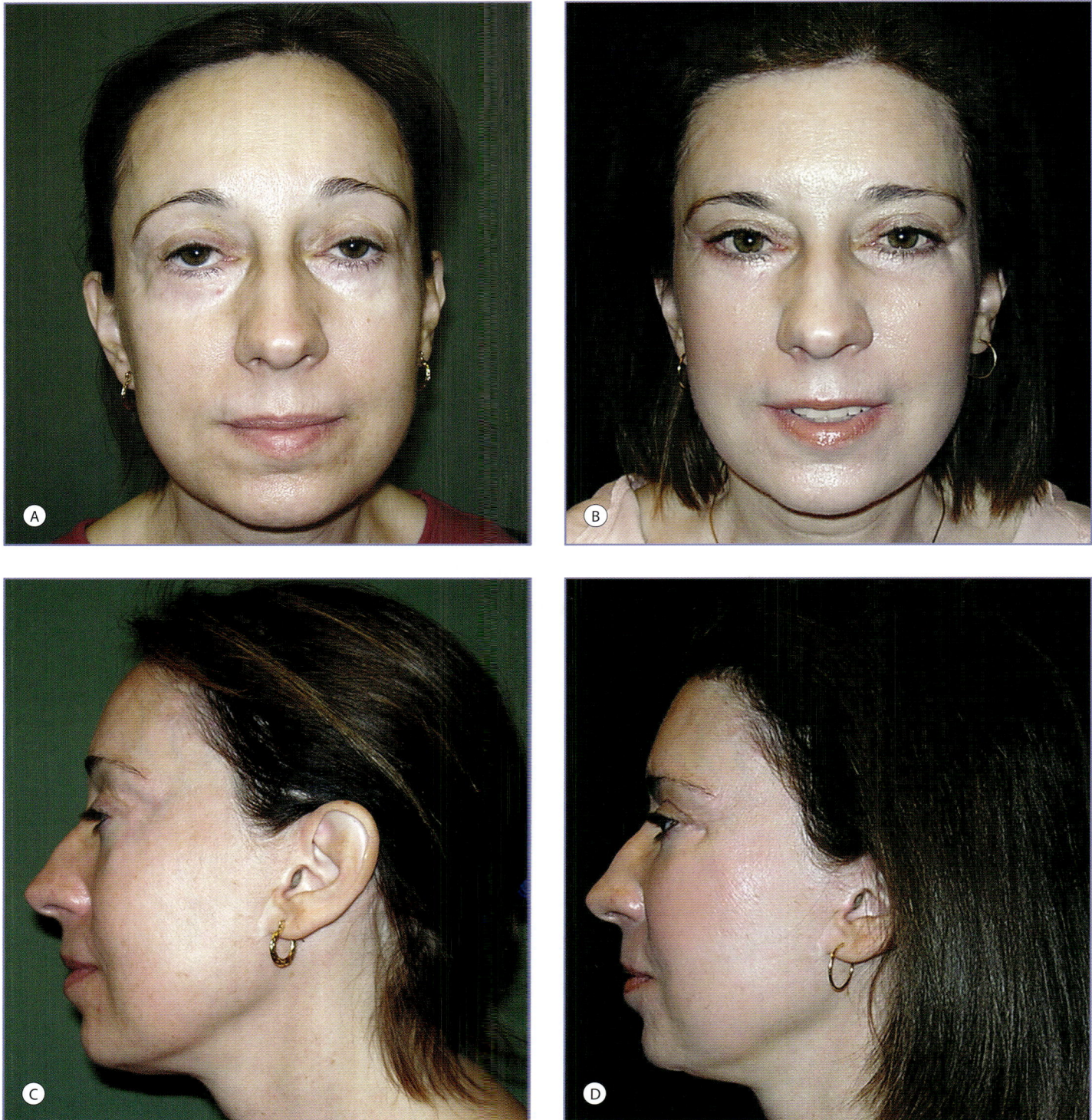

Figure 6.20 A 52-year-old woman had undergone previous brow lift, rhytidectomy, and upper and lower lid blepharoplasty. Lower lid retraction was treated by multiple canthopexies, spacer grafts, and full-thickness skin grafts. Dry eye symptoms persisted. Infraorbital rim augmentation, midface lift, and lateral canthopexy resolved her symptoms. Her brows and hairline were repositioned. (**A**) Preoperative and (**B**) postoperative frontal views. (**C**) Preoperative and (**D**) postoperative lateral views.

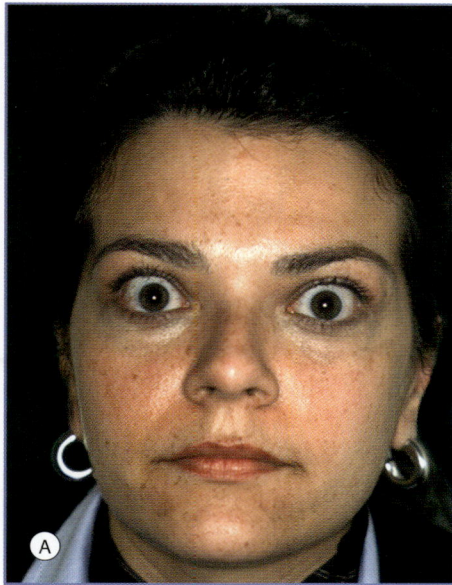

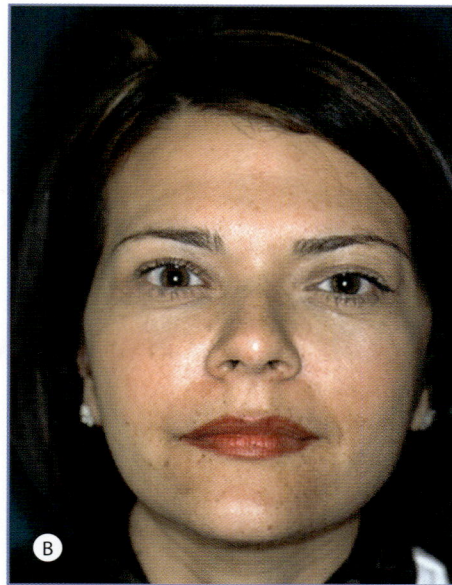

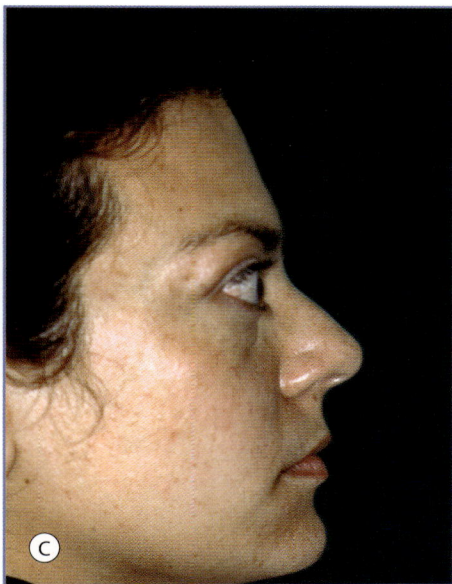

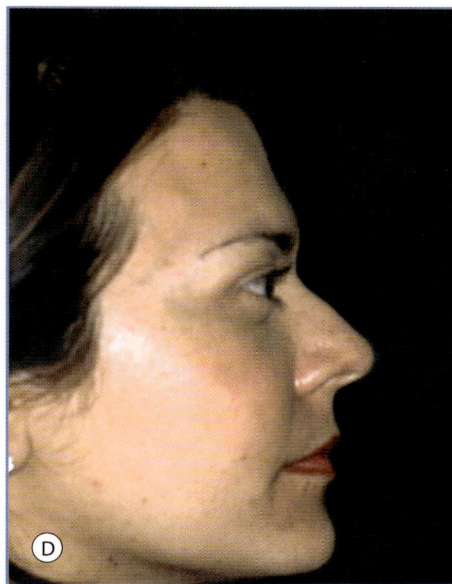

Figure 6.21 A 30-year-old woman with Graves disease underwent medial and lateral orbital decompression with preservation of the lateral orbital rim. The orbital floor was not manipulated, to avoid problems with globe displacement and dystopia. Globe–rim relations were further improved by augmenting the infraorbital rim, elevating the midface soft tissue, and performing lateral canthopexy. In this patient, a transconjunctival incision with lateral canthotomy was used. Note the distortion in the lateral canthal appearance on the right side due to improper lateral canthal realignment. Dry eye symptoms were relieved. (**A**) Preoperative and (**B**) postoperative frontal views. (**C**) Preoperative and (**D**) postoperative lateral views. (**E**) Diagrammatic representation of procedure. (Panels A–D from Yaremchuk 2004,[9] with permission.)

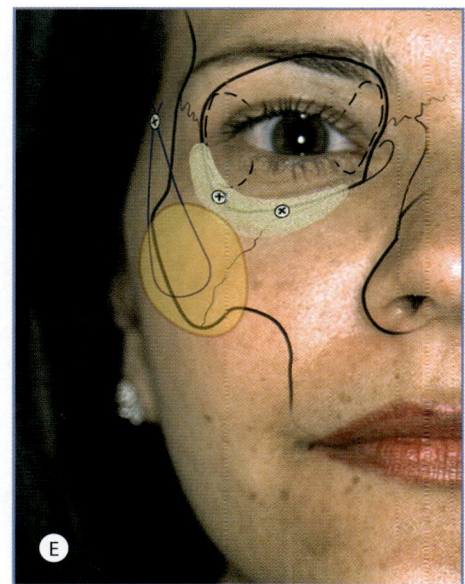

REFERENCES

1. Mulliken JB, Goodwin SL, Pracharktam N, et al. The concept of the sagittal orbital–globe relationship in craniofacial surgery. Plast Reconstr Surg 1996; 97(4):700–706.

2. Whitaker LA, Morales L Jr, Farkas LG. Aesthetic surgery of the supraorbital ridge and forehead structures. Plast Reconstr Surg 1986; 78(1):23–32.

3. Pessa JE, Desvigne LD, Lambros VS, et al. Changes in ocular globe-to-orbital rim position with age: implications for aesthetic blepharoplasty of the lower eyelids. Aesthetic Plast Surg 1999; 23(5):337–342.

4. Farkas LG, Hreczko TA, Katic JJ. Appendix A. Craniofacial norms in North American Caucasians from birth (one year) to adulthood. In: Farkas LG, ed. Anthropometry of the head and face. 2nd edn. New York: Raven Press; 1995.

5. Migliori ME, Gladstone GJ. Determination of the normal range of exophthalmometric values for black and white adults. Am J Ophthalmol 1984; 98(4):438–442.

6. Hirmand H, Codner MA, McCord CD, et al. Prominent eyes: operative management in lower lid and midface rejuvenation the morphologic classification system. Plast Reconstr Surg 2002; 11:620.

7. Yaremchuk MJ. Subperiosteal and full thickness skin rhytidectomy. Plast Reconstr Surg 2001; 107(4):1045–1058.

8. Yaremchuk MJ. Restoring palpebral fissure shape after previous lower blepharoplasty. Plast Reconstr Surg 2003; 111(1):441–450.

9. Yaremchuk MJ. Improving periorbital appearance in the 'morphologically prone'. Plast Reconstr Surg 2004; 114:980–987.

10. Rees TD, LaTrenta GS. The role of Schirmer's test and orbital morphology in predicting dry-eye syndrome after blepharoplasty. Plast Reconstr Surg 1988; 82(4):619–625.

11. Jelks GW, Jelks EB. The influence of orbital and eyelid anatomy on the palpebral aperture. Clin Plast Surg 1991; 18:193.

12. Yaremchuk MJ. Infraorbital rim augmentation. Plast Reconstr Surg 2001; 107(6):1585–1592.

13. McCord CD Jr. Eyelid surgery: principles and techniques. Philadelphia: Lippincott-Raven; 1995:95.

14. McCord CD Jr. The correction of lower lid malposition following lower blepharoplasty. Plast Reconstr Surg 1999; 103(3):1036–1039.

15. Baylis HI, Goldberg RA, Groth MJ. Complications of lower blepharoplasty. In: Putterman AM, ed. Cosmetic oculoplastic surgery: eyelid, forehead and facial techniques. 3rd edn. Philadelphia: Saunders; 1999:446.

16. Yaremchuk MJ, Kim WK. Soft-tissue alterations with acute, extended open reduction and internal fixation of orbital fractures. J Craniofac Surg 1992; 3(3):134–140.

17. Yaremchuk MJ. Orbital deformity after craniofacial fracture repair: avoidance and treatment. J Craniomaxillofac Trauma 1999; 5(2):7–16.

18. Phillips JH, Gruss JS, Wells MD, et al. Periosteal suspension of the lower eyelid and cheek following subciliary exposure of facial fractures. Plast Reconstr Surg 1991; 88(1):145–148.

19. Stuzin JM, Wagstrom L, Kawamoto HK, et al. Anatomy of the frontal branch of the facial nerve: the significance of the temporal fat pad. Plast Reconstr Surg 1989; 83(2):265–271.

20. Whitaker LA. Selective alterations of palpebral fissure form by lateral canthopexy. Plast Reconstr Surg 1984; 74(5):611–619.

21. Flowers RS. Canthopexy as a routine blepharoplasty component. Clin Plast Surg 1993; 20(2):351–365.

22. Shorr N, Fallor MK. 'Madam Butterfly' procedure: combined cheek and lateral canthus suspension procedure for post-blepharoplasty: 'round eye' and lower eyelid retraction. Ophthalmic Plast Reconstr Surg 1985; 1:229.

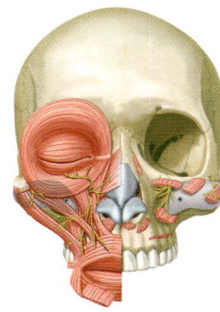

Chapter 7

Malar

Prominent malar bones are considered attractive.[1] Hence the malar area is frequently augmented with implants. Although not documented in the literature, personal experience with primary and secondary malar implant surgery has shown me that there is a significant incidence of patient dissatisfaction with this surgery. Patients presenting for secondary surgery have three main complaints: implant asymmetry; displeasing implant contours—too wide, too large, too low, or too prominent with time; and symptoms of infraorbital nerve compression.[2] Concepts and techniques presented in this chapter hope to optimize results and avoid these problems.

PREOPERATIVE PLANNING

A domelike shape with an absence of easily defined landmarks that are projected to the surface of the skin precludes anthropometric or cephalometric analysis of the malar area. The resultant paucity of objective data describing the malar area has inevitably made implant augmentation of this area more subjective. Because it is difficult to define what is average or normal for the malar area, selection of implant shape, implant size, and implant position for malar augmentation can be problematic.

Anthropometric data

The only anthropometric landmark for analysis of the malar area is zygion, which allows measurement of the bizygomatic distance or width of the midface (Fig. 7.1).[3] Several landmarks lie adjacent to or involve portions of the malar bone, but there are none defining an area of maximum malar prominence.

> **PEARL**
>
> There are no anthropometric or cephalometric landmarks defining malar prominence.

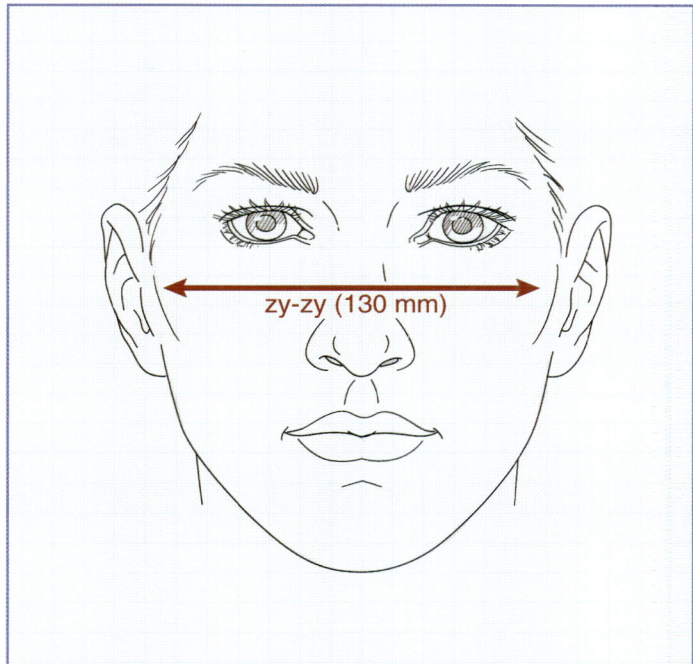

Figure 7.1 The only anthropometric measurement relative to the malar bone is zy–zy, which measures midface width. Similarly, there are no cephalometric landmarks to assess malar projection (zy), zygion.

Subjective analyses

Several surgeons, working without quantitative data, have suggested techniques to identify the malar prominence as a guide to malar augmentation. Their techniques use fixed relations to various anatomical landmarks to determine an ideal position of malar prominence.

Hinderer

Hinderer, one of the first to advocate the use of alloplastic implants for aesthetic surgery,[4] divided the malar area into quadrants formed by two intersecting lines. One is drawn from the ala to the tragus, and the other from the oral commissure to the lateral canthus. He advocated placing the implant in the upper outer quadrant formed by these intersecting lines (Fig. 7.2).

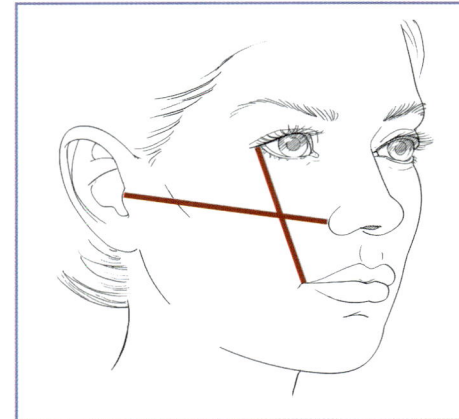

Figure 7.2 Hinderer's lines are two intersecting lines. One is drawn from the ala to the tragus, and the other from the oral commissure to the lateral canthus. He advocated placing the implant in the upper outer quadrant formed by these intersecting lines.[4]

Silver

Silver devised a triangle to determine the ideal position for the malar prominence (Fig. 7.3).[5] The Frankfort horizontal forms the base of the triangle. A vertical line from the lateral limbus with the eyes in a neutral position will bisect the base of the triangle. The point where this vertical line intersects a horizontal line placed between the subnasion and the vermilion border determines the apex of the triangle. A line is then drawn from the apex to the Frankfort horizontal equal in length to the other side. This point of intersection marks the malar prominence.

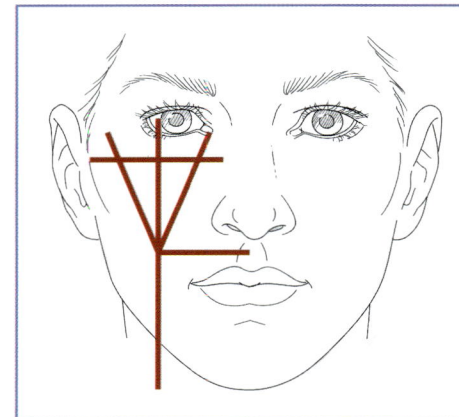

Figure 7.3 Silver devised a triangle to determine the ideal position for the malar prominence. The Frankfort horizontal forms the base of the triangle. A vertical line from the lateral limbus with the eyes in a neutral position will bisect the base of the triangle. The point where this vertical line intersects a horizontal line placed between the subnasion and the vermilion border determines the apex of the triangle. A line drawn from the medial canthus to the apex forms one side of the triangle. The other wall of the triangle is a line drawn from the apex to the Frankfort horizontal equal in length to the other side. The point of intersection between this line and the Frankfort horizontal marks the malar prominence.[5]

Wilkinson

Wilkinson proposed a method for determining the point of maximum malar projection by dropping a line vertically to the mandible border, then dividing it into thirds. The malar prominence should lie just lateral to the point one-third down from the canthus (Fig. 7.4).[6]

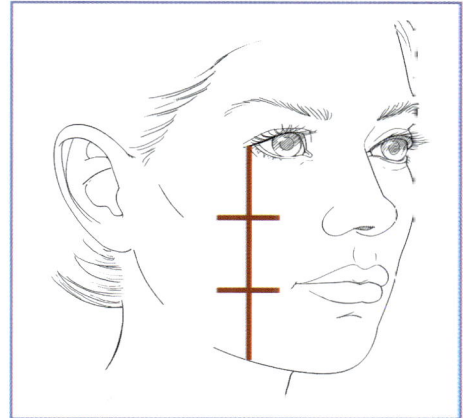

Figure 7.4 Wilkinson proposed a method for determining the point of maximum malar projection. He dropped a line vertically from the lateral canthus to the mandibular border, then divided it into thirds. The malar prominence should lie just lateral to the point one-third down from the canthus.[6]

Powell

Powell also defined the malar prominence relative to the Frankfort horizontal. He drew a line from the lateral canthus to the ala, and a second line from the oral commissure parallel to the first. The malar prominence was defined as the point where this second line intersected the Frankfort horizontal. This places the malar prominence 1.5–2 cm lateral to the lateral canthus (Fig. 7.5).[7]

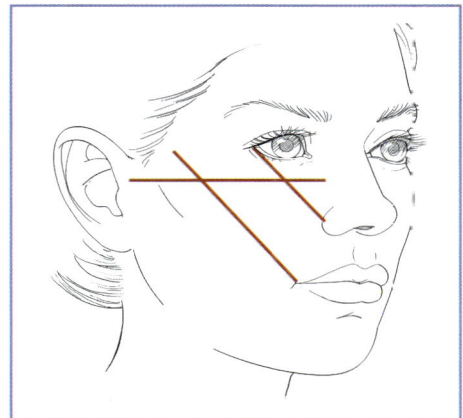

Figure 7.5 Powell defined the malar prominence relative to the Frankfort horizontal. He drew a line from the lateral canthus to the ala, and a second line from the oral commissure parallel to the first. The malar prominence was defined as the point where this second line intersected the Frankfort horizontal. This places the malar prominence 1.5–2 cm lateral to the lateral canthus.[7]

PEARL

Techniques used to define an area of malar prominence are based on subjective analyses.

123

Prendergast and Schoenrock

Prendergast and Schoenrock drew a line from the oral commissure to the lateral canthus. They determined the malar prominence to be on this line at a point one-third of the distance from the canthus (Fig. 7.6).[8]

The lack of consensus regarding the most projecting point of the malar prominence reflects the clinician's dilemma. Of the five analyses presented here, it is my aesthetic judgment that all the analyses, save for Prendergast and Schoenrock's, place the point of maximum malar projection too lateral. This placement will increase the bizygomatic distance, already the widest part of the face, and exaggerate any midface hypoplasia (a common skeletal morphology in patients receiving malar implants).

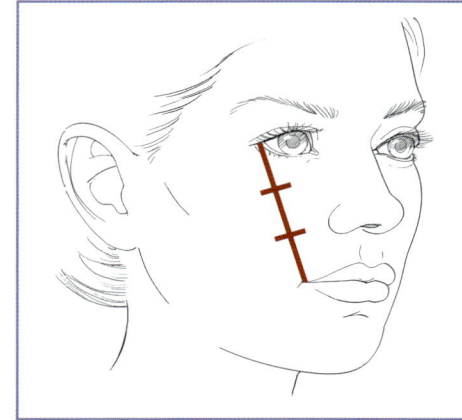

Figure 7.6 Prendergast and Schoenrock drew a line from the oral commissure to the lateral canthus. They determined the malar prominence to be on this line at a point one-third of the distance from the canthus.[8]

Whitaker

Whitaker's analysis of the malar midface considered three zones in the malar–midface complex: a medial paranasal area, a central malar area, and a lateral zygomatic arch area (Fig. 7.7).[9] It did not define an area of maximum malar prominence. The division of the midface into anatomical zones, also advocated—but divided differently—by Terino,[10] has been extremely helpful in visualizing and correcting not only malar, but also other areas of midface deficiency.

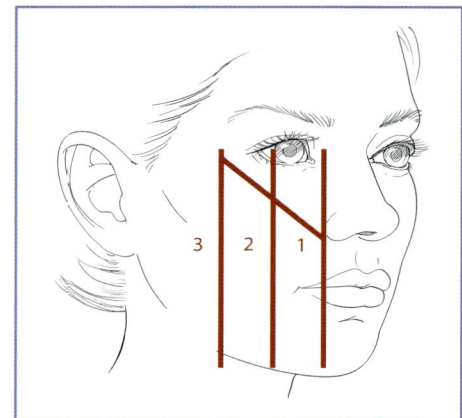

Figure 7.7 Whitaker divided the malar–midface complex into three anatomical zones: a medial paranasal, a central malar, and a lateral arch area. This complex forms an angle of approximately 45° from the vertical, as measured from the lateral orbit to the alar lobule.[9]

As the most prominent and surgically accessible portion of the midface and, until recently, the only area of the midface for which implants were available, many patients receive malar implants when the entire midface or another midface area is deficient. This may exaggerate the facial imbalance. For example, malar augmentation, particularly when it extends far on to the zygomatic arch, may exaggerate the appearance of prominent eyes due to midface hypoplasia. These patients are better served with augmentation of the infraorbital rim alone or in combination with malar augmentation and other soft tissue manipulations (see Ch. 9).[11]

Because full cheeks are associated with youth, malar augmentation is often performed to provide a youthful appearance.[12,13] This may provide an aesthetic benefit if there is a relative malar hypoplasia, or if the implants are of modest size and projection. This skeletal augmentation is not equivalent to a soft tissue augmentation or resuspension (see Ch. 1). Similarly, malar implants are often advocated as a means to obliterate lower eyelid wrinkles or secondary bags. Malar augmentation impacts poorly on these surface irregularities. More often, they detract from periorbital aesthetics by contributing to lower lid malposition, particularly when placed through an eyelid approach.

Certain implant designs do not mimic the contours of the midface skeleton. For example, submalar implants are designed to be placed over and below the origin of the masseter muscle—a location where there is no midface skeleton— in an attempt to provide cheek fullness. It is often performed as an adjunct to or as an alternative to a face-lift.[13] The result is an unnatural midface—one with too much lower midface fullness, which actually detracts from malar definition and projection (see Fig. 7.16).

In summary, the lack of anthropometric and cephalometric landmarks precludes the availability of normative data, making analysis and augmentation of the malar area largely subjective. Malar deficiency is often part of a generalized midface deficiency for which malar augmentation alone may be inadequate or even inappropriate. Clinical experience has shown that when malar projection is deemed inadequate, malar augmentation is most effective when it recreates the contours of a normal skeleton with prominent anterior projection. Malar skeletal augmentation is not a substitute for soft tissue augmentation or repositioning.

PEARL

Midface augmentation should be specific to the area of skeletal deficiency.

PEARL

Skeletal augmentation is not a substitute for soft tissue augmentation or resuspension.

SURGICAL ANATOMY

The anatomical structures relevant to implant augmentation of the malar area are presented below (Fig. 7.8).

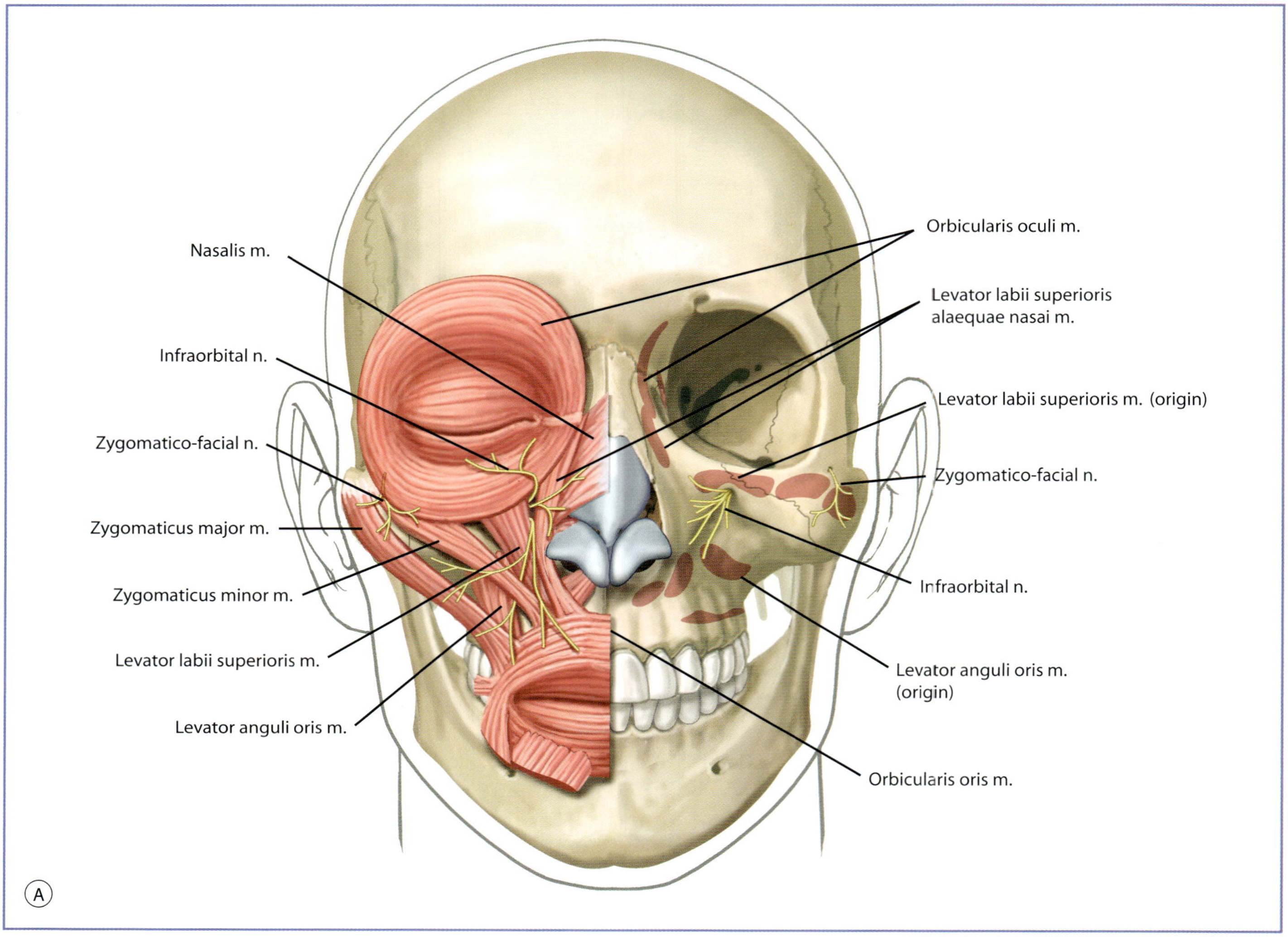
Nasalis m.
Infraorbital n.
Zygomatico-facial n.
Zygomaticus major m.
Zygomaticus minor m.
Levator labii superioris m.
Levator anguli oris m.
Orbicularis oculi m.
Levator labii superioris alaequae nasai m.
Levator labii superioris m. (origin)
Zygomatico-facial n.
Infraorbital n.
Levator anguli oris m. (origin)
Orbicularis oris m.
A

Figure 7.8 The malar midface anatomy. (**A**) Frontal views.

Skeleton

The zygomatic or malar bone forms the prominence of the cheek. It also forms part of the lateral wall and floor of the orbit, as well as parts of the temporal and infratemporal fossae. The zygoma sends a frontal process upward along the lateral margin of the orbit to articulate with the frontal bone, and a temporal process backward to form the anterior end of the zygomatic arch. The zygoma articulates with the maxilla medially and presents malar, orbital, and temporal surfaces. The malar surface is convex, and is perforated in its midaspect by the zygomaticofacial foramen for the passage of the zygomaticofacial nerve and vessels. Just below this foramen is a slight elevation of the bone, from which the zygomaticus major and the levator labii superioris arise.

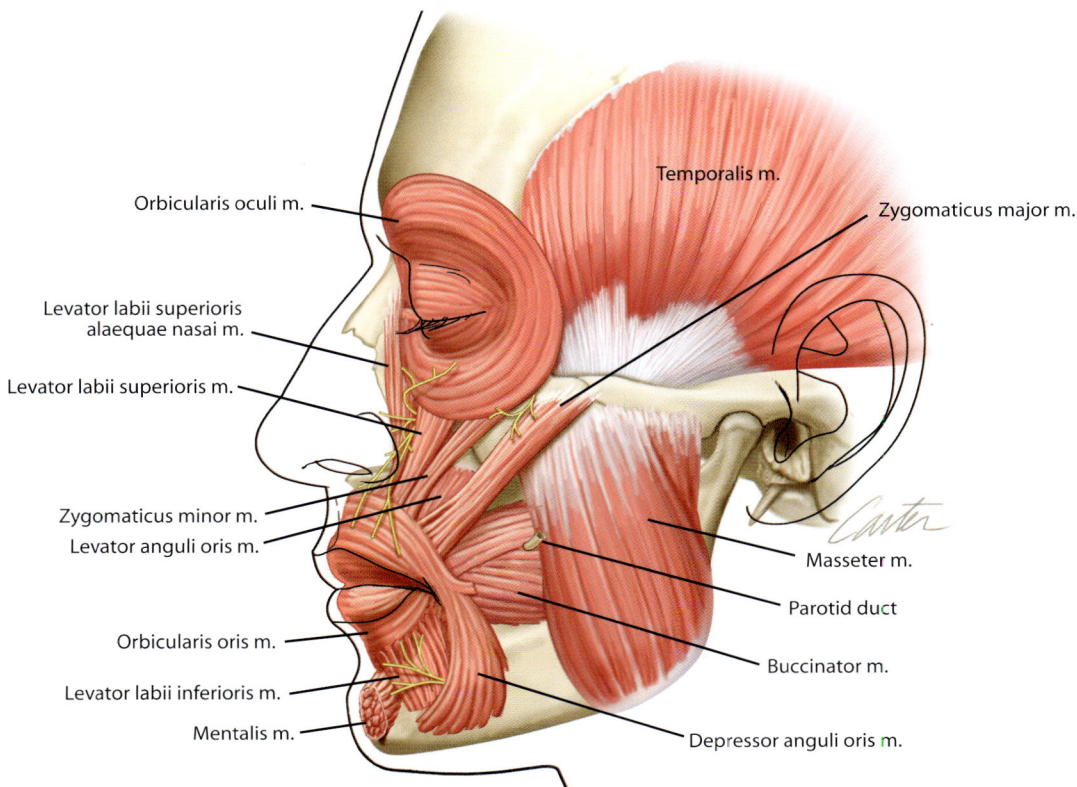

Figure 7.8 (*Cont'd*) The malar midface anatomy. (**B**) Lateral views.

Muscles

The muscles of the midface largely provide facial expression. They arise from the bones of the face and insert into the skin. These muscles seldom remain distinct throughout their length; rather, they tend to merge with their neighbor where they terminate. Those that are freed from their origins during malar augmentation elevate the upper lip and are described below.

The zygomaticus major muscle originates from the lateral surface of the zygoma just medial to the zygomaticotemporal suture, and sometimes intermingles with the orbicularis oculi. It passes obliquely downward and forward to the corner of the mouth, where it inserts into skin and mucosa.

The zygomaticus minor lies medial to the zygomaticus major. It originates from the malar surface of the zygoma immediately lateral to the zygomatico-maxillary suture, and passes downward and medially to insert into the lip just medial to the corner of the mouth.

The levator labii superioris originates from the lower margin of the orbit just above the infraorbital foramen. It travels downward and medially to insert into the orbicularis oris as well as the skin of the lip.

The levator anguli oris (caninus) lies deep to the above muscles. It arises from the canine fossa of the maxilla immediately inferior to the infraorbital foramen. It inserts into the angle of the mouth. The facial vessels travel across its lower border. Branches of the infraorbital nerve travel in the connective tissue between it and the overlying musculature.

127

Sensory nerves

The infraorbital nerve exits the maxilla through the infraorbital foramen, and travels beneath the levator superioris and above the levator anguli oris. Its branches supply the skin of the lower lid, the side of the nose, and most of the cheek and upper lip. This nerve must be identified and preserved. The zygomaticofacial nerve exits through a small foramen located on the lateral aspect of the malar bone. It supplies a small portion of the skin of the upper cheek. It is routinely sacrificed during malar augmentation.

IMPLANT DESIGN

A malar implant should reproduce the normal contours of the facial skeleton. Morales's modification of Whitaker's design can fulfill this requisite.[9] It extends from just beyond the zygomaticotemporal suture, over the malar area, passing just below the infraorbital foramen, to the canine fossa and the piriform aperture. Its shape mimics the contours of a normal skeleton (Fig. 7.9). I have never used this large implant without modifying it. It is contoured to meet the specific needs of each patient.

Although implants with greater projection are available, I rarely provide more than 3 mm of augmentation at the point of maximum projection. Larger implants will become obvious with time as the overlying soft tissues atrophy and sag. The capsule formation that accompanies smooth-surfaced implants further exaggerates the tendency toward implant visibility (see Fig. 7.15).

In my experience, implants with large surface areas do not mimic natural skeletal topography and cause unnatural, implant-dictated contours.

> **PEARL**
>
> Extending a malar implant on to the zygomatic arch has a profound impact on midfacial width.

> **PEARL**
>
> Large malar implants will become visible with time.

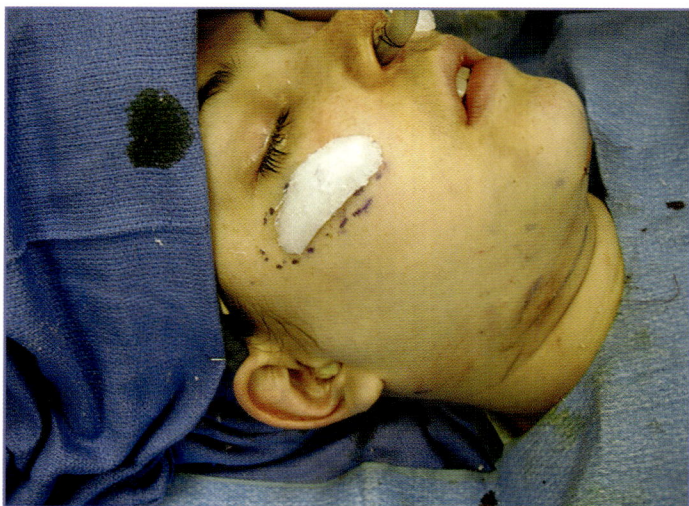

Figure 7.9 Morales's modification of a Whitaker-style implant (Porex Surgical, Fairburn, Georgia) is the preferred implant for malar augmentation. This implant is always carved to meet the needs of the patient. Most often, its length is adjusted so that it extends from the zygomaticotemporal suture to just beneath the infraorbital foramen. This intraoperative view shows how this implant design was modified to meet the needs of the patient.

OPERATIVE TECHNIQUE: PRIMARY SURGERY (Fig. 7.10)

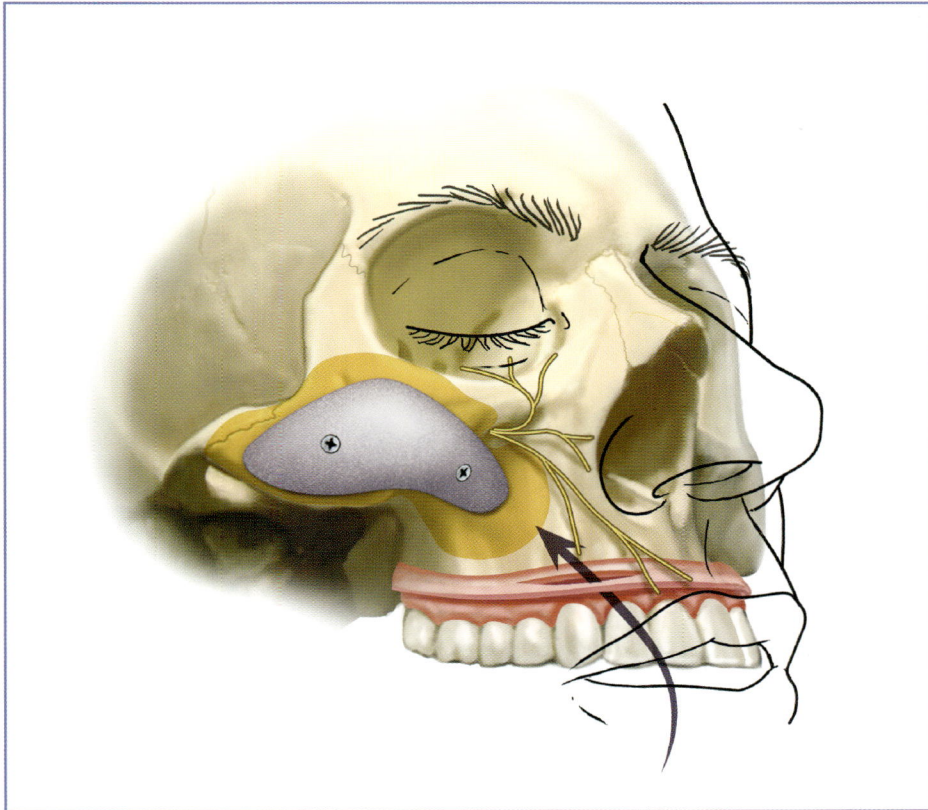

Figure 7.10 Overview of the operative technique for malar augmentation. The upper buccal sulcus incision is at least 1 cm above the apex so that sufficient tissue is available for closure. Taking care to identify the infraorbital nerve, the subperiosteal dissection is carried over the malar eminence and on to the zygomatic arch just beyond the zygomaticotemporal suture. It is useful to identify or create landmarks (e.g. scoring the zygoma relative to the infraorbital foramen) to allow symmetric placement of the implants. Implants are fixed with titanium screws for immobilization, and for the obliteration of dead space between the posterior surface of the implant and the anterior surface of the facial skeleton. The implants are contoured so that they are identical in size and shape, are appropriate for the area to be augmented, and merge imperceptibly with the native skeleton. A trocar-attached suction drain is placed. It exits through temporal hair-bearing scalp. The buccal sulcus incision and the area of subperiosteal dissection are shown. The implant usually extends from the temperozygomatic suture on the zygomatic arch to just below the foramen of the infraorbital nerve. It does not extend beyond the malar bone into the submalar area.

Prior to the induction of anesthesia, the area desired for augmentation is determined with the patient. This is marked on the surface of the skin.

Malar augmentation can be performed under local or general anesthesia. My preference is to use general endotracheal or nasotracheal anesthesia. This allows optimal preparation of the operative site and control of the airway. A long-acting local anesthetic mixed with 1:200 000 adrenaline (epinephrine) is infiltrated at the surgical site. This solution reduces general anesthetic requirements and postoperative discomfort while it provides hemostasis.

An upper gingivobuccal sulcus incision is made over the premolars. The incision is made at least 1 cm above the sulcus to provide an adequate inferior cuff of mucosa for closure. The lip elevators can be seen after the mucosa is incised. These muscles are not divided, but rather separated in their longitudinal orientation and retracted during the exposure of the zygoma and lower maxilla.

Subperiosteal dissection exposes the area to be augmented. Laterally, the dissection extends just beyond the zygomaticotemporal suture. Medially, at this level, it extends to the infraorbital foramen. This requires elevation of the zygomaticus major and zygomaticus minor muscles from their origins, and usually sacrifice of the zygomaticofacial nerve. The levator anguli oris (caninus) lies deep to the above muscles. Its origins are usually separated from the canine fossa of the maxilla immediately inferior to the infraorbital foramen. The lip elevators and the infraorbital nerve are retracted to provide exposure.

After skeletal exposure, the implants are carved to provide the desired augmentation as guided by the preoperative skin markings. Three maneuvers ensure symmetric placement and desired augmentation. The implants are carved so as to create mirror images of one another. Using the drill, the skeleton may be marked at measured locations to provide points of orientation for implant placement. For example, using a caliper, the skeleton is scored 5 mm medial to the infraorbital foramen and 5 mm inferior to the infraorbital foramen as orienting points for implant placement.

Finally, the implant is fixed with titanium screws to permanently ensure this intraoperative position. Gaps between the surface of the skeleton and the undersurface of the implant can equal or exceed the thickness of the implant. These gaps, which would result in unanticipated increases in augmentation, are obliterated by screw fixation of the implant to the skeleton (Fig. 7.11).

A suction drain is placed. Using a trocar guide, it exits the face in hair-bearing preauricular scalp. Before the incision is closed in layers, the infraorbital nerve is identified to be confident that any early postoperative complaints of decreased sensation in the distribution of the infraorbital nerve can be attributed to the trauma of soft tissue retraction, and not implant compression.

> **PEARL**
>
> Use skeletal reference points to ensure symmetric malar implant placement.

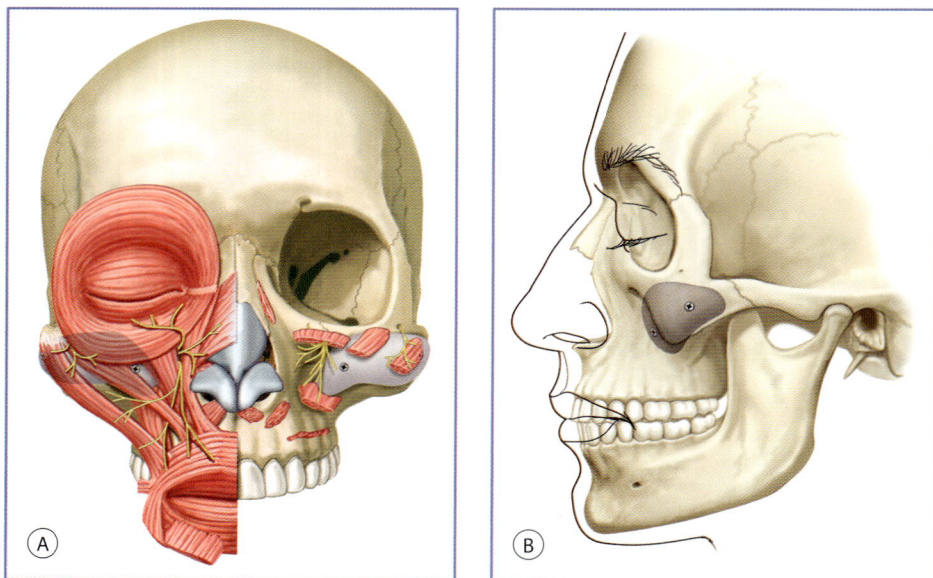

Figure 7.11 Typical placement of a malar implant relative to the skeleton and overlying musculature. (**A**) Frontal and (**B**) lateral views.

Clinical examples
Patients who have undergone malar augmentation are shown in Figures 7.12–7.14.

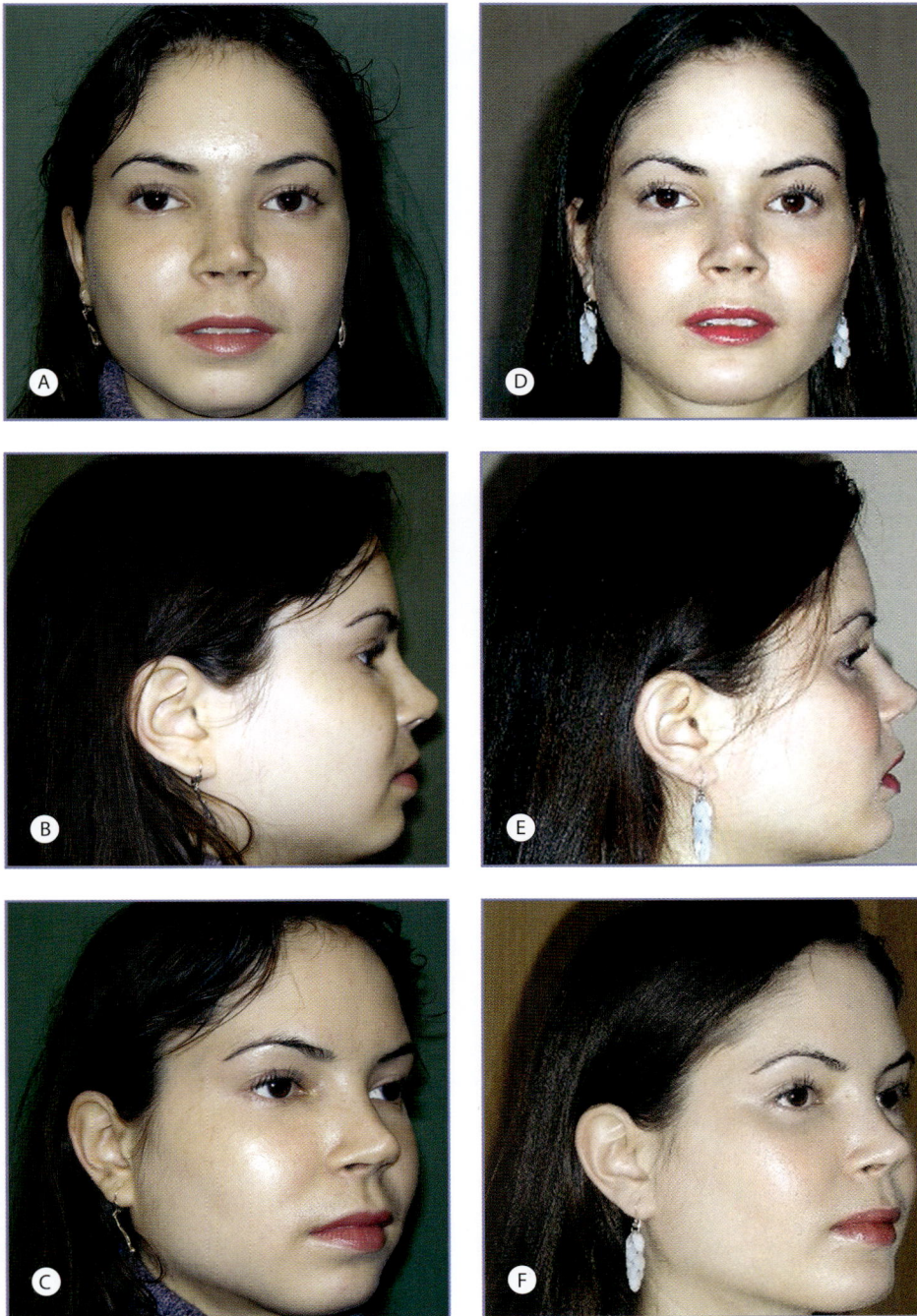

Figure 7.12 A 24-year-old woman underwent malar augmentation, chin augmentation, and submental lipectomy. (**A–C**) Preoperative frontal, lateral, and oblique views. (**D–F**) Postoperative frontal, lateral, and oblique views.

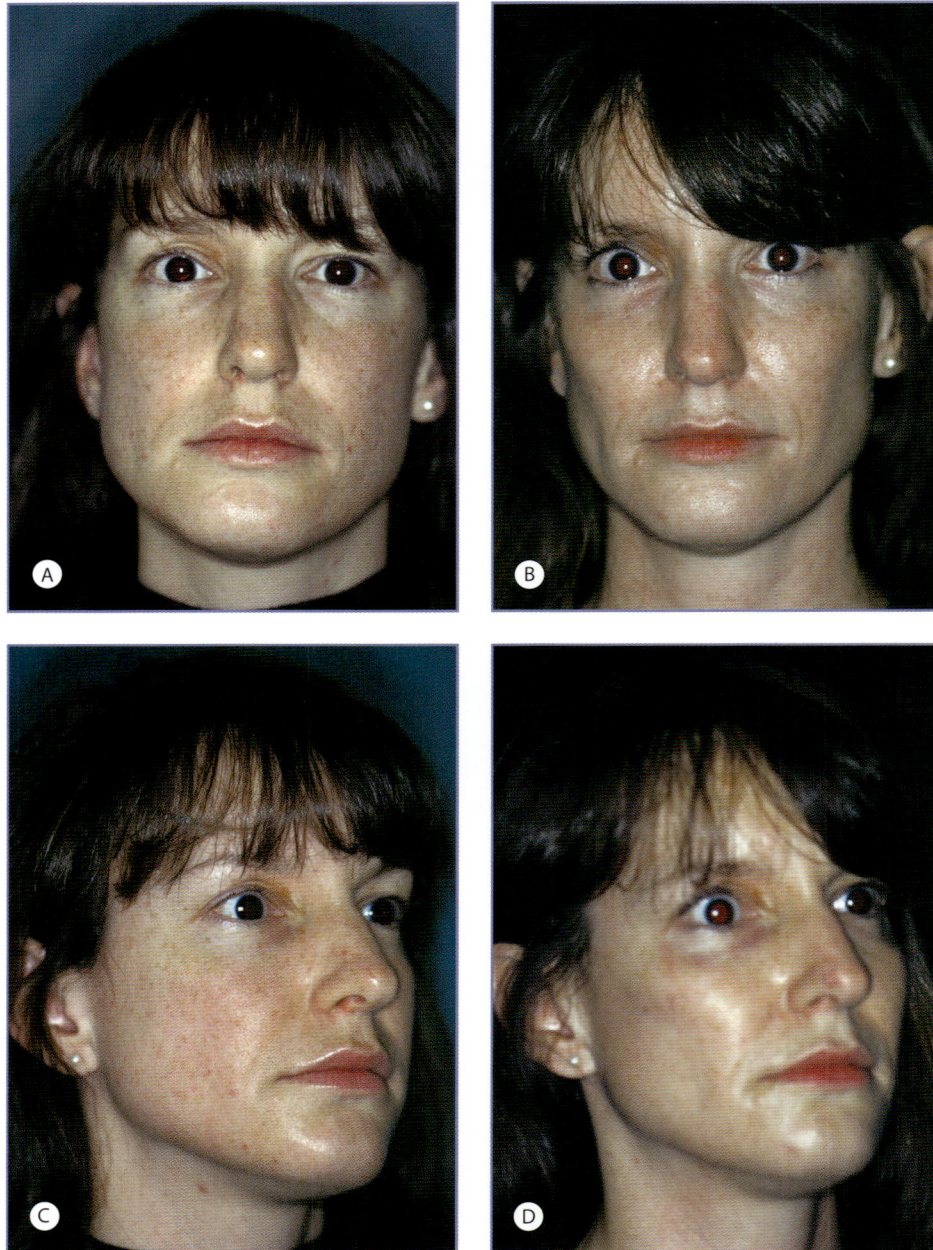

Figure 7.13 A 34-year-old woman underwent malar augmentation with screw-immobilized porous polyethylene implants. (**A**) Preoperative and (**B**) postoperative frontal views. (**C**) Preoperative and (**D**) postoperative oblique views.

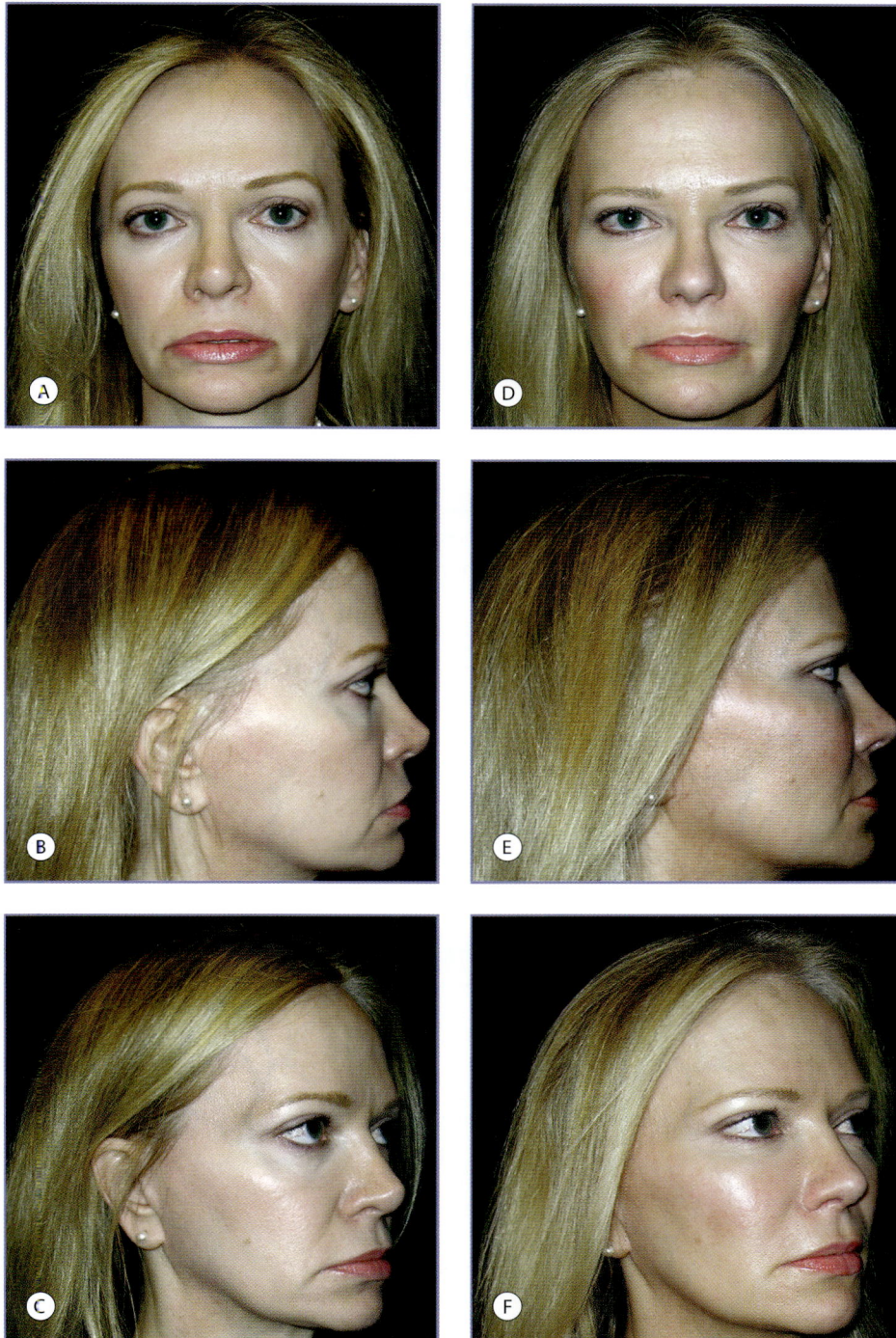

Figure 7.14 A 50-year-old woman had undergone bilateral upper and lower lid blepharoplasty, brow lift, and rhytidectomy 5 years prior to presentation. In addition to infraorbital rim and malar augmentation, midface elevation, and lateral canthopexy, the hairline and brows were lowered. The chin was lengthened, and a secondary rhinoplasty was performed by another surgeon. (**A–C**) Preoperative frontal, lateral, and oblique views. (**D–F**) Postoperative frontal, lateral, and oblique views.

OPERATIVE TECHNIQUE: SECONDARY SURGERY

Inadequate exposure of the complex curvatures of the midface skeleton is a common error in primary surgery, predisposing to implant malposition, implant asymmetry, and infraorbital nerve impingement at the infraorbital foramen. Lack of adequate exposure of the area to be augmented and its relation to the implant similarly limits the effectiveness of revisional surgery. Similar to primary surgery, failure to fix the implant to the facial skeleton with a screw at the time of revisional surgery may lead to asymmetry or implant malposition. Screw fixation prevents perioperative movement of the implant. Screw fixation also applies the posterior surface of the implant to the surface of the bone. This obliterates any gaps between the implant and the skeleton. Gaps result in unanticipated increases in the projection of the implant.

The conduct of revisional surgery is determined by the patient's concerns and the time interval between implant placement and patient presentation. If revisional surgery is pursued within months of the original surgery, implant repositioning or replacement alone is appropriate. Wide exposure of both malar areas allows symmetric implant repositioning or replacement. Screw fixation ensures maintenance of the intraoperative position.

When implants have been in place long enough to be well encapsulated, surgery is more complex. Implant encapsulation distorts the soft tissue envelope. The capsule, scar tissue mimicking the contours of the implant, permanently distorts the soft tissue envelope. Its impact on the appearance of the cheek will depend on the size of the implant, the projection of the implant, and the thickness of the overlying subcutaneous tissue. The removal of a large, overly projecting implant in a patient whose subcutaneous tissues are beginning to thin with age will inevitably impart a relief of the implant in the cheek soft tissues (Fig. 7.15). This soft tissue distortion can be camouflaged by repositioning the soft tissues. After implant removal, an appropriately sized and shaped implant is placed, and a subperiosteal midface lift is performed to redistribute the cheek soft tissues (see Ch. 6). This maneuver has been effective in improving midface contour and lessening the implant-related soft tissue distortions.

> **PEARL**
>
> When reoperating to correct implant asymmetry, expose both sides to compare implant position.

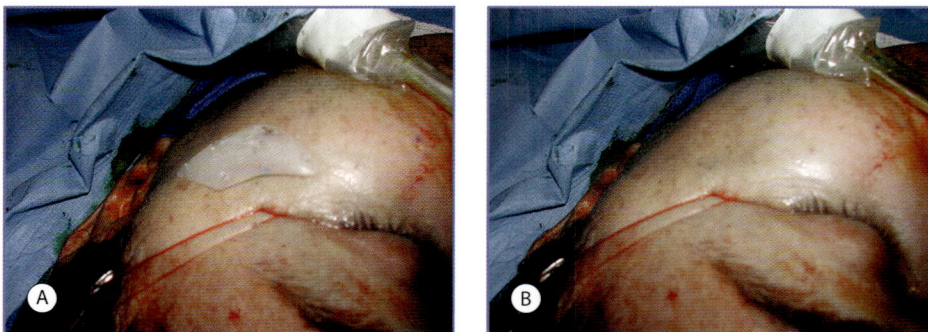

Figure 7.15 Intraoperative view showing silicone malar implant removed at surgery (**A**) and the soft tissue depression left after its removal (**B**).

Clinical examples

Patients who have undergone surgery to correct malar implant-related deformities are presented in Figures 7.16 and 7.17.

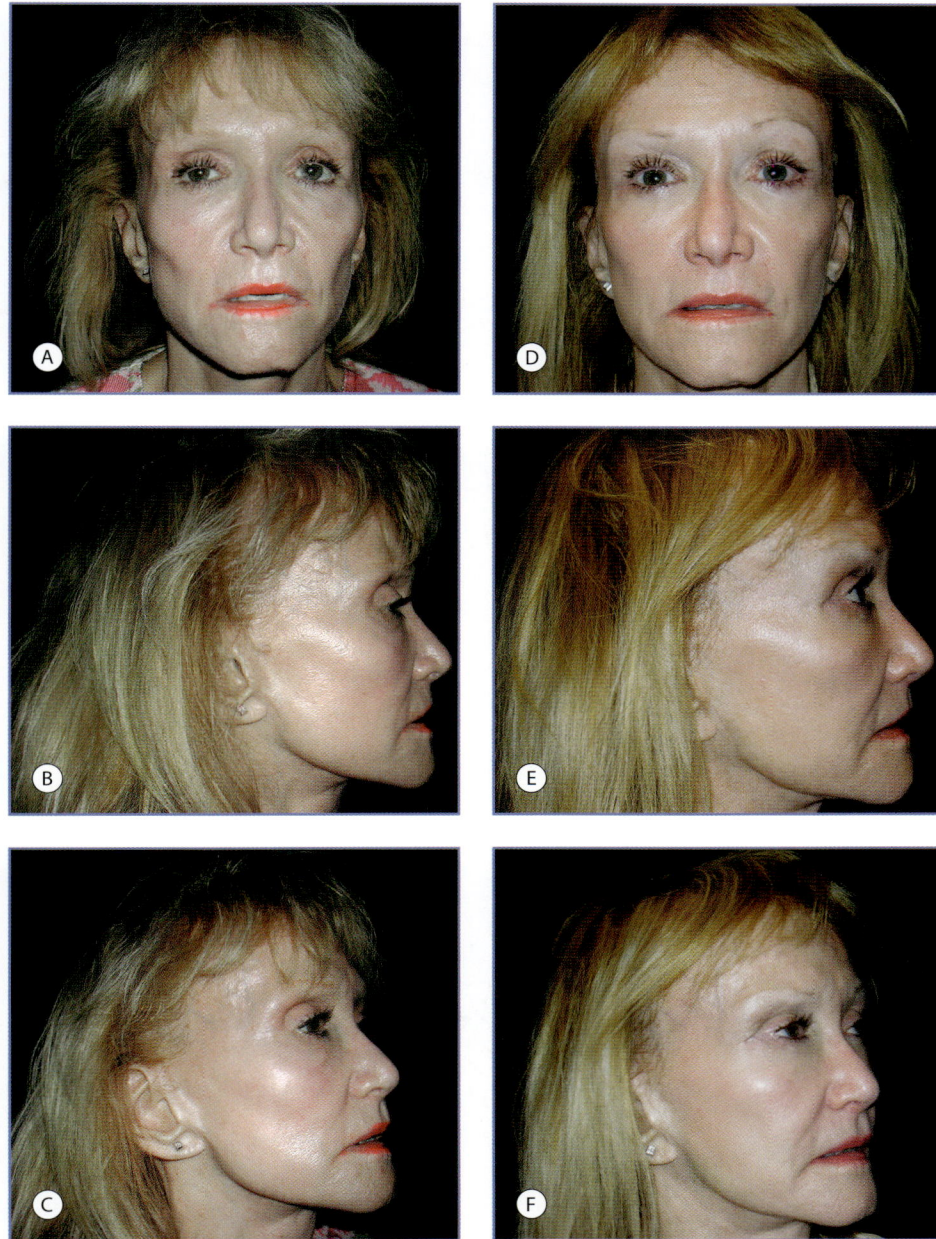

Figure 7.16 A 64-year-old woman underwent surgery for her malar implant-induced midface deformity. The combination of capsule formation around a large, smooth-surfaced implant and soft tissue atrophy resulted in an overly prominent, unnatural contour. The patient had also had upper and lower lid blepharoplasty and rhytidectomy in the past. Her lower lid retraction was symptomatic. Corrective surgery included implant removal, subperiosteal midface elevation, and lateral canthopexy. (**A–C**) Preoperative frontal, lateral, and oblique views. (**D–F**) Postoperative frontal, lateral, and oblique views.

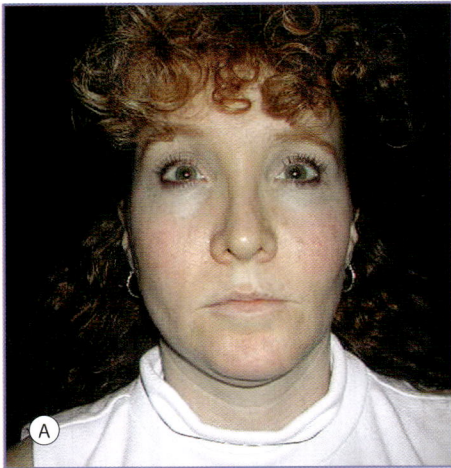

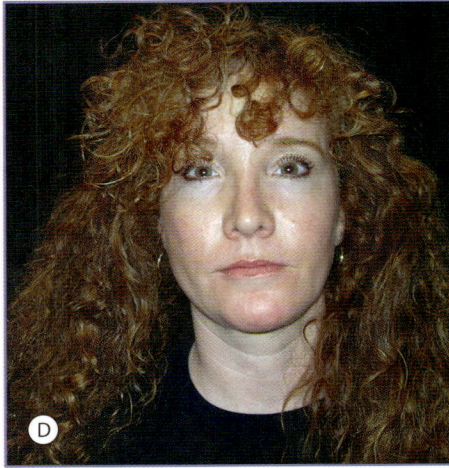

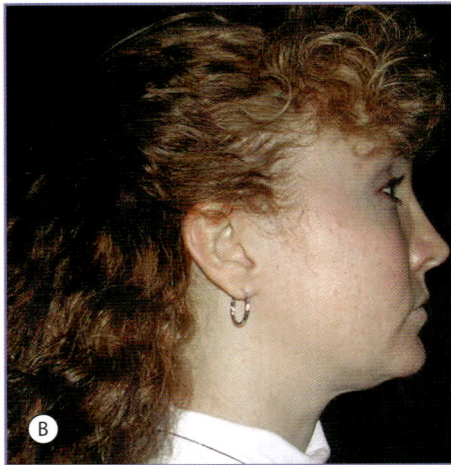

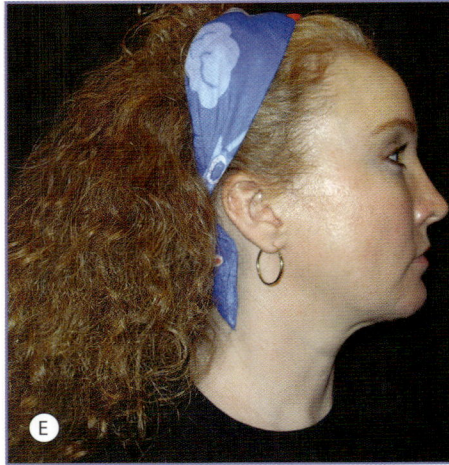

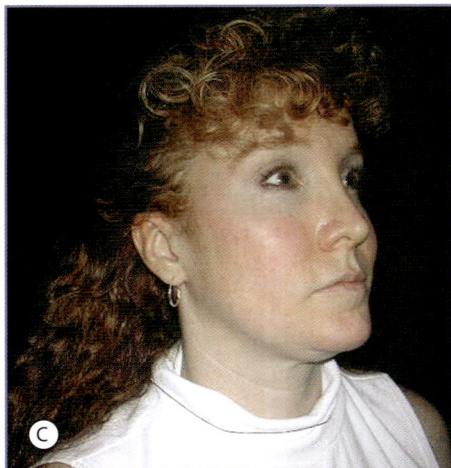

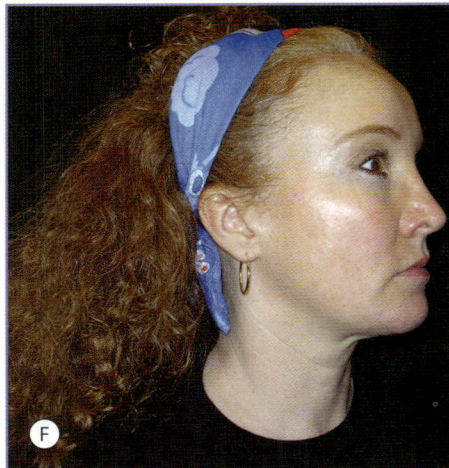

Figure 7.17 A 40-year-old woman had undergone endoscopic brow lift, malar augmentation, and sliding genioplasty in the past. She was displeased with her appearance. At revisional surgery, her brow was repositioned, her malar implants were removed, a subperiosteal midface lift was performed, the depressions at the chin osteotomy sites were filled with porous polyethylene, and her chin pad was resuspended. (A–C) Preoperative frontal, lateral, and oblique views. (D–F) Postoperative frontal, lateral, and oblique views. (G) Intraoperative view. The implant removed at revisional surgery had been placed in a submalar position.

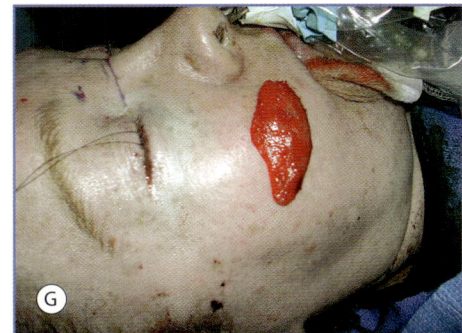

REFERENCES

1. Perrett DI, May KA, Yoshokawa S. Facial shape and judgment of female attractiveness. Nature 1994; 368:239–242.
2. Yaremchuk MJ. Avoidance and treatment of malar implant deformities. Presented at the American Society of Plastic Surgeons Annual Meeting, Chicago, September 2005.
3. Farkas LG, Hreczko TA, Katic MJ. Appendix A. Craniofacial norms in North American Caucasians from birth (one year) to adulthood. In: Farkas LG, ed. Anthropometry of the head and face. 2nd edn. New York: Raven Press; 1994.
4. Hinderer UT. Malar implants for the improvement of facial appearance. Plast Reconstr Surg 1975; 56:157–165.
5. Silver WE. The use of alloplastic material in contouring the face. Facial Plast Surg 1986; 3:81–98.
6. Wilkinson TS. Complications in aesthetic malar augmentation. Plast Reconstr Surg 1987; 80:337–346.
7. Powell NB, Riley RW, Lamb DR. A new approach to evaluation and surgery of the malar complex. Ann Plast Surg 1988; 20:206–214.
8. Prendergast M, Schoenrock LD. Malar augmentation. Arch Otolaryngol Head Neck Surg 1989; 115:964–969.
9. Whitaker LA. Aesthetic augmentation of the malar midface structures. Plast Reconstr Surg 1987; 80:337–346.
10. Terino EO. Alloplastic contouring by zonal principles of skeletal anatomy. Clin Plast Surg 1992; 19(2):487–510.
11. Yaremchuk MJ. Making concave faces convex. Aesthetic Plast Surg 2005; 29(3):141–147.
12. May JW, Zenn MR, Zingarelli P. Subciliary malar augmentation and cheek advancement: a 6-year study on 22 patients undergoing blepharoplasty. Plast Reconstr Surg 1995; 96(7):1553–1559.
13. Binder WJ. Submalar augmentation. An alternative to face-lift surgery. Arch Otolaryngol Head Neck Surg 1989; 115:797–801.

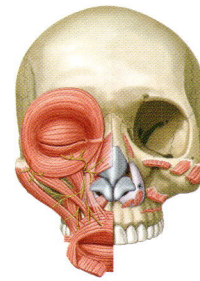

Chapter 8

Piriform aperture

A relative deficiency in lower midface projection may be congenital or acquired, particularly after cleft surgery and maxillary fractures. Patients with satisfactory occlusion and lower midface concavity can have their aesthetic desires satisfied with skeletal augmentation. Implantation of alloplastic material in the paranasal area can simulate the visual effect of LeFort I advancement and other skeletal manipulations.[1] Augmentation of the piriform aperture is often a useful adjunct during the rhinoplasty procedure. Augmenting the skeleton in this area can alter the projection of the nasal base, the nasolabial angle, and the vertical plane of the lip.

The implant design and surgical techniques described here are extensions of others' previous efforts to improve paranasal aesthetics. Severe cases of the nasomaxillary deficiency, seen with Binder syndrome, have been treated with bone and cartilage grafts alone or together with osteotomies.[2–3] Lower midface deficiency has also been treated with cartilage grafts or silicone implants as adjuncts to aesthetic rhinoplasty.[9–11]

PREOPERATIVE EVALUATION

Anthropometric data

Because the majority of white faces are convex, midface concavity is often considered less attractive. Augmentation of the piriform aperture area is usually performed to move the lower midface profile from one of concavity to relative convexity. Figure 8.1 shows the average midface inclination of North American white persons, as determined by Farkas.[12]

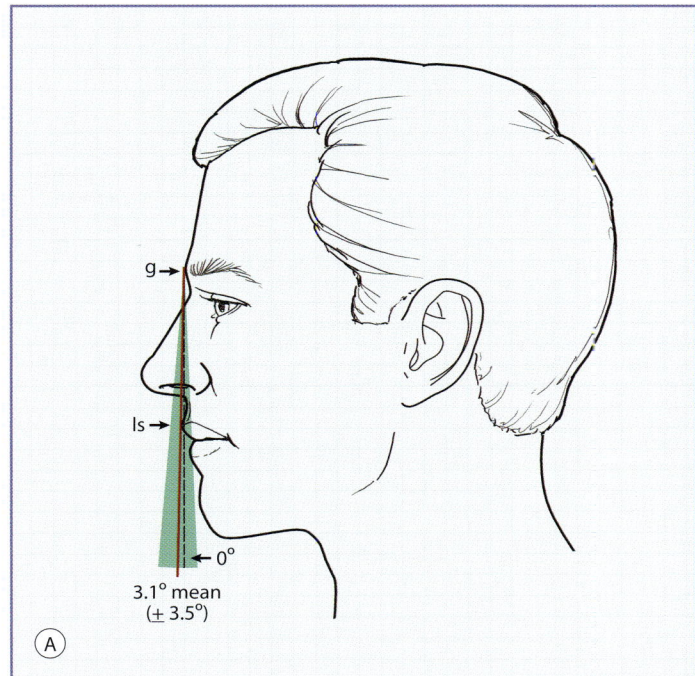

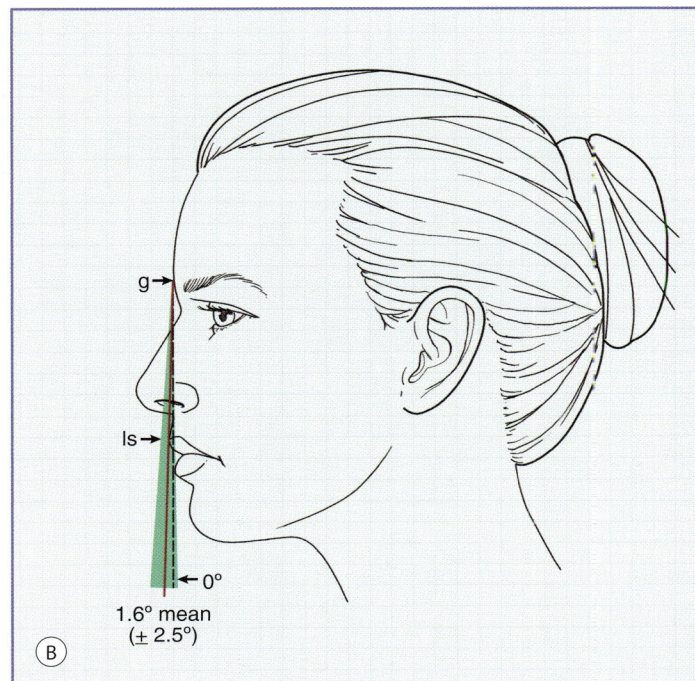

Figure 8.1 The inclination of the midface (glabella, g, to upper lip, ls) in men and women. (**A**) The inclination of the midface (g–ls) in men is 1.3 ± 3.5° (**B**) The inclination of the midface (g–ls) in women is 1.6 ± 2.5°. (After Farkas et al. 1994,[12] with permission.)

When used as an adjunct to rhinoplasty, augmentation latter to the piriform aperture will increase the projection of the nasal base. Augmentation of the maxillary alveolus below the piriform aperture will increase the nasolabial angle and the vertical plane of the lip. Figure 8.2 shows the average nasolabial angle in North American white persons, as determined by Farkas.

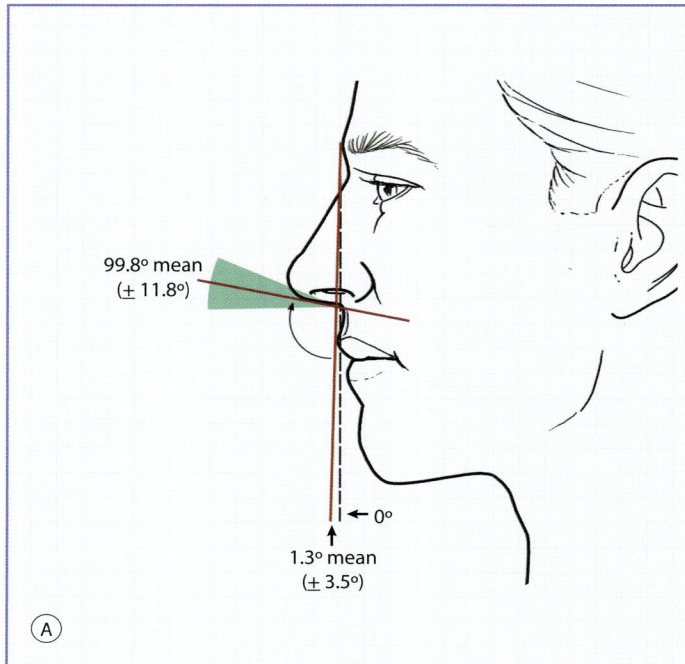

Figure 8.2 The nasolabial angle in men and women. (**A**) The nasolabial angle in men is 99.8 ± 11.8°. (**B**) The nasolabial angle in women is 104.2 ± 9.8°. (After Farkas et al. 1994,[12] with permission.)

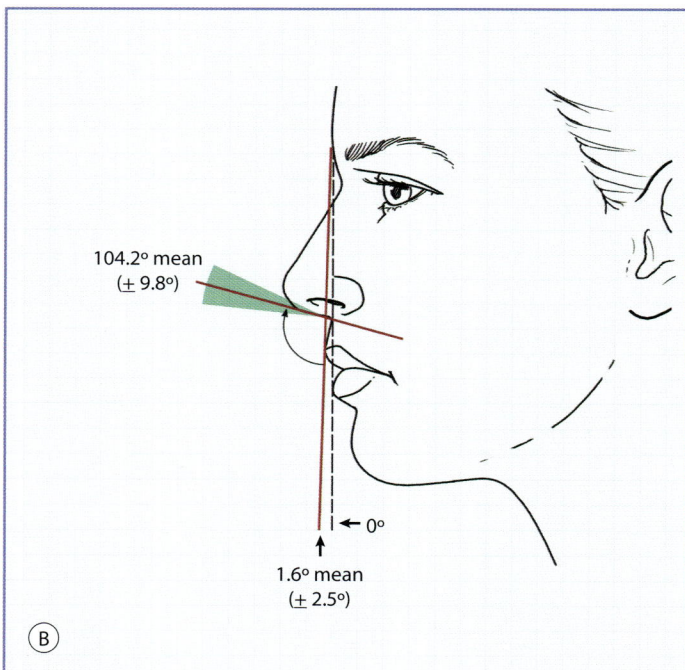

SURGICAL ANATOMY (Fig. 8.3)

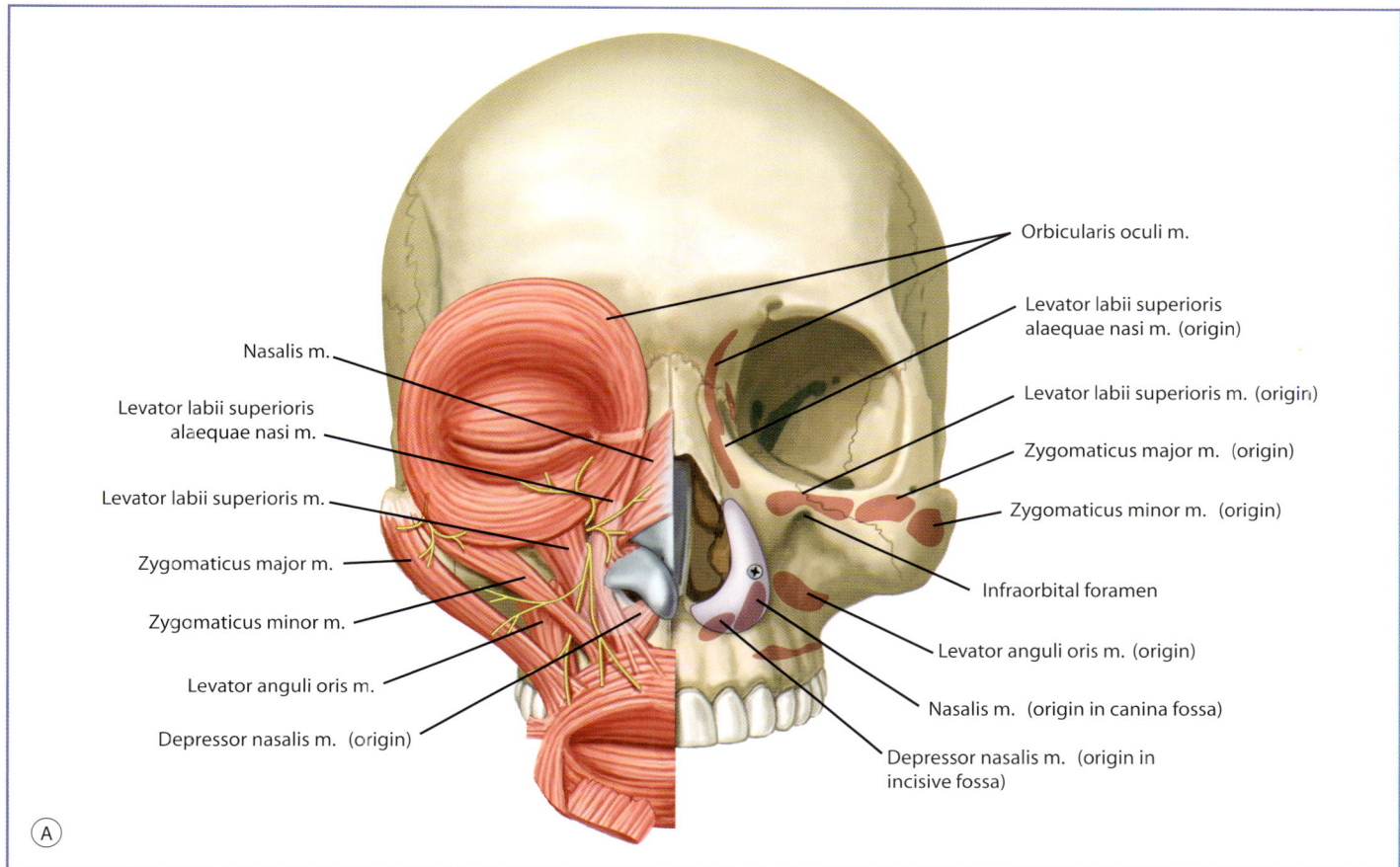

Orbicularis oculi m.

Levator labii superioris alaequae nasi m. (origin)

Levator labii superioris m. (origin)

Zygomaticus major m. (origin)

Zygomaticus minor m. (origin)

Infraorbital foramen

Levator anguli oris m. (origin)

Nasalis m. (origin in canina fossa)

Depressor nasalis m. (origin in incisive fossa)

Nasalis m.

Levator labii superioris alaequae nasi m.

Levator labii superioris m.

Zygomaticus major m.

Zygomaticus minor m.

Levator anguli oris m.

Depressor nasalis m. (origin)

(A)

Figure 8.3 Midface anatomy (see text). (**A**) Frontal views.

The anterior or facial surface of the maxilla is very irregular. Inferiorly, this is due to a series of eminences and corresponding depressions reflecting the apices of the teeth. The incisive fossa is the depression above the prominent incisors. This depression gives rise to the origin of the depressor septi. The canine tooth forms a vertical ridge that separates the incisive fossa from the canine fossa, which is deeper and larger than the incisive fossa. The canine fossa gives rise to the levator anguli oris. The infraorbital foramen is located just above the canine fossa. It allows exit of the infraorbital nerve and vessels. They travel beneath the levator superioris and above the levator anguli oris. The infraorbital nerve supplies the skin of the lower lid, the side of the nose, and most of the cheek and upper lip. Medial to the infraorbital foramen is the nasal notch, which is a concavity whose margin gives rise to the dilator naris as it ends below as the anterior nasal spine.

The deeply located levator anguli oris (caninus), dilator naris, and depressor septi, as well as portions of the maxillary origins of the buccinator, are separated from the maxilla during implant placement. The lip elevators and the infraorbital nerve are retracted to provide exposure. As a result of these manipulations, there is usually temporary dysfunction of these structures postoperatively.

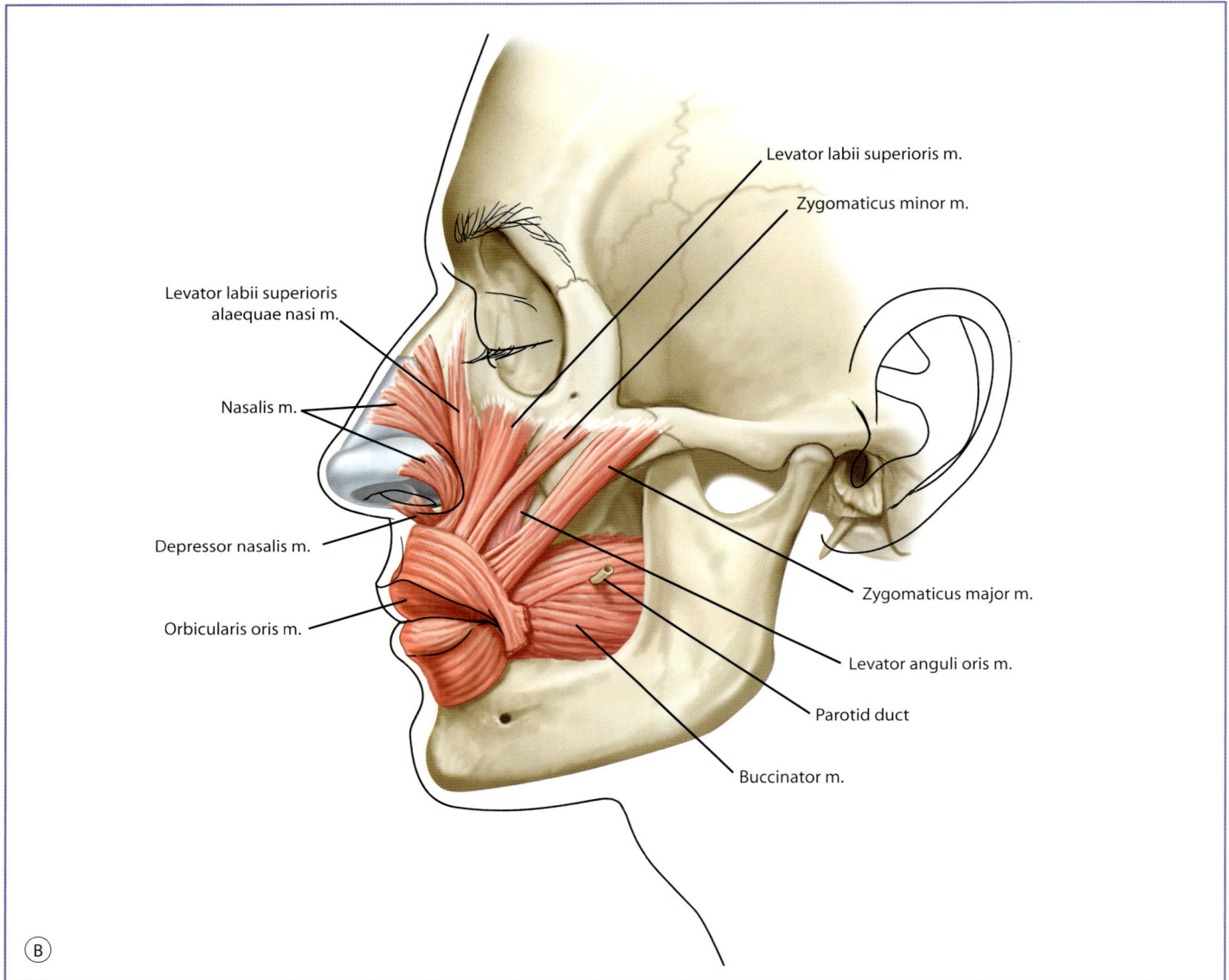

Figure 8.3 (*Cont'd*) Midface anatomy (see text). (**B**) Lateral views.

THE IMPLANT

Piriform aperture (or paranasal) implants are available from Porex Surgical (Fairburn, Georgia). They are designed as right and left crescents and come in two sizes. The smaller implant is 27 mm long by 25 mm high, and provides 4.5 mm of projection. The larger implant, which is 30 mm long by 28 mm high, provides 7 mm of projection. These implants are designed to be tailored to the patient's particular aesthetic needs. The implant is positioned to sit flush on the bone. The patient's anatomy will determine whether the entire crescent or just the horizontal or vertical limb of the crescent will be used (Fig. 8.4).

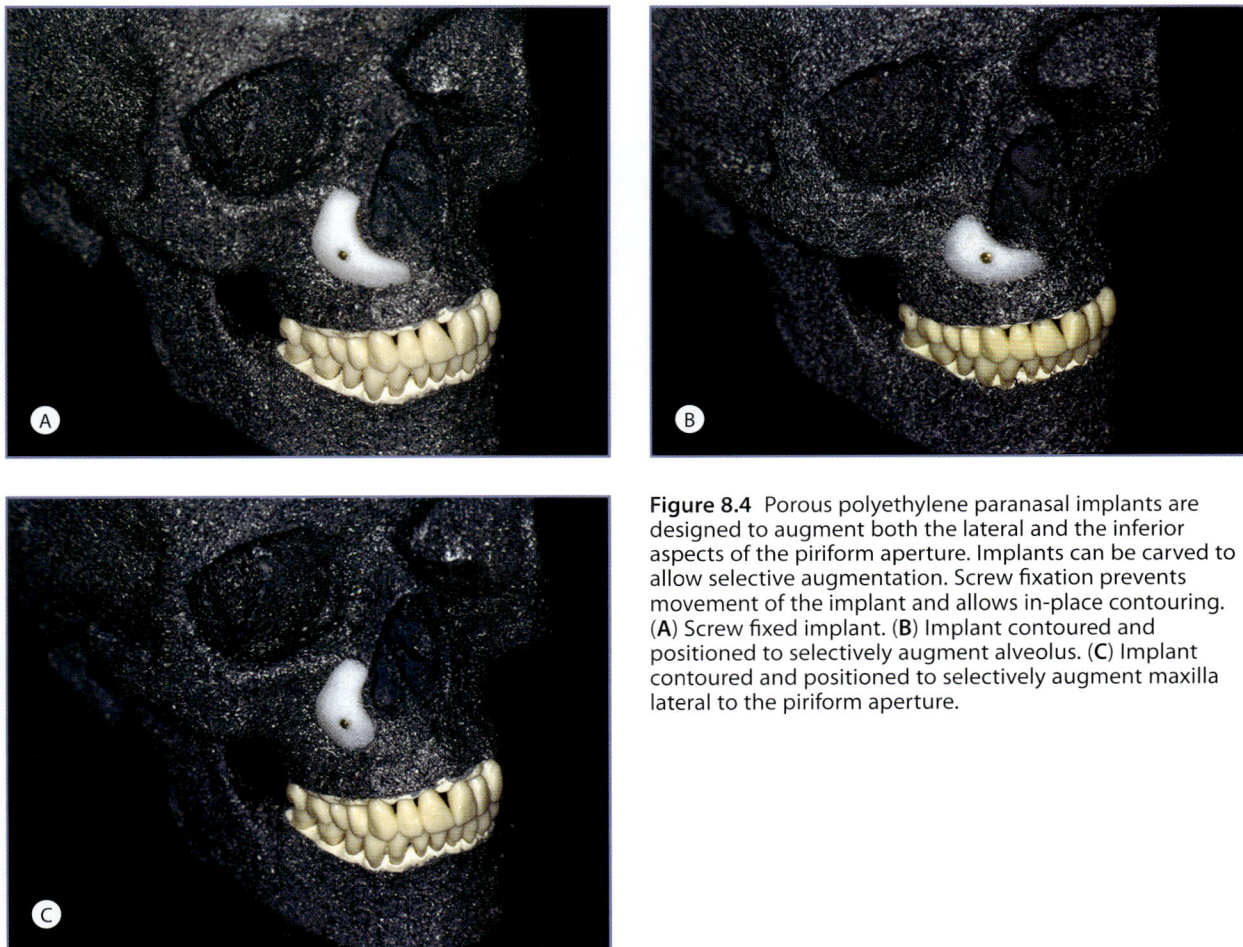

Figure 8.4 Porous polyethylene paranasal implants are designed to augment both the lateral and the inferior aspects of the piriform aperture. Implants can be carved to allow selective augmentation. Screw fixation prevents movement of the implant and allows in-place contouring. (**A**) Screw fixed implant. (**B**) Implant contoured and positioned to selectively augment alveolus. (**C**) Implant contoured and positioned to selectively augment maxilla lateral to the piriform aperture.

OPERATIVE TECHNIQUE (Figs 8.5 and 8.6)

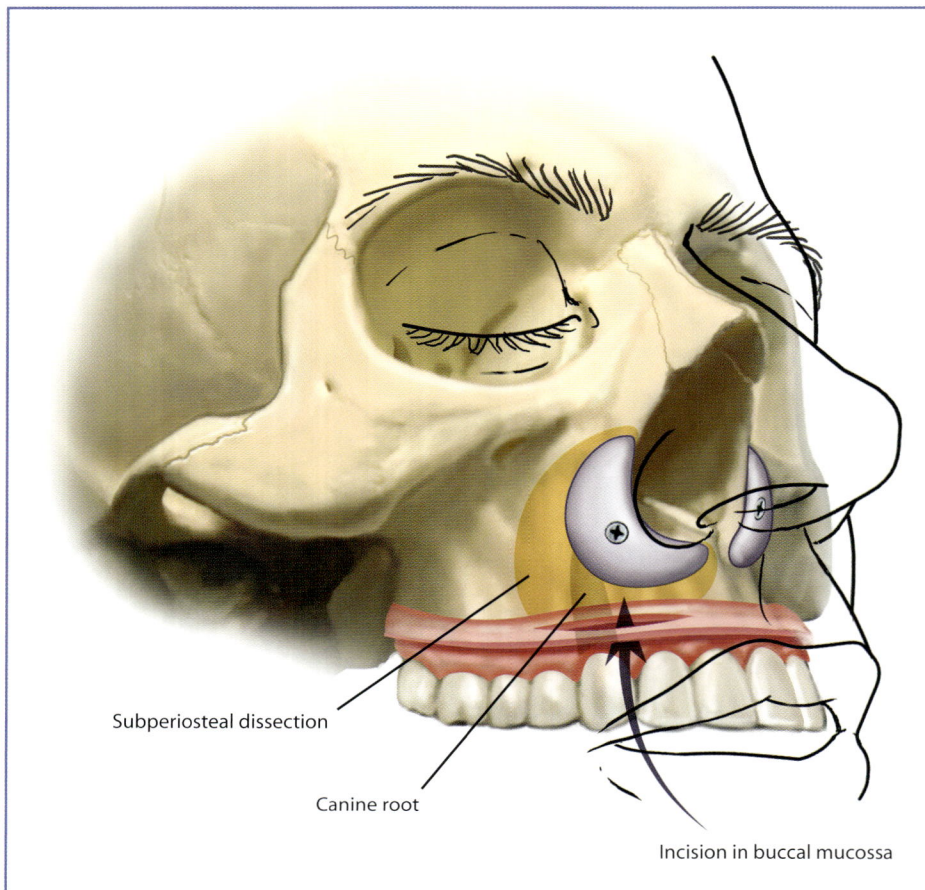

Subperiosteal dissection

Canine root

Incision in buccal mucossa

Figure 8.5 Overview of paranasal implant surgery. The incision is made on the labial side of the buccal sulcus. The gold area indicates the area of subperiosteal dissection. Note the proximity of the infraorbital nerve. Note that the root of the canine tooth lies below the area to be augmented. It must be avoided during screw immobilization of the implant.

Paranasal augmentation can be done under local or general anesthesia. After sterile preoperative preparation and draping, a local anesthetic with 1:200 000 adrenaline (epinephrine) is infiltrated at the surgical site. An upper gingivobuccal sulcus incision is made just lateral to the piriform aperture to avoid placing incisions directly over the implant. The incision is made at least 1 cm above the sulcus to provide an adequate cuff of mucosa inferiorly to allow layered closure. The lip elevators can be seen after the mucosa is incised. These muscles are not divided, but rather retracted during the exposure of the maxilla.

Subperiosteal dissection exposes the area to be augmented. The levator anguli oris (caninus) and maxillary origins of the buccinator are separated from the maxilla during implant placement. The lip elevators and the infraorbital nerve are retracted to provide exposure. The borders of the piriform aperture, the infraorbital nerve, and the root of the canine tooth should be identified during surgery. Defining the bony edges of the piriform aperture provides bony landmarks facilitating precise and symmetric implant placement.

PEARL

Avoid making the incision directly over the area to be augmented.

The implant may compromise the nasal airway if positioned beyond the bony edge of the aperture. Identification of the nerve avoids inadvertent retractor or implant damage to the structure. The root of the canine tooth will be visible as a distinct bulge just lateral to the piriform aperture. The implant will, in part, lie directly over it. The surgeon must avoid damaging these structures if screw fixation is used to immobilize the implant.

The incision is closed in layers. Because of the relatively small area of dissection, no drains are used.

PEARL

The implant may compromise the nasal airway if malpositioned.

PEARL

Avoid the root of the canine tooth during screw fixation of the implant.

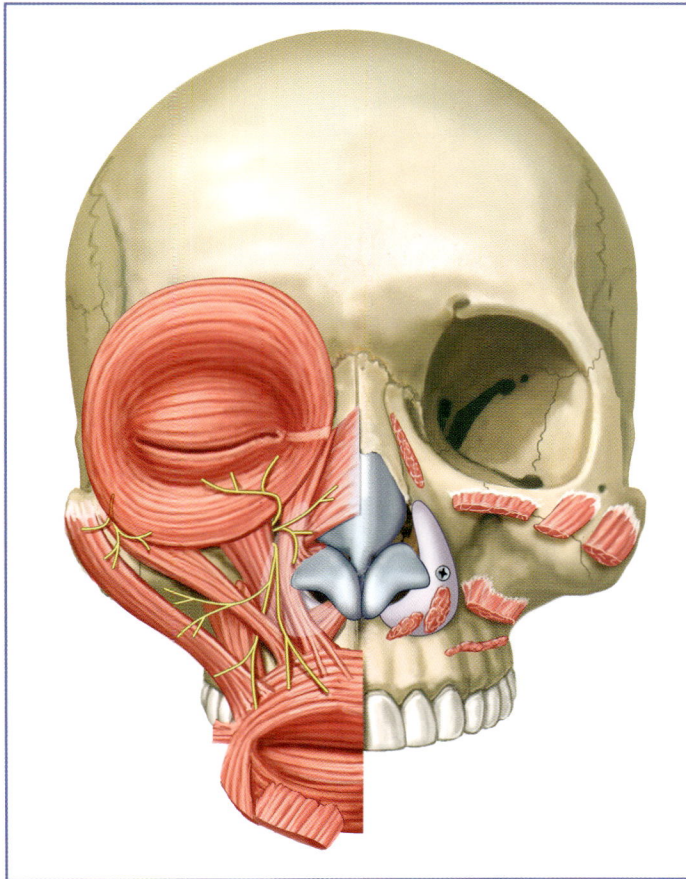

Figure 8.6 Position of implant relative to paranasal musculature and underlying skeleton.

145

CLINICAL EXAMPLES

A deficiency in lower midface projection is common in patients with surgically corrected clefts. Both the alteration of soft tissue skeletal relationships during surgical repair and the growth-retarding forces of scarring are believed to restrict palatal and maxillary growth after cleft repair. As shown diagrammatically in Figure 8.7 and clinically in Figure 8.8, augmentation of the alveolus and lower lateral paranasal area will improve lip and nasal relationships and overall facial balance.

> **PEARL**
>
> Piriform aperture augmentation increases the projection of the nasal base and therefore opens the nasolabial angle.

> **PEARL**
>
> Piriform aperture augmentation increases the convexity of the lower midface.

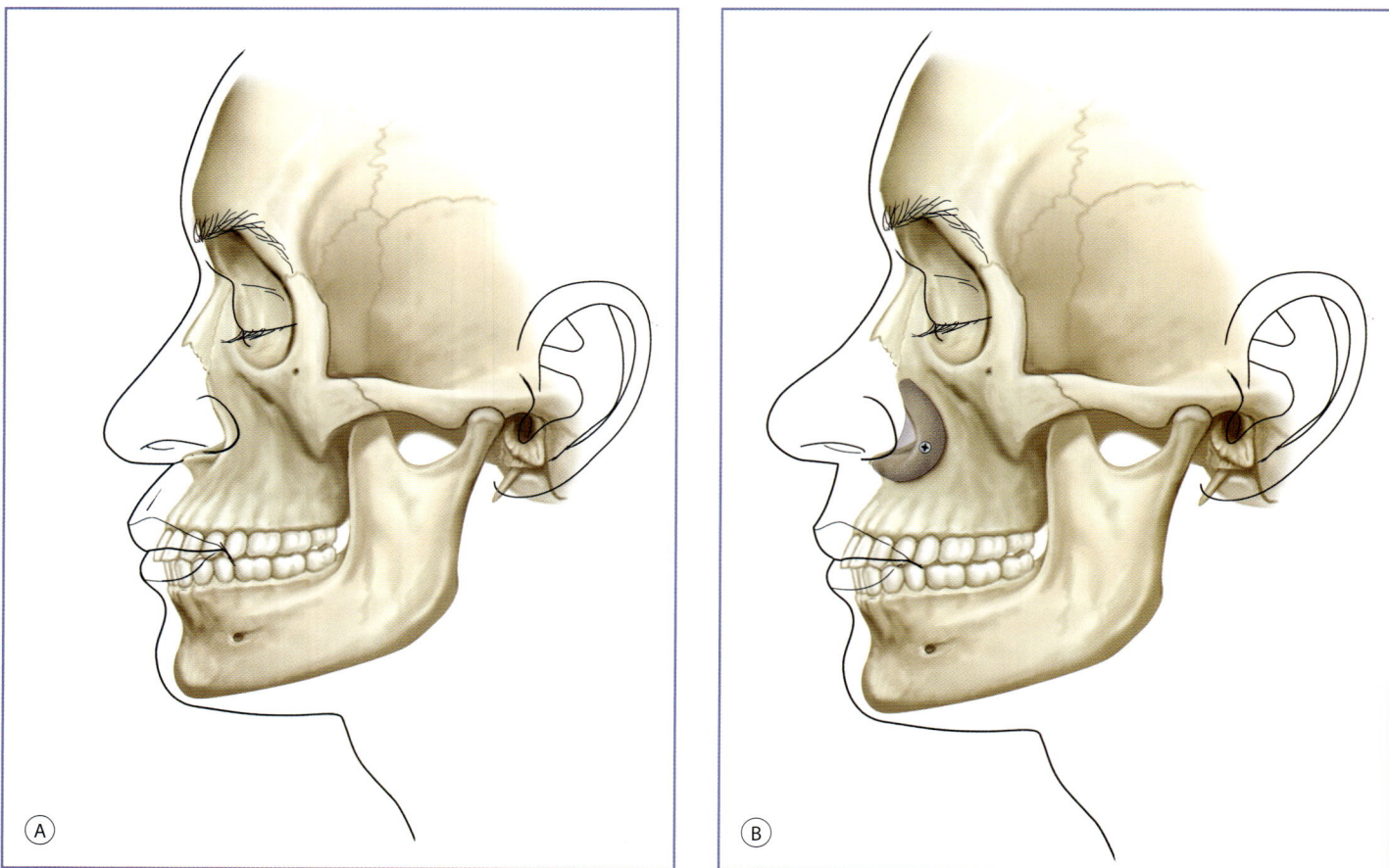

Figure 8.7 The impact of an implant relative to profile and nasolabial angle. (**A**) Profile view of patient with lower midface concavity and acute nasolabial angle. (**B**) Profile view shows that augmentation of the piriform aperture area creates a convex profile and opens the nasolabial angle.

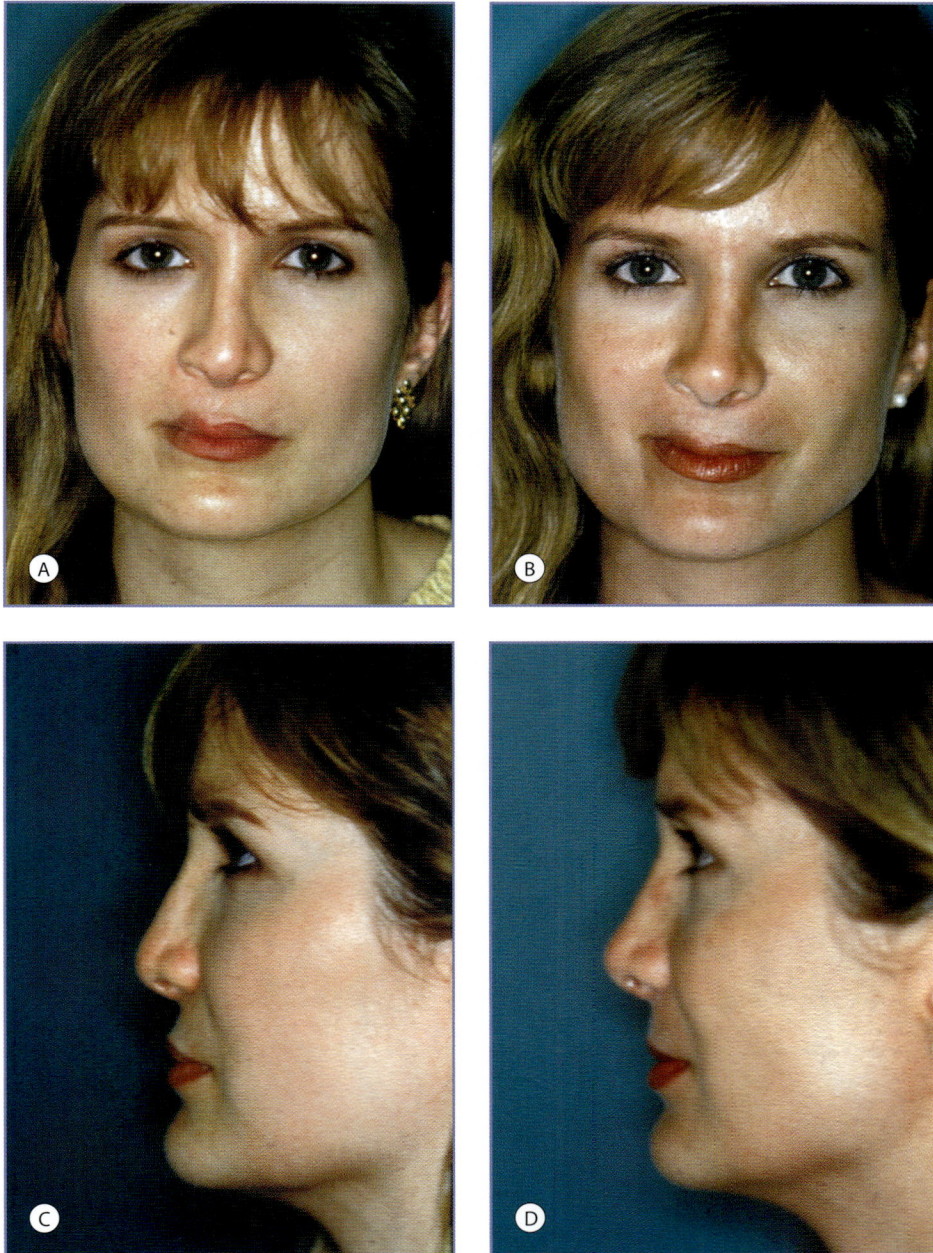

Figure 8.8 A 31-year-old woman, after remote cleft lip repair, cleft palate repair, and two rhinoplasties, underwent rhinoplasty with a tip graft, alar base repositioning, and paranasal augmentation. A larger implant was placed on the cleft side. (**A**) Preoperative and (**B**) postoperative frontal views. (**C**) Preoperative and (**D**) postoperative lateral views.

Patients who have been treated for extensive midface or panfacial fractures may present with relative midface deficiency but normal occlusion. This 'dish face' deformity occurs when preinjury maxillary anatomy is not restored or not maintained. Retrusion of the lower midface may occur when upper and lower jaw fractures are reduced with respect to occlusion only, and not to preinjury three-dimensional skeletal anatomy above the occlusal level. It may also occur after comminuted maxillary fracture reduction and fixation if the surgery is inadequate to resist soft tissue deformity forces accompanying massive edema. As seen in Figure 8.9, paranasal augmentation can help restore the preinjury contour.

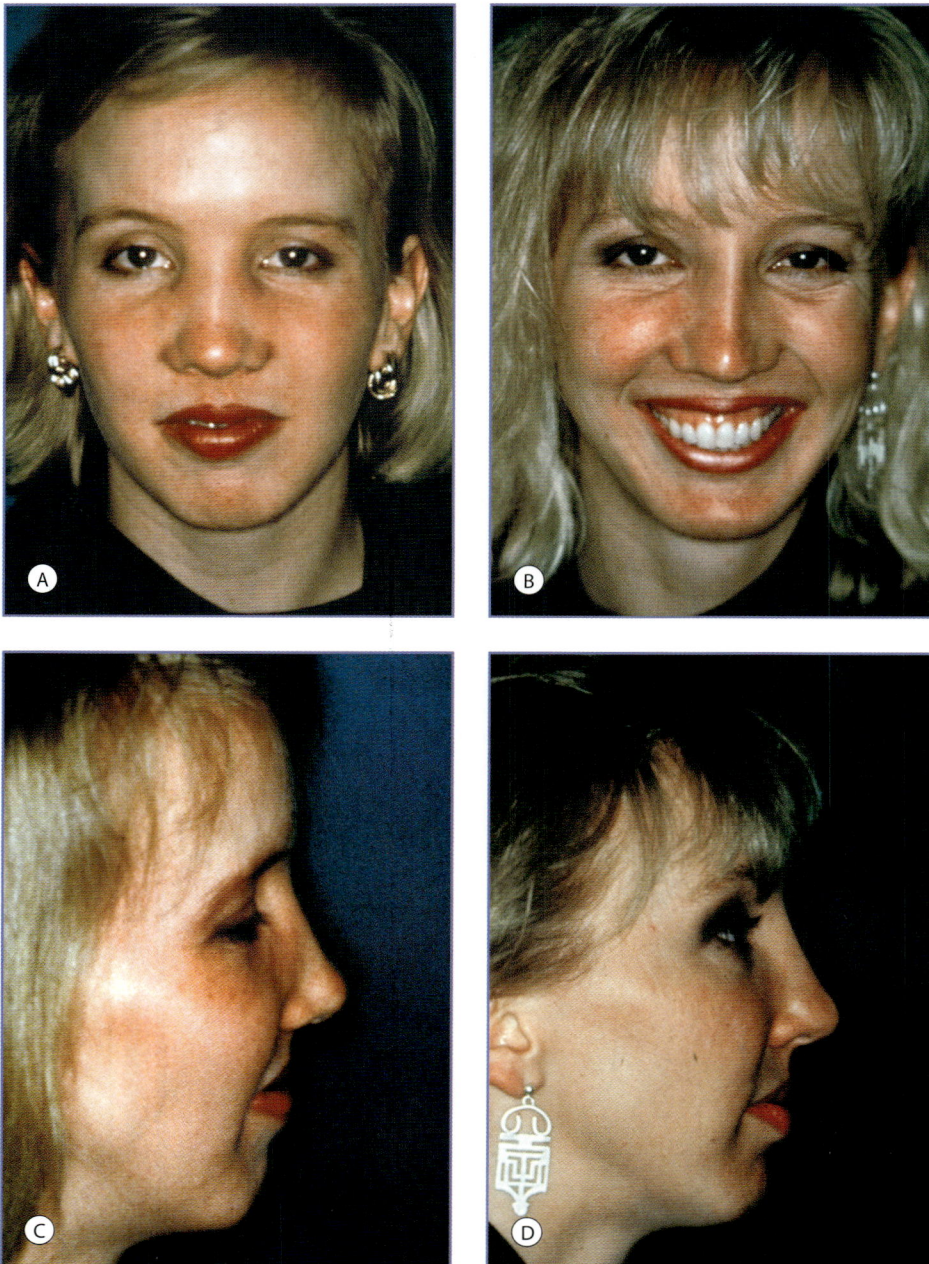

Figure 8.9 A 26-year-old woman presented after secondary repair of panfacial fractures. Central maxillary and nasal medial orbital osteotomies were performed, and a cantilever cranial bone graft was placed to correct the nasoethmoid orbital deformity. The internal orbits were reconstructed. Six months later, paranasal implants were placed and a sliding genioplasty was performed. (**A**) Preoperative and (**B**) postoperative frontal views. (**C**) Preoperative and (**D**) postoperative lateral views.

Another major group of patients is made up of people who were born with relative midface lower deficiency.

These facial skeletal characteristics are noted more commonly in certain ethnic groups, including Asian and black people, in whom relative maxillary hypoplasia can result in concave midface profile. Piriform aperture augmentation often benefits those patients during rhinoplasty where, depending on implant placement, it can increase the projection of the nasal base, efface the acute nasolabial angle, and straighten the vertical plane of the lip (Figures 8.10–8.12). The patient in Figure 8.13 had nasal aesthetics improved with piriform aperture augmentation without rhinoplasty.

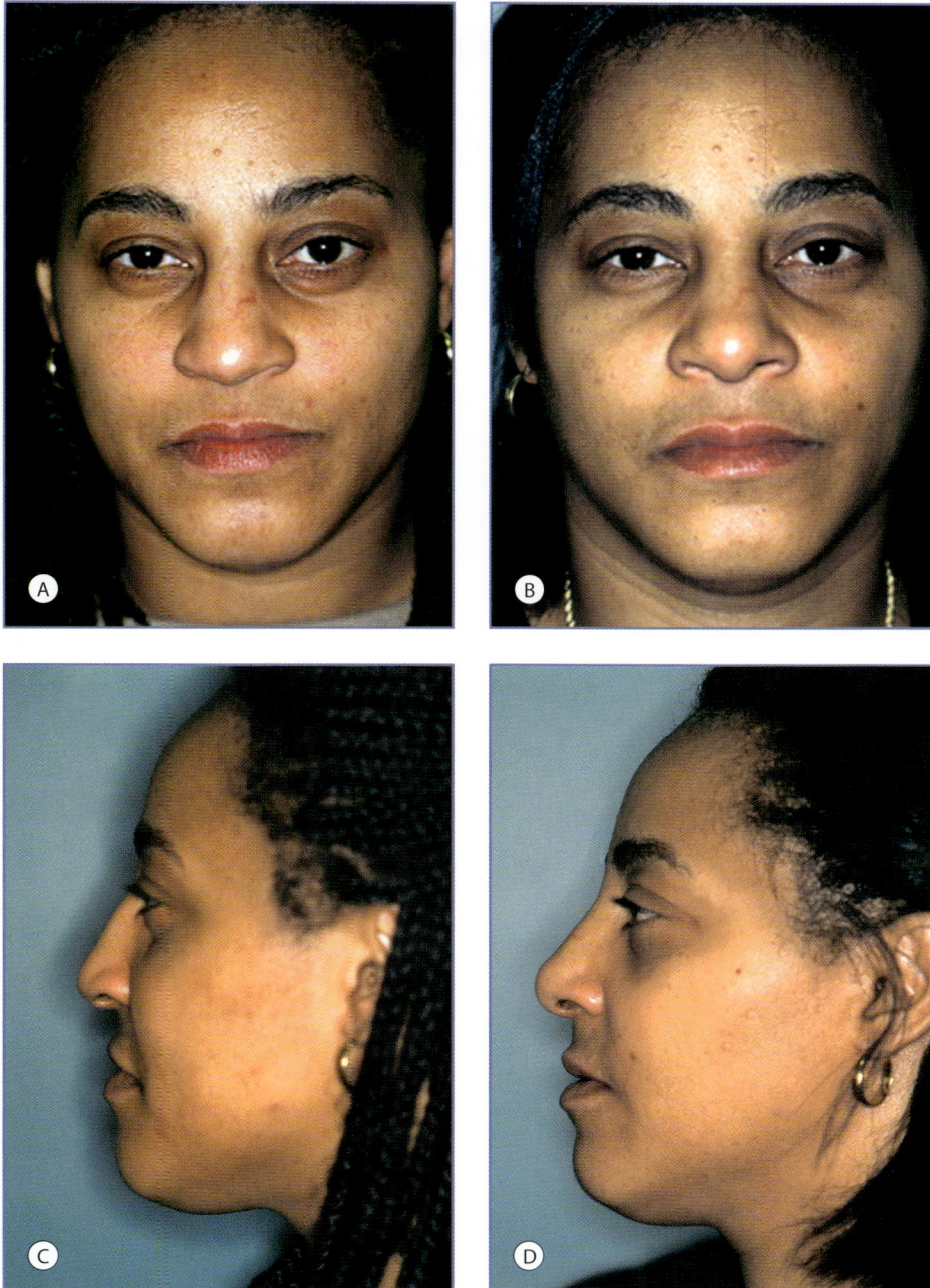

Figure 8.10 A 44-year-old woman presented for rhinoplasty. An open rhinoplasty with tip graft, submucous resection, and paranasal augmentation were performed. (**A**) Preoperative and (**B**) postoperative frontal views. (**C**) Preoperative and (**D**) postoperative lateral views.

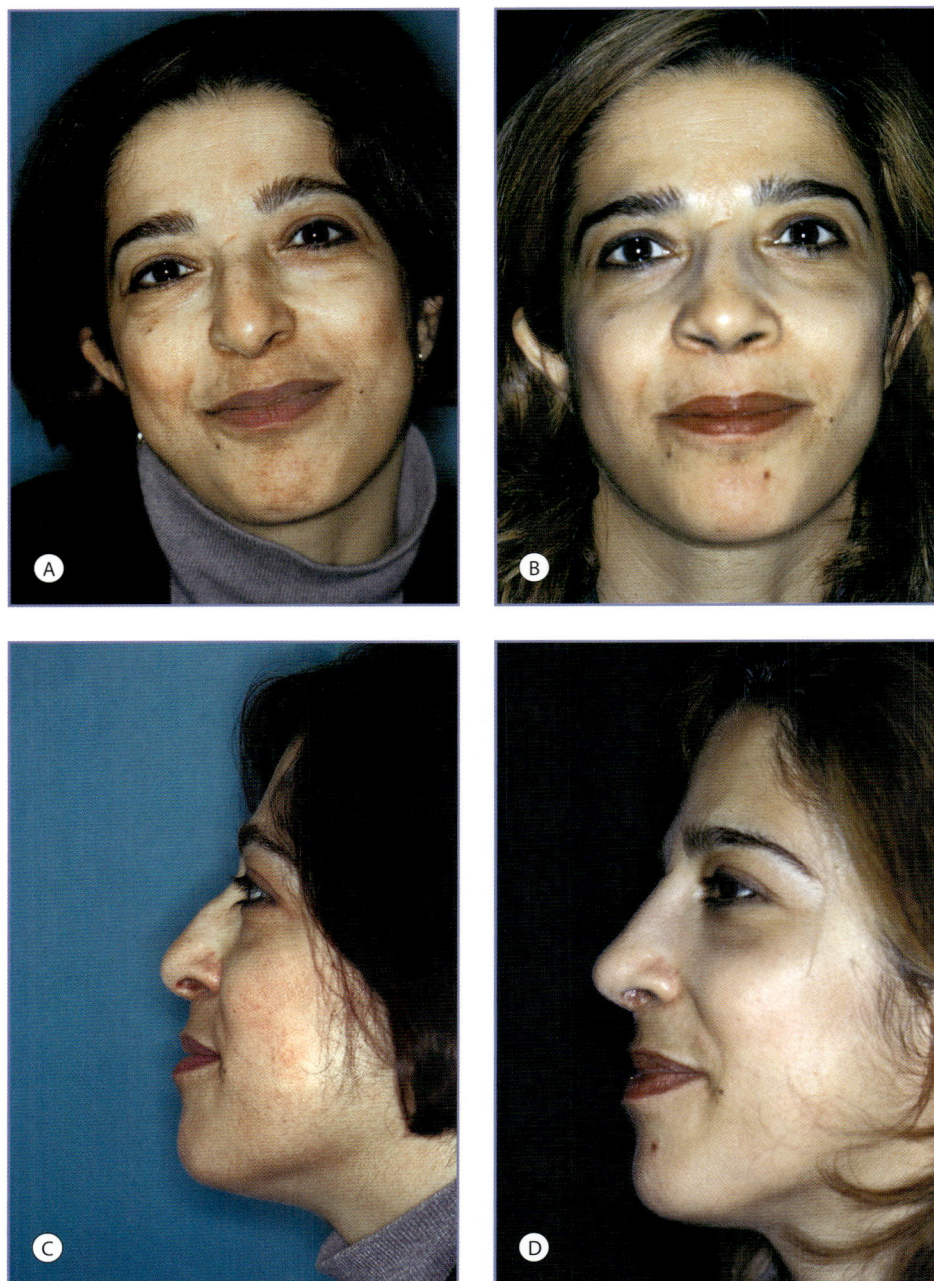

Figure 8.11 A 34-year-old woman presented for rhinoplasty. An open rhinoplasty with tip graft, submucous resection, and paranasal augmentation was performed. (**A**) Preoperative and (**B**) postoperative frontal views. (**C**) Preoperative and (**D**) postoperative lateral views.

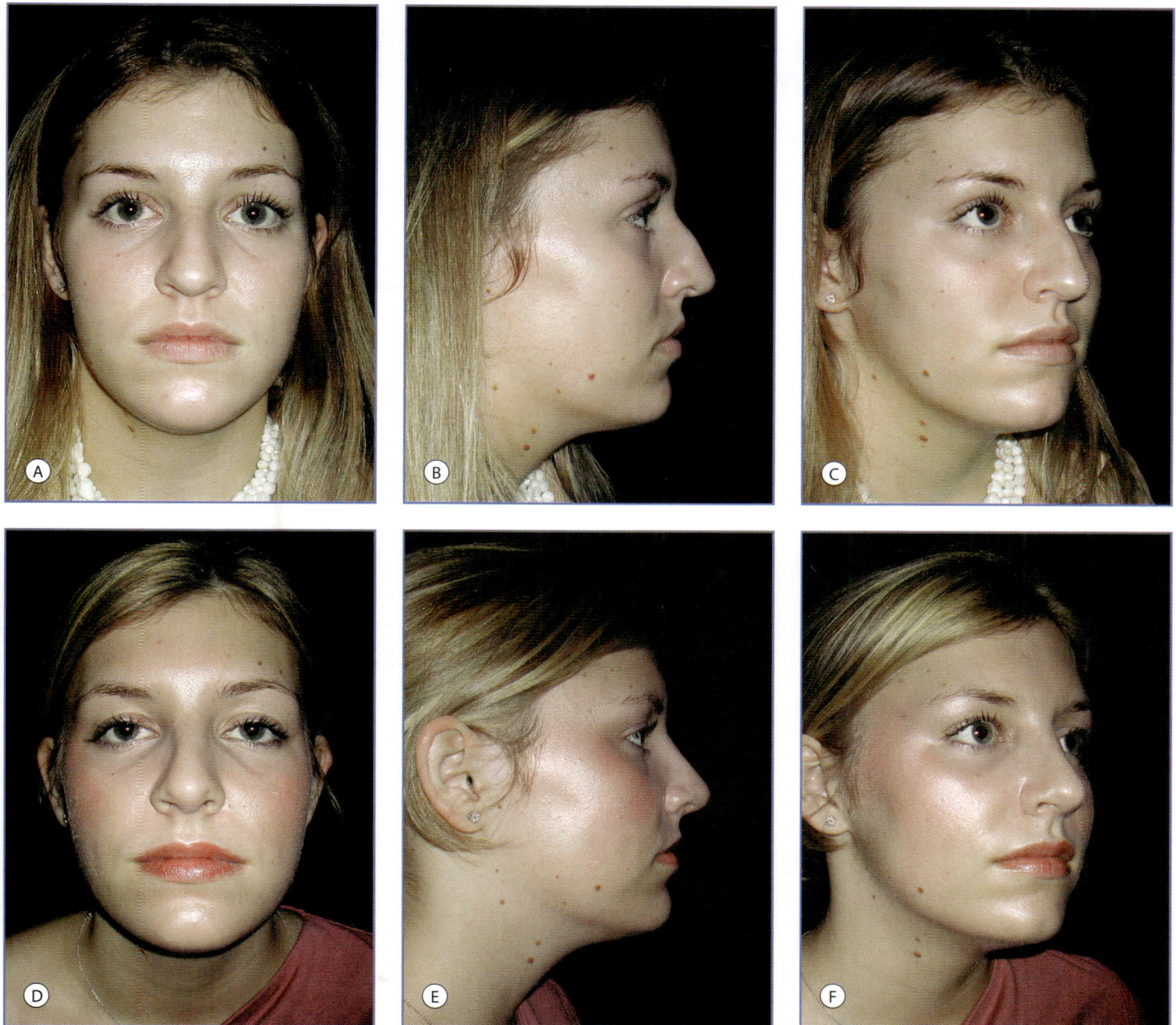

Figure 8.12 This 20-year-old woman underwent rhinoplasty and paranasal augmentation. (**A–C**) Preoperative frontal, lateral, and oblique views. (**D–F**) Postoperative frontal, lateral, and oblique views.

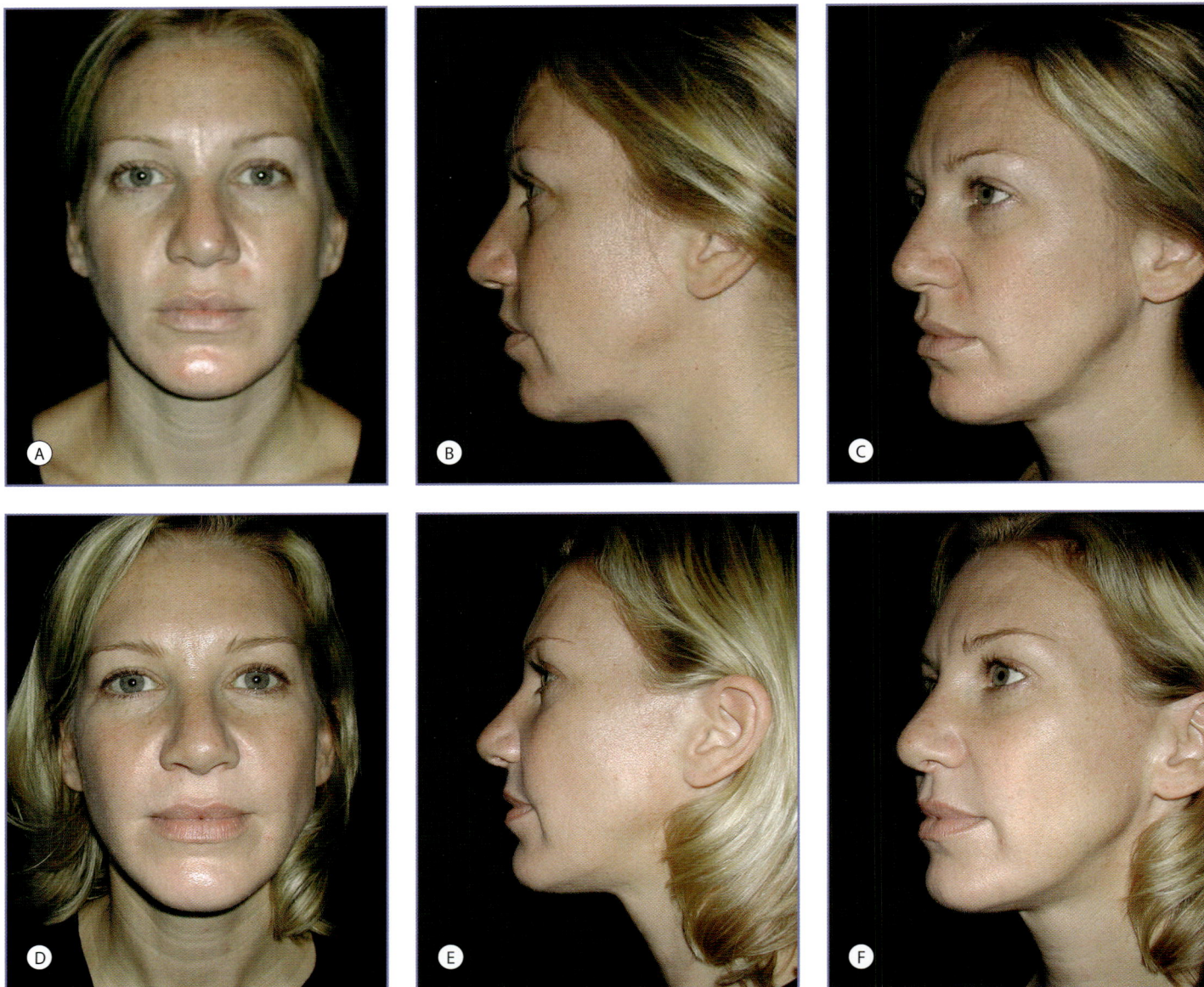

Figure 8.13 A 30-year-old woman underwent paranasal augmentation. A subperiosteal midface lift was also performed. (**A–C**) Preoperative frontal, lateral, and oblique views. (**D–F**) Postoperative frontal, lateral, and oblique views.

REFERENCES

1. Yaremchuk MJ, Israeli D. Paranasal implants for correction of midface concavity. Plast Reconstr Surg 1998; 102(5):1676–1684.
2. Converse JM. Techniques of bone grafting for contour restoration of the face. Plast Reconstr Surg 1954; 14(5):332–346.
3. Converse JM, Horowitz SL, Valauri AJ, et al. Treatment of nasomaxillary hypoplasia. Plast Reconstr Surg 1970; 45:427.
4. Jackson IT, Moos KF, Sharpe DT. Total surgical management of Binder's syndrome. Ann Plast Surg 1981; 7(1):25–34.
5. Obwegeser HL. Surgical correction of small or retrodisplaced maxillae. Plast Reconstr Surg 1969; 43(4):351–365.
6. Ortiz-Monasterio F, Molina F, McClintock JS. Nasal correction in Binder's syndrome: the evolution of a treatment plan. Aesthetic Plast Surg 1997; 21(5):299–308.
7. Psillakis JM, Lapa F, Spina V. Surgical correction of mid-facial retrusion (nasomaxillary hypoplasia) in the presence of normal dental occlusion. Plast Reconstr Surg 1973; 51(1):67–70.
8. Ragnell A. A simple method of reconstruction in some cases of dish-face deformity. Plast Reconstr Surg 1952; 10(4):227–237.
9. Caronni E. A new method to correct the nasolabial angle in rhinoplasty. Plast Reconstr Surg 1972; 50(4):338–340.
10. Guerrerosantos J. Nose and paranasal augmentation: autogenous fascia and cartilage. Clin Plast Surg 1991; 18(1):65–86.
11. Hinderer UT. Nasal base, maxillary, and infraorbital implants—alloplastic. Clin Plast Surg 1991; 18(1):87–105.
12. Farkas LG, Hreczko TA, Katic MJ. Appendix A. Craniofacial norms in North American Caucasians from birth (one year) to adulthood. In: Farkas LG, ed. Anthropometry of the head and face. 2nd edn. New York: Raven Press; 1994.

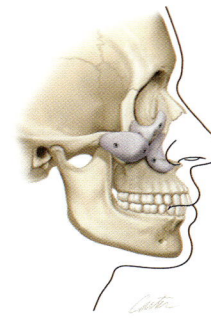

Chapter 9

Multiple midface implants

On average, most young adult white men and women have convex faces (Fig. 9.1).[1] Perhaps because they are not as common, concave faces are often considered not as attractive as convex ones.[2-4] Furthermore, the lesser midface skeletal projection intrinsic to concave faces poorly supports the midface soft tissues, resulting in premature lower lid and cheek descent, as well as visible bags.[5-7] These faces are also 'morphologically prone' to further lower lid descent after blepharoplasty.[7-10] Finally, a concave midface also makes the eyes and nose appear more prominent.

Severe midface concavity is often seen with the craniofacial dysostoses of Apert and Crouzon. It may not only result in occlusal disharmony, but also compromise globe protection and airway adequacy. Patients with this morphology require skeletal osteotomies, usually at the LeFort III and sometimes at the LeFort I level to remedy ocular, respiratory, and occlusal dysfunction as well as to improve facial aesthetics.

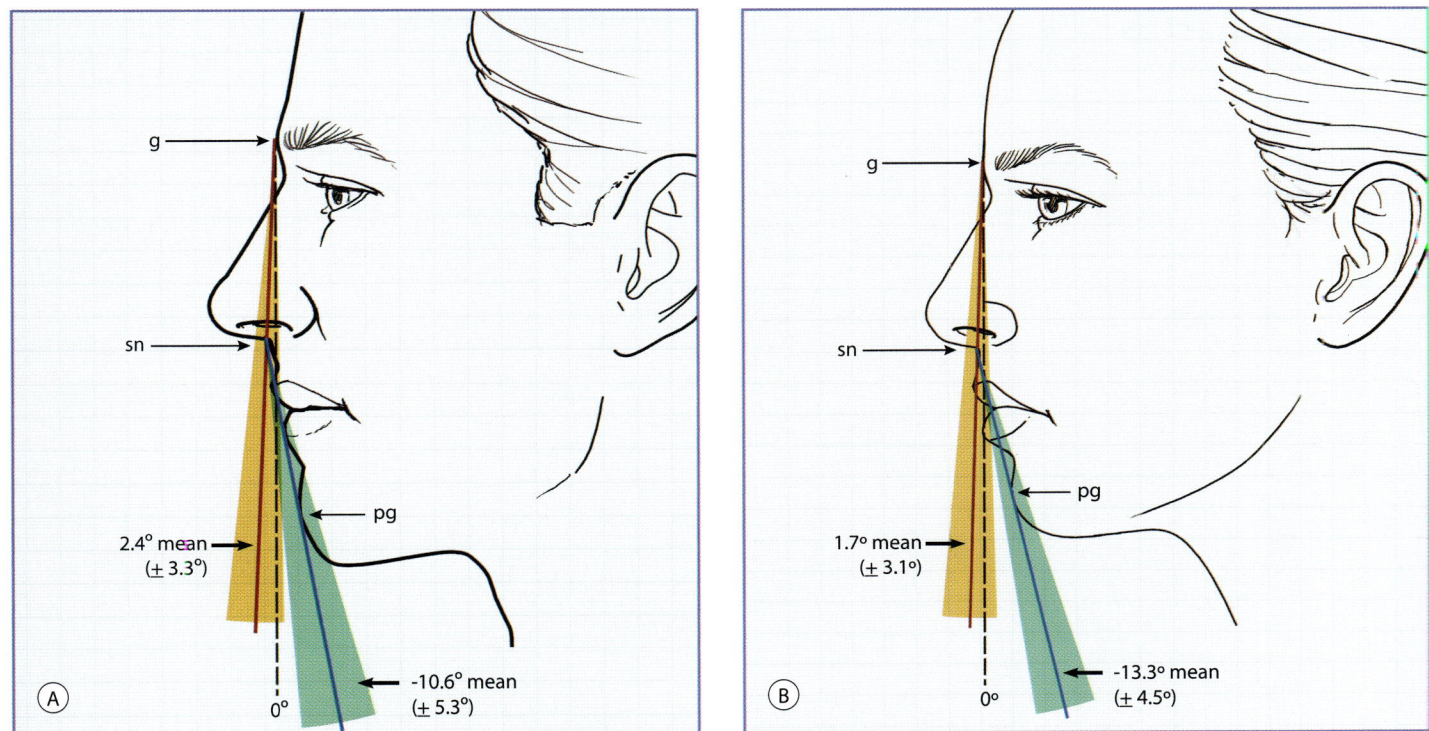

Figure 9.1 Average inclinations of the upper face profile (glabella, g, to subnasale, sn) and lower face profile (subnasale, sn, to pogonion, pg) in young adult North American white men and women. (**A**) The mean inclination of the upper face profile for men (n = 109) was 2.4 ± 3.3°. The mean inclination of the lower face profile for men (n = 109) was −10.6 ± 5.3°. (**B**) In women, these figures were 1.7 ± 3.1° (n = 200) and −13.3 ± 4.5° (n = 200), respectively. (After Farkas et al. 1994,[1] with permission.)

Less severe midface hypoplasia is a common facial skeletal variant.[10] In patients with this morphology; occlusion is normal or has been compensated by orthodontics. They have neither respiratory nor ocular compromise. In skeletally deficient patients whose occlusion is normal or has been previously normalized by orthodontics, skeletal repositioning would necessitate additional orthodontic tooth movement. Such a treatment plan is time-consuming, costly, and potentially morbid. It is therefore appealing to few patients. It is in this population that midface skeletal augmentation with multiple implants can simulate the visual effects of skeletal osteotomy and advancement (Fig. 9.2).

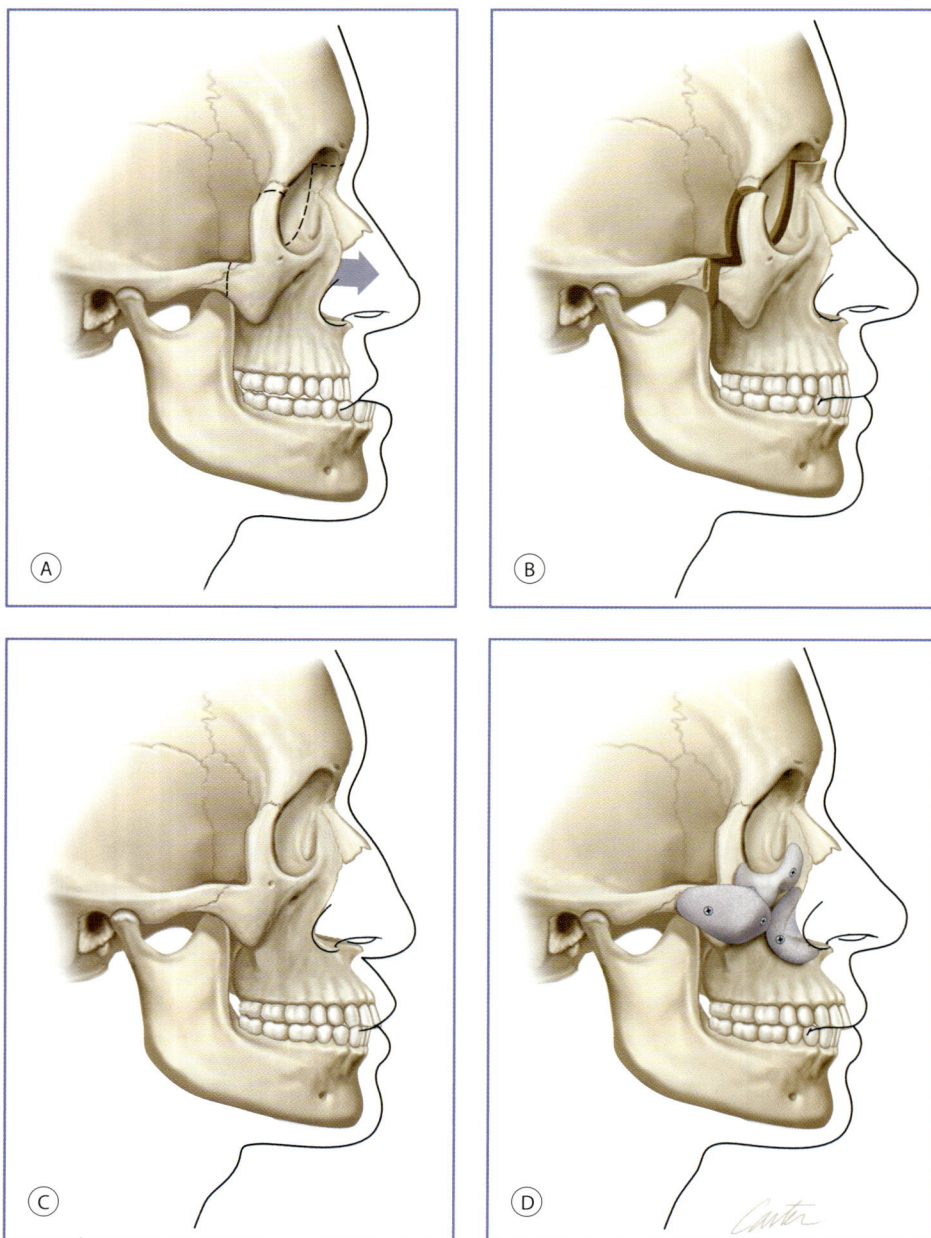

Figure 9.2 Multiple implant augmentation of the midface skeleton can simulate the appearance of LeFort III osteotomy and advancement without altering dental occlusion. (**A**) Midface concavity and class III malocclusion. (**B**) Osteotomy and advancement at the LeFort III level provide midface projection and class I occlusion. (**C**) Midface concavity and class I occlusion. (**D**) Multiple midface implants provide the visual effect of LeFort III osteotomy and advancement but do not alter occlusion.

The implants used to effect these changes include ones that augment the infraorbital rim,[6] the piriform aperture,[11] and the malar area.[12] These implants are all modified so as to meet the specific needs of the patient. Multiple implants are used so that the infraorbital nerve is not compromised and so that the complex curvature of the midface skeleton can be mimicked.

Free fat grafting can be an effective means of augmenting midface contour.[13–15] This technique is intuitive for the restoration of soft tissue volume loss due to senile atrophy. In my experience, fat injection has a limited role in simulating the effect of an increase in skeletal projection. Whereas augmenting the facial skeleton results in an increase in the projection of the soft tissue envelope, augmenting the soft tissue volume results in an inflation of the soft tissue envelope. Overaugmentation of either component brings home the point. If overly large implants were placed on the skeleton, the appearance would be too defined and ultimately skeletal. If too much fat were placed in the soft tissue envelope, an increasingly spherical and otherwise undefined shape would result (see Figs 1.11 and 1.12).

Repositioning midface soft tissues has several benefits. It restores cheek fullness and recreates a cheek–lid interface with a relatively shortened lower lid, while narrow-ing the palpebral fissure shape by raising the lower lid margin.[6,16]

This chapter presents the rationale and surgical technique for transforming a concave face into a convex one. It requires the use of multiple implants, together with a subperiosteal midface soft tissue resuspension.

SURGICAL ANATOMY

The anatomy of the midface skeleton and overlying soft tissues has been presented in Chapters 6–8.

THE IMPLANTS

Three implants are usually required to increase the projection of the midface skeleton. The use of multiple implants allows more precise mimicry of each skeleton's unique and complex contours. The implants are placed around the infraorbital nerve, which would inevitably be impinged on by a single implant.

The most important implant is one specifically designed to augment the projection of the infraorbital rim.[6] This implant can provide up to 5 mm of anterior projection. It is trimmed to meet the specific needs of the patient. A small flange allows it to rest on the most anterior aspect of the orbital floor. This flange allows easier positioning of the implant and a possible area for screw fixation to the skeleton. A paranasal implant has been designed to augment the piriform aperture.[11] Usually, implants are carved from a malar design to augment the area below the lateral aspect of the rim implant and the area lateral to the paranasal implant. All implants are immobilized with titanium screws. The implants are trimmed so that there are imperceptible transitions between the implants and the native skeleton.

OPERATIVE TECHNIQUE

Overview

A diagrammatic overview of the operation is presented in Figure 9.3. Access to the midface skeleton is obtained through lower lid and intraoral incisions. The entire midface is freed in the subperiosteal plane. The midface skeleton is augmented with a combination of porous polyethylene implants immobilized with screws. The midface soft tissue envelope is elevated and fixed with sutures tied to the infraorbital rim, the infraorbital rim implant, and/or the lateral orbital rim.

Anesthesia

A general anesthetic administered through nasotracheal intubation is preferred. The nasotracheal intubation protects the airway during the surgery and allows optimal intraoral preparation and surgical access.

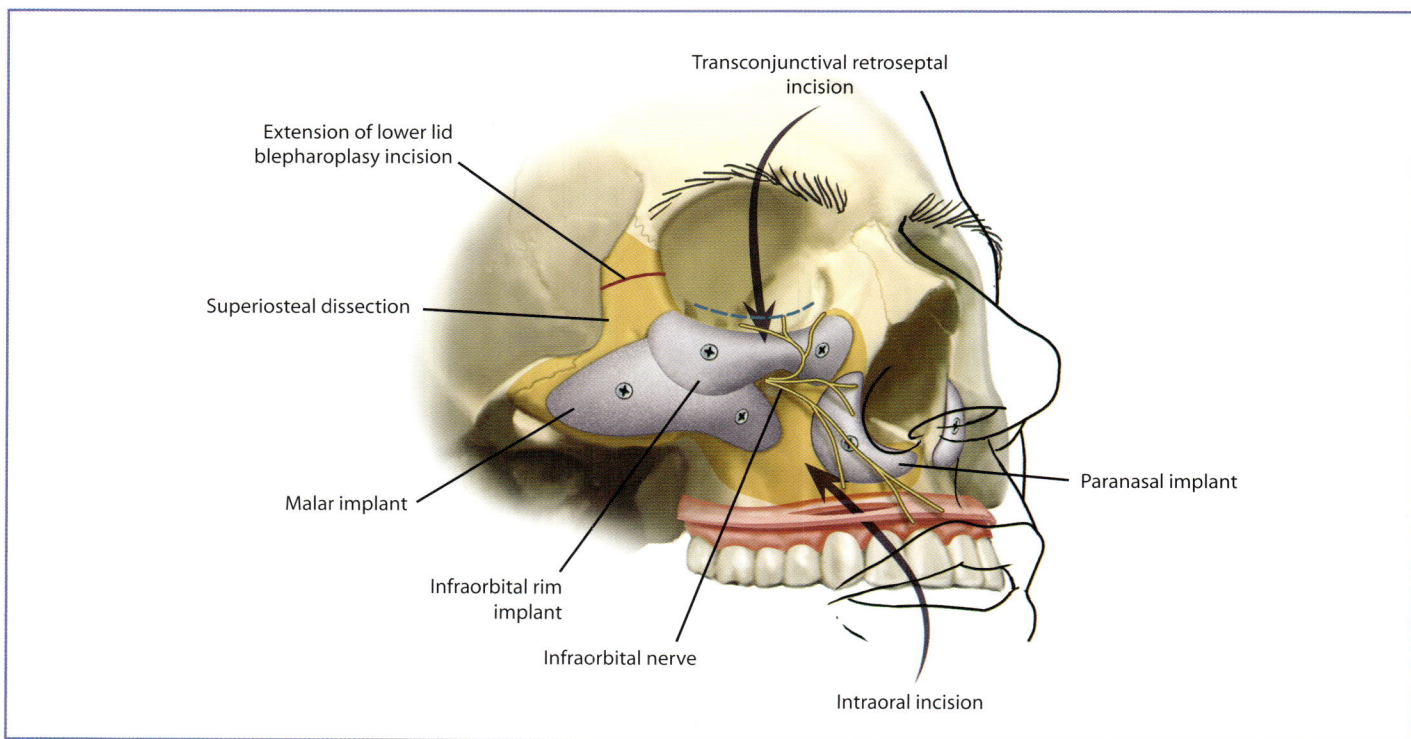

Transconjunctival retroseptal
incision

Extension of lower lid
blepharoplasy incision

Superiosteal dissection

Malar implant

Infraorbital rim
implant

Infraorbital nerve

Intraoral incision

Paranasal implant

Figure 9.3 The surgical procedure. Arrows indicate major access to midface skeleton through transconjunctival and intraoral sulcus incisions. The lateral extent of a lower lid blepharoplasty incision facilitates implant and soft tissue fixation in this area. Infraorbital rim, paranasal, and malar implants are applied to the midface skeleton. They are immobilized with titanium screws. Implants are custom contoured to the patient's specific needs and to provide imperceptible implant–native skeleton and implant–implant transitions. The midface soft tissue envelope, freed by subperiosteal dissection, is elevated and secured by sutures to the infraorbital rim or rim implant and to drill holes made in the lateral orbital rim, similar to that shown in Figure 6.11.

Incisions

To accurately position the infraorbital rim implant, a combination of periorbital and intraoral incisions is used. So as not to distort palpebral fissure shape, it is my preference to avoid, if possible, violating the lateral canthus and to avoid delaminating and relaminating the lower lid. For that reason, a trans-conjunctival retroseptal incision alone, or in combination with the lateral extent of the lower lid blepharoplasty incision, is preferred to access the upper midface skeleton. The entire midface skeleton, including the zygomatic arch, is separated from its overlying soft tissues by subperiosteal dissection.

Soft tissue elevation

Through the intraoral incision, a figure-of-eight suture purchases the cheek soft tissues approximately 3 cm beneath the pupil, while a second suture purchases the soft tissues approximately 3 cm beneath the lateral canthus. The sutures are used to elevate the midface soft tissues. They are tied to the infraorbital rim implant or are fastened to a drill hole in the lateral orbital rim.[7]

A suction drain is placed between the implants and the overlying soft tissues. It usually exits from the temporal scalp. The transconjunctival incision is approximated but not sutured. The intraoral incision is closed with absorbable sutures. A temporary tarsorrhaphy suture is often placed to minimize chemosis. The patient is administered intravenous antibiotics intraoperatively and oral antibiotics for 5 days postoperatively.

CLINICAL EXAMPLES

Patients who have had this surgery are shown in Figures 9.4–9.8.

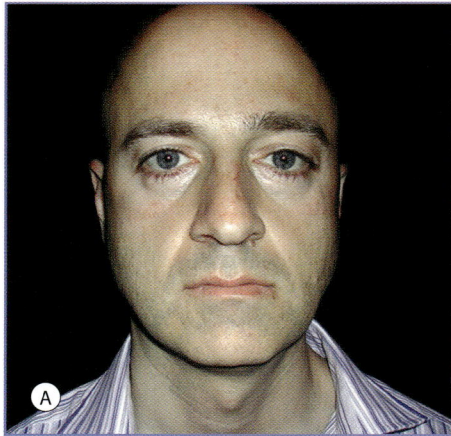

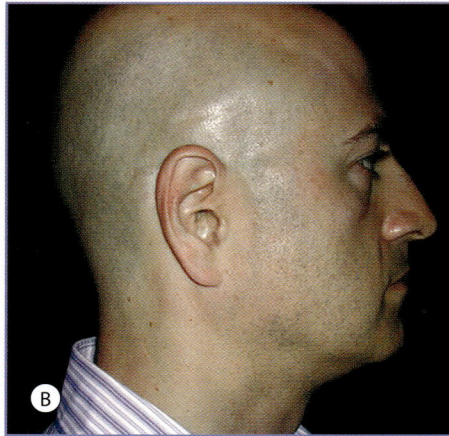

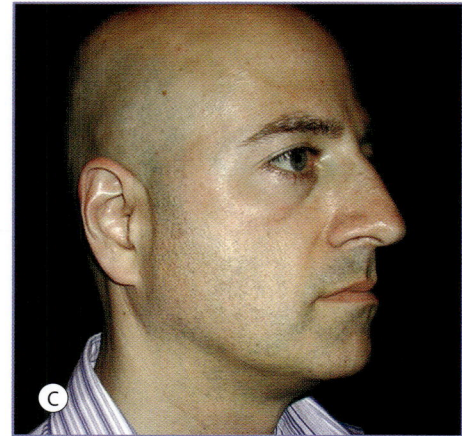

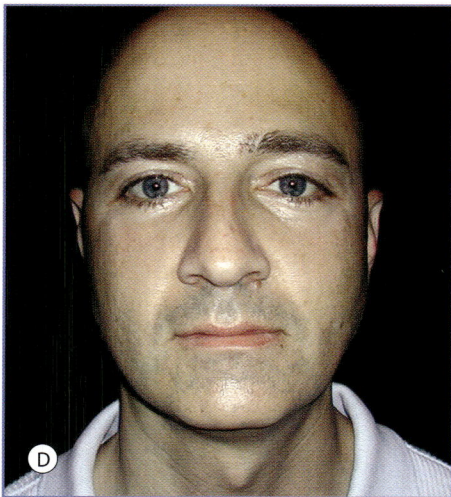

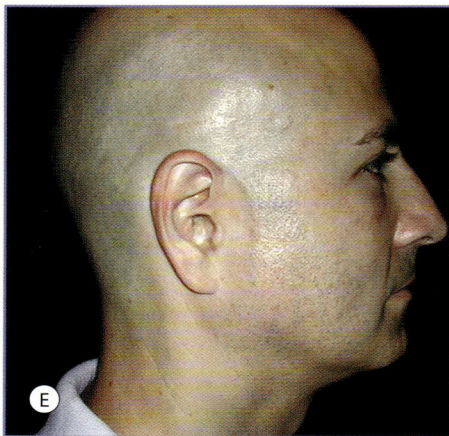

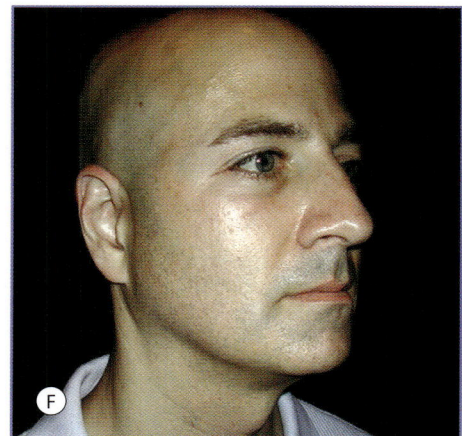

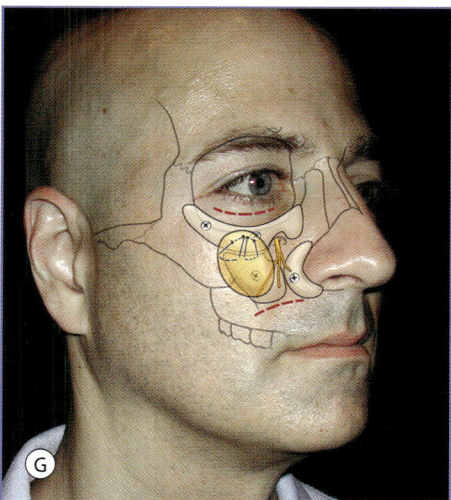

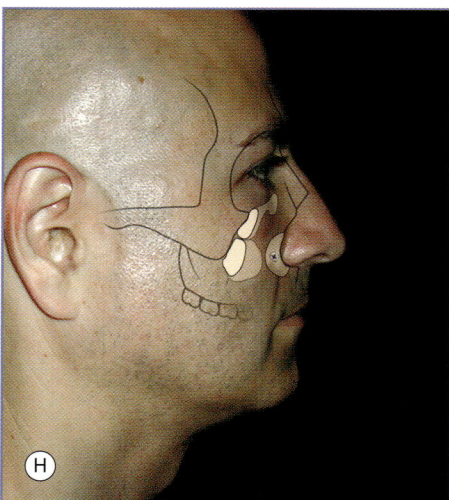

Figure 9.4 A 42-year-old man had multiple implant midface augmentation and subperiosteal midface elevation. (**A–C**) Preoperative frontal, lateral, and oblique views. (**D–F**) Postoperative frontal, lateral, and oblique views. (**G**) Artist's depiction of procedure: an oblique view shows position of implants and midface elevation. (**H**) Lateral view shows how implants increase midface projection. (Figures A–G from Yaremchuk 2005,[18] with permission.)

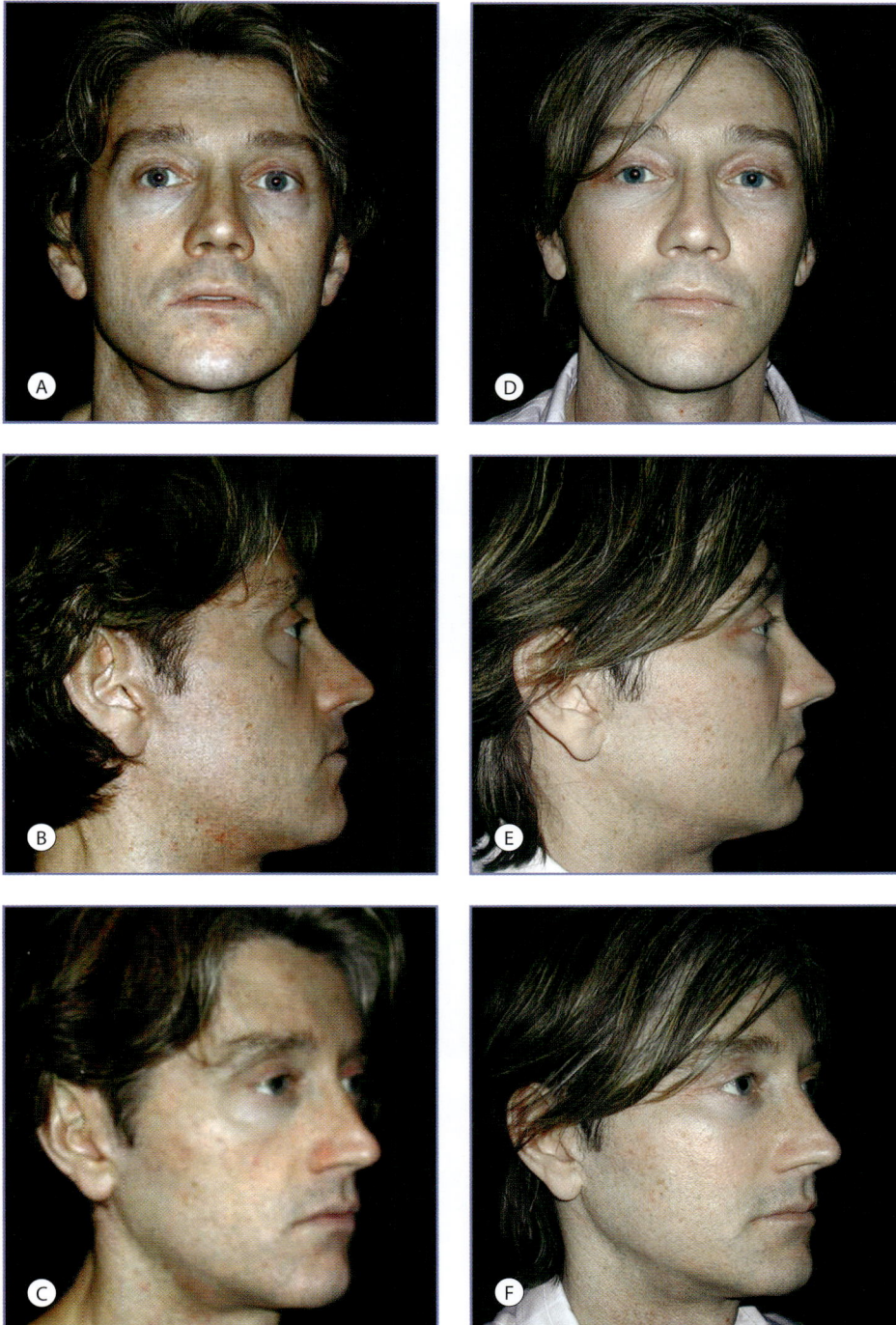

Figure 9.5 A 47-year-old man had multiple midface implants placed as well as midface elevation. Rhytidectomy, upper and lower lid blepharoplasty, and a brow lift had been performed by other surgeons in the past. (**A–C**) Preoperative frontal, lateral, and oblique views. (**D–F**) Postoperative frontal, lateral, and oblique views. (From Yaremchuk 2005,[18] with permission.)

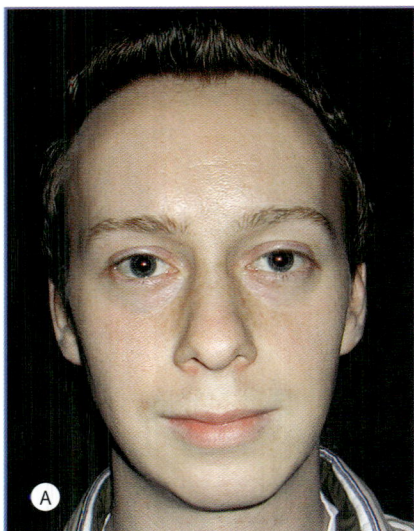

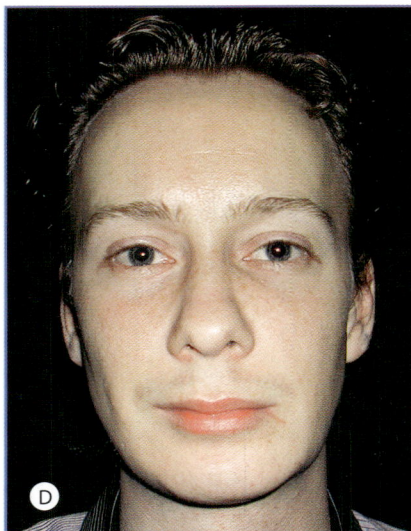

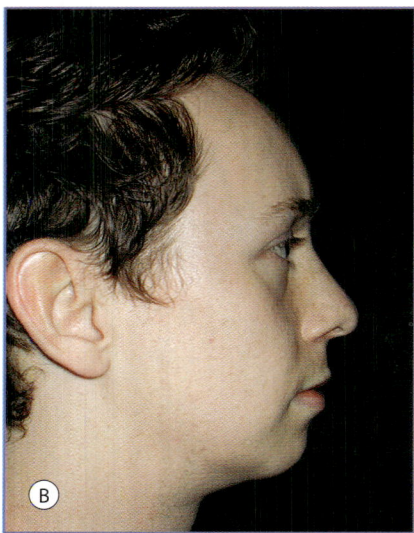

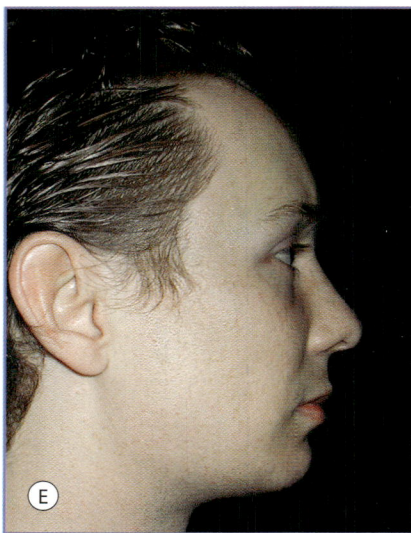

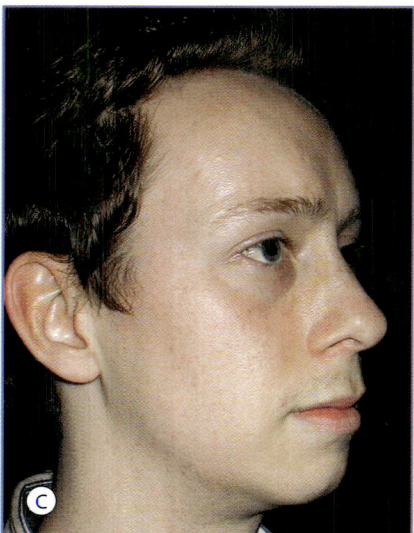

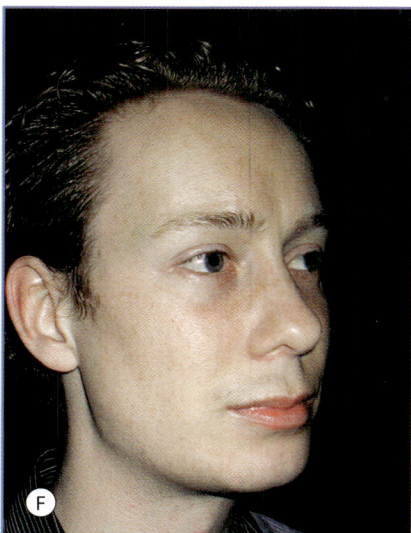

Figure 9.6 A 28-year-old man had multiple midface implants and midface elevation performed. During the same operation, chin and mandible implants were placed and the vertical height of the chin was reduced. (**A–C**) Preoperative frontal, lateral, and oblique views. (**D–F**) Postoperative frontal, lateral, and oblique views. (**G**) Artist's depiction of implant placement. (From Yaremchuk 2005,[18] with permission.)

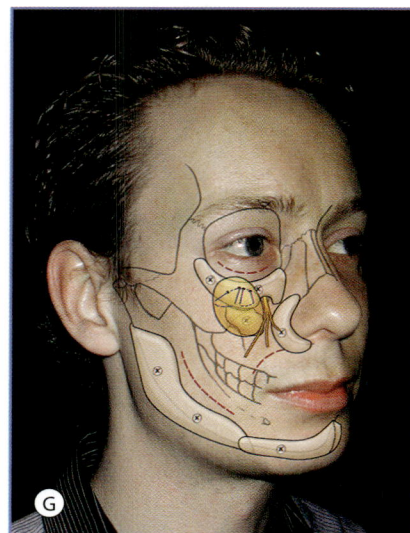

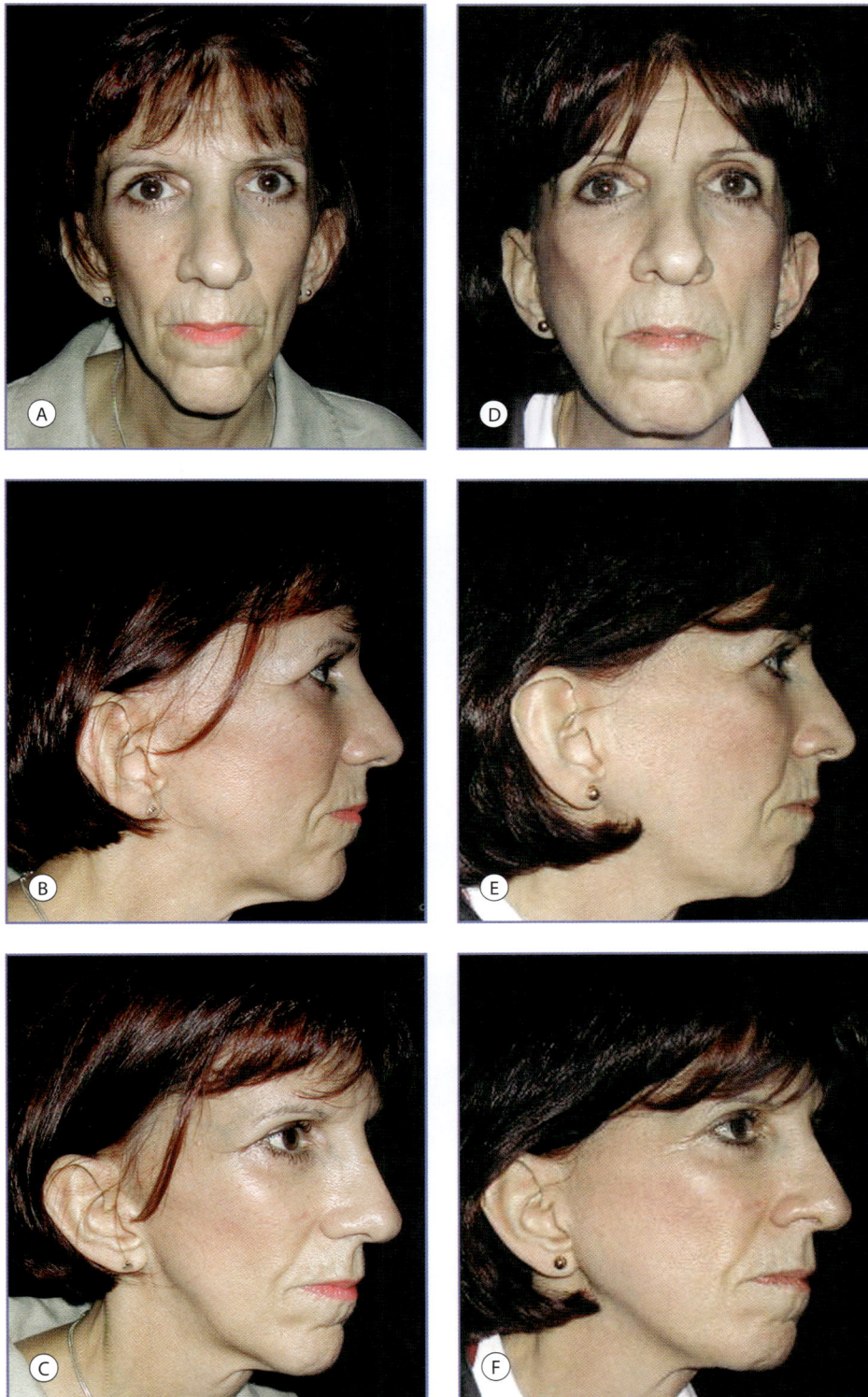

Figure 9.7 A 50-year-old woman had multiple midface implants and midface elevation performed. In addition, a lateral canthopexy and mandibular body and angle implants were placed. In the past, the patient had undergone upper and lower lid blepharoplasty as well as chin augmentation performed by other surgeons. (**A–C**) Preoperative frontal, lateral, and oblique views. (**D–F**) Postoperative frontal, lateral, and oblique views.

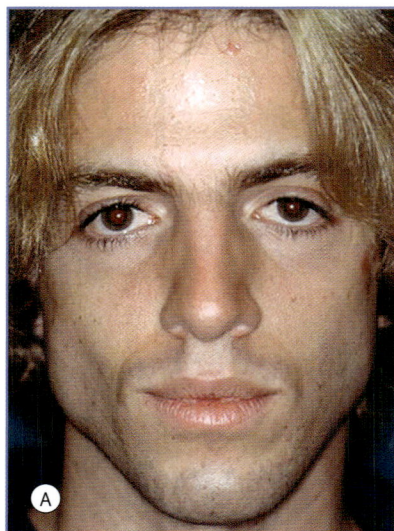

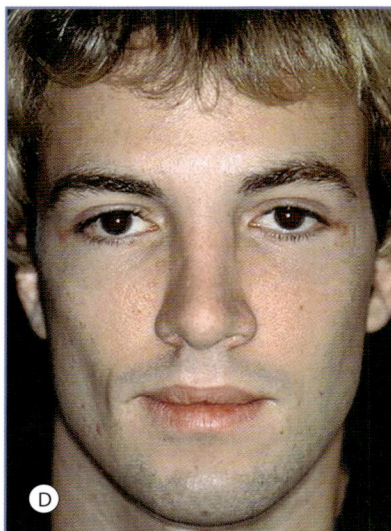

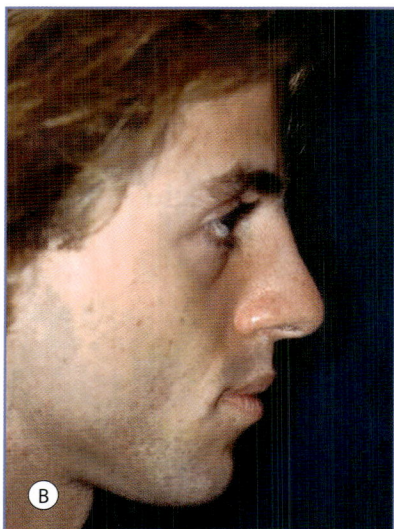

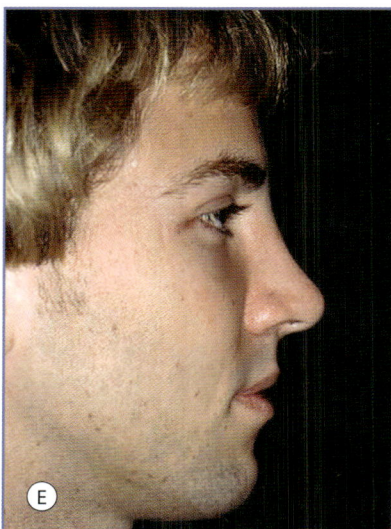

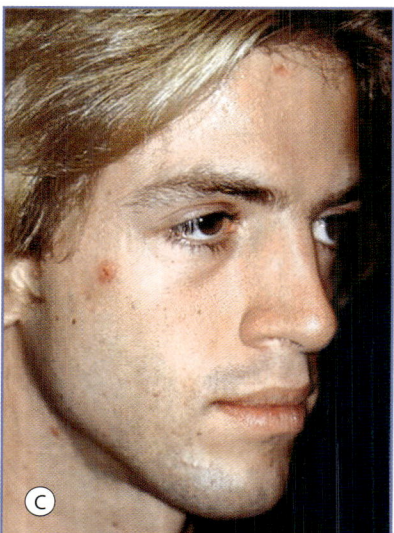

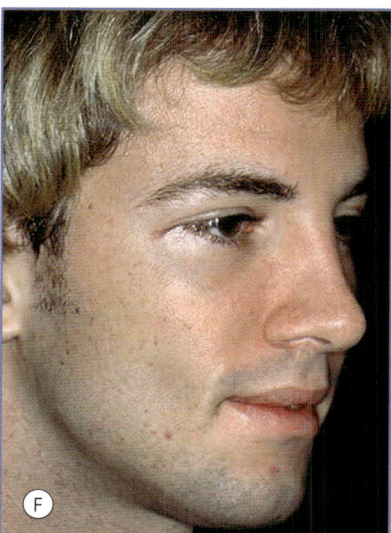

Figure 9.8 A 24-year-old man requested several changes in his facial contour. Two operations were performed, 18 months apart. In the first operation, malar and infraorbital rim implants were placed and a rhinoplasty was performed, through bicoronal, intraoral, and intranasal incision. In the second operation, paranasal and mandibular body implants were placed, the rhinoplasty was revised, and a midface lift and lateral canthopexies were performed. (A–C) Preoperative frontal, lateral, and oblique views. (D) Postoperative frontal views. (E–F) Postoperative lateral, and oblique views. (G) Diagrammatic representation of implant placement. (From Yaremchuk 2003,[17] with permission.)

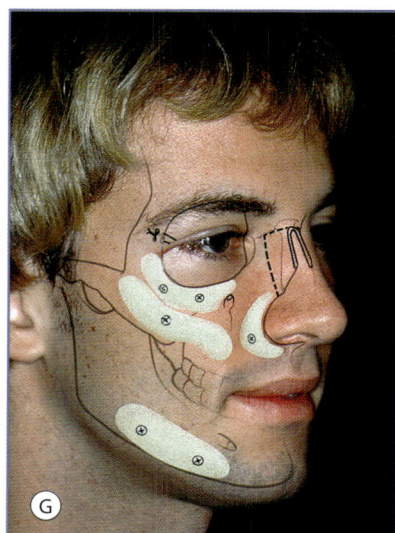

REFERENCES

1. Farkas LG, Hreczko TA, Katic MJ. Appendix A. Craniofacial norms in North American Caucasians from birth (one year) to adulthood. In: Farkas LG, ed. Anthropometry of the head and face. 2nd edn. New York: Raven Press; 1994.
2. Freihofer HPM. Reversing segmental osteotomies of the upper jaw. Plast Reconstr Surg 1995; 96:86–91.
3. Rosen HM. Maxillary advancement for mandibular prognathism. Indications and rationale. Plast Reconstr Surg 1991; 87:823–828.
4. Rosen HM. Facial skeletal expansion. Treatment strategies and rationale. Plast Reconstr Surg 1992; 89:798–803.
5. Pessa JE, Desvigne LD, Lambros VS, et al. Changes in ocular globe-to-orbital rim position with age: implications for aesthetic blepharoplasty of the lower eyelids. Aesthetic Plast Surg 1999; 23:337–342.
6. Yaremchuk MJ. Infraorbital rim augmentation. Plast Reconstr Surg 2001; 107:1585–1590.
7. Yaremchuk MJ. Improving periorbital appearance in the 'morphologically prone'. Plast Reconstr Surg 2004; 114:980–987.
8. Hirmand H, Codner MA, McCord CD, et al. Prominent eyes: operative management in lower lid and midface rejuvenation—the morphologic classification system. Plast Reconstr Surg 2002; 11:620–625.
9. Jelks GW, Jelks EB. The influence of orbital and eyelid anatomy on the palpebral aperture. Clin Plast Surg 1991; 18:193–204.
10. Rees TD, LaTrenta GS. The role of the Schirmer's test and orbital morphology in predicting dry-eye syndrome after blepharoplasty. Plast Reconstr Surg 1988; 82:619–624.
11. Yaremchuk MJ, Israeli D. Paranasal implants for correction of midface concavity. Plast Reconstr Surg 1998; 102:1676–1684.
12. Whitaker LA. Aesthetic augmentation o the malar–midface structures. Plast Reconstr Surg 1987; 90:337–341.
13. Carraway JH, Mellon CG. Syringe aspiration and fat concentration: a simple technique for autologous fat injection. Ann Plast Surg 1990; 24:293–296.
14. Coleman SR. The technique of periorbital lipoinfiltration: operative techniques. Plast Reconstr Surg 1994; 1:120–134.
15. Guerreosantos J, Haidar F, Paillet JC. Aesthetic facial contour augmentation with microprofiling. Aesthetic Surg J 2003; 23:239–247.
16. Yaremchuk MJ. Subperiosteal and full thickness skin rhytidectomy. Plast Reconstr Surg 2001; 107:1045–1058.
17. Yaremchuk MJ. Facial skeletal reconstruction using porous polyethylene implants. Plast Reconstr Surg 2003; 111:1818–1827.
18. Yaremchuk MJ. Making concave faces convex. Aesthetic Plast Surg 2005; 29(3):141–147.

Section 4 Lower Face

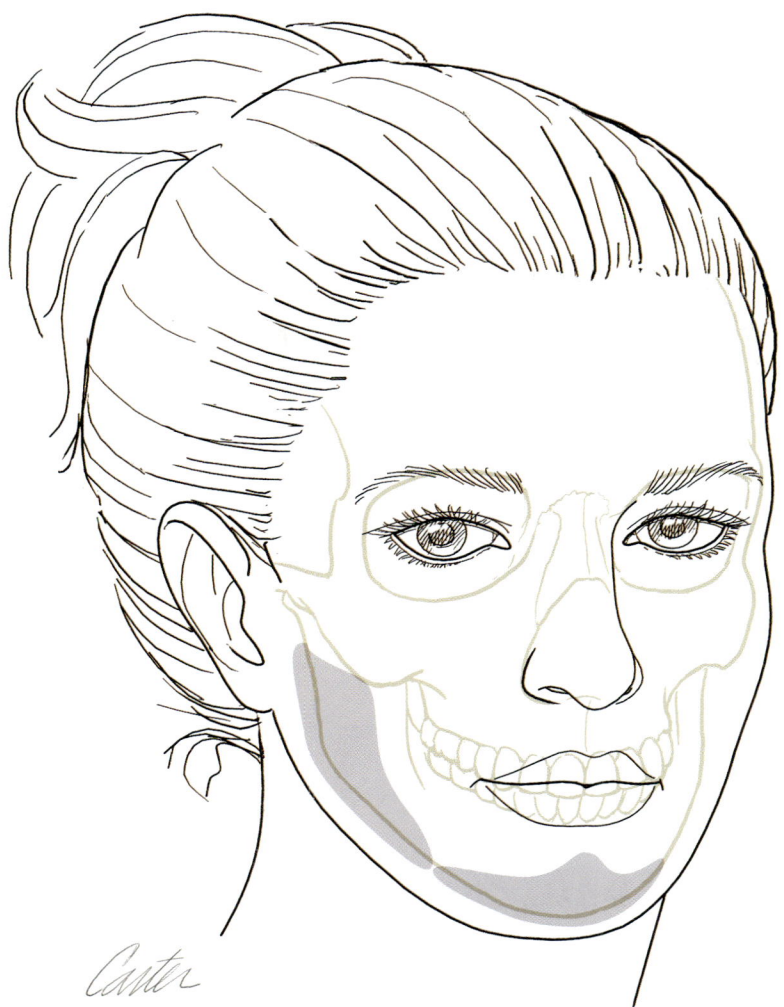

Carter

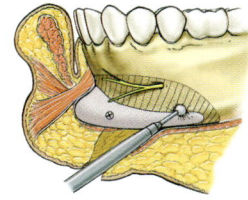

Chapter 10

Chin

Chin augmentation with implants is the most frequently performed facial implant surgery. It has long been considered a simple procedure, often done in the office setting, and one that always gives gratifying results.[1-3] Unfortunately, outcomes after chin augmentation are often less than ideal. It is not uncommon for the augmented chin to be asymmetric, to be too large (especially in women), to have a poor transition with the native mandible, or to negatively impact on the adjacent and overlying soft tissues.[3,4] Optimization of the aesthetic results after alloplastic chin augmentation requires careful preoperative analysis as well as refinements in surgical technique and implant design.

EVALUATION AND PLANNING

Effective preoperative planning requires understanding of the patient's desires, recognition of the impact of previous facial surgery or orthodontic treatment on the patient's appearance, and careful facial examination. When chin augmentation is considered as an adjunct to rhinoplasty or neck rejuvenation,[5,6] the preoperative analysis should be as rigorous as it is when chin deficiency alone is the presenting complaint.

Physical examination
Physical examination must include analysis of both the skeleton and its soft tissue envelope. The lower one-third of the face must relate appropriately to the upper two-thirds. Within the lower one-third, the position of the lips and depth of the labiomental sulcus are impacted by the projection of the chin.

X-rays
Unlike orthognathic surgery, where cephalometric x-ray studies are intrinsic to the preoperative planning, preoperative x-rays can be helpful but are not mandatory for implant surgery. Plain x-rays may be particularly helpful during revisional surgery after previous osteotomies.

Three-dimensional computed tomography (CT) scans and the models that can be generated from their data can be useful for planning surgery to ameliorate facial skeletal asymmetries. Custom implants can be made using these data.

Anthropometric data
Normative data are helpful in analyzing the chin, not only in its sagittal but also in its vertical and horizontal projections. These dimensions and their potential change with chin augmentation should all be considered in the context of lip projection and the depth of the labiomental angle. Although these data derive from large numbers reflecting a heterogeneous population and cannot be applied to every individual, average values of the normal face should not be discounted and should be used in the evaluation process.

Sagittal projection (profile)

The anthropometric studies of Farkas et al. showed that the mean inclination of the facial profile, as defined by a line from the glabella to the pogonion, was $-3.0 \pm 3.4°$ in men and $-4.1 \pm 3.0°$ in women (Fig. 10.1).[7] These data show that men's chins project more than women's, and that 'normal' chin projection is considerably less than that determined ideal by subjective criteria. This does not mean that augmentation beyond one standard deviation would be unattractive in any given individual, but that it is more likely to look too large, especially in a woman.

PEARL

Placing a large chin implant in a woman may masculinize her lower face.

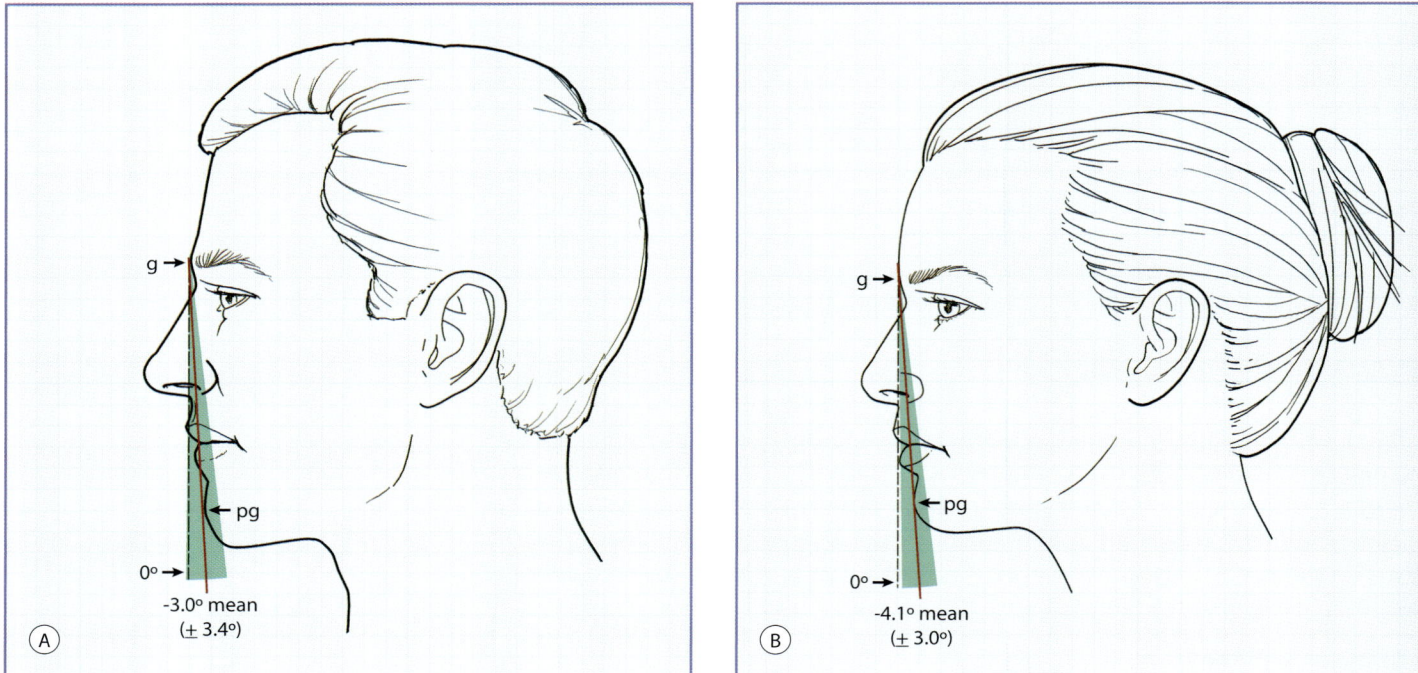

Figure 10.1 The inclination of the facial profile as defined by a line from the glabella (g) to the pogonion (pg). The broken line is drawn perpendicular to the Frankfort horizontal at the inclination of 0°. The solid red line represents the mean inclination of the study group. The shaded area encompasses 1 SD. (**A**) The mean inclination in 100 young North American white men was $-3.0 \pm 3.4°$. (**B**) The mean inclination in 100 young North American white women was $-4.1 \pm 3.0°$. In both men and women, note that the chin rests slightly posterior to the lower lip and that the lower lip lies slightly posterior to the upper lip. (After Farkas et al. 1994,[7] with permission.)

Lip–chin relations

Suggested ideal relationships between the chin and the lips, based on normative cephalometric data by different authors,[8–12] are in consensus that the chin should rest slightly posterior to the lower lip and the lower lip posterior to the upper lip (Fig. 10.1).

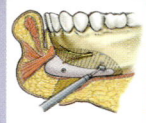

Labiomental angle

The inclination of the labiomental angle must be evaluated when considering an increase in the sagittal projection of the chin. There is a considerable variability in this inclination. In general, the inclination is more acute in men (113 ± 21°) than it is in women (121 ± 14°) (Fig. 10.2).

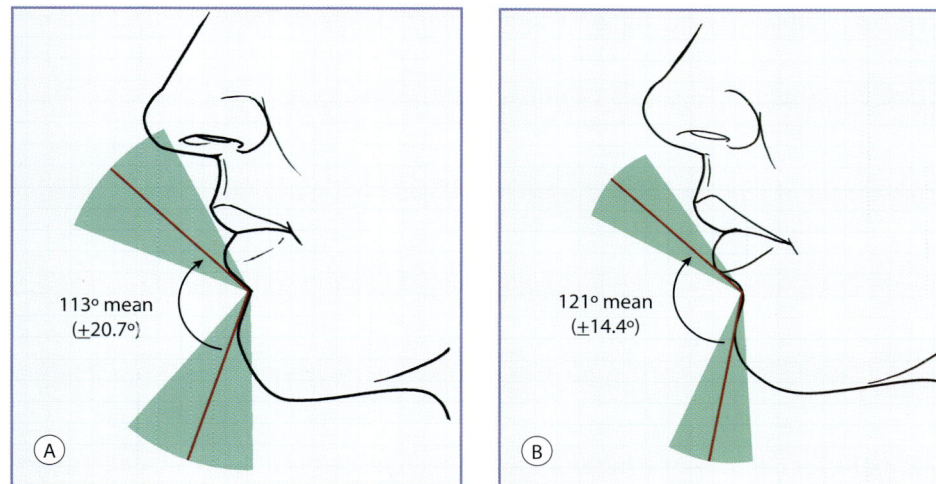

113° mean (±20.7°)

A

121° mean (±14.4°)

B

Figure 10.2 Labiomental angle has considerable variability. The inclination is more acute in men (−113 ± 21°) (**A**) than it is in women (−121 ± 14°) (**B**). (After Farkas et al. 1994,[7] with permission.)

When the angle is already acute, chin augmentation will make it more acute, thereby deepening the labiomental angle. Such deepening is usually dysesthetic. Certain patients with retrognathia have their upper central incisors abutting on their lower lip, thrusting it forward and creating a deep sulcus (Fig. 10.3). These patients are better served with repositioning of the entire mandible by sagittal split osteotomy.[3,13]

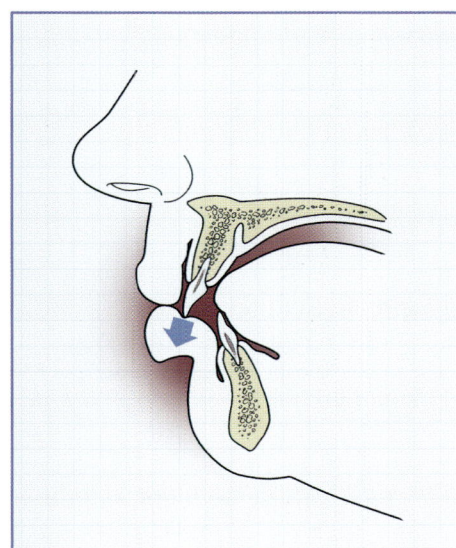

Figure 10.3 In patients with severe mandibular deficiency and overbite, the upper incisors may thrust the lower lip forward, resulting in acute labiomental angle after Flowers.[13] Chin augmentation in such patients will further decrease the labiomental angle.

Subjective criteria

Subjective criteria for an ideal profile are at variance from those obtained by objective analyses. When McCarthy and Ruff[14] and Farkas et al.[15] compared the profiles of young North American white adults to classical art and medical illustrations, they found that artists usually portray a larger chin than normally exists in reality.

A frequently cited ideal chin projection is adapted from Gonzalez-Ulloa.[16,17] His ideal facial plane was a vertical line that extended downward from the nasion to meet the Frankfort horizontal (which extends from the upper margin of the external auditory meatus to the lower orbital ridge). This was determined from his analysis of 'contemporary beautiful faces and faces known as beautiful through history'.[16] It is redrawn in Figure 10.4. This ideal is beyond the upper limit of normal for women (as determined by the data of Farkas et al.[7]), does not take into account sexual dimorphism, and is at variance with ideal lip–chin relations derived from cephalometric studies.[8–12]

Vertical projection (height)

Figure 10.5 shows average dimensions of both attractive male and attractive female faces. On average, the distance from the base of the nose (subnasion, sn) to the mouth opening (stomion, sto) is half the distance from sn to gnathion (gn). In other words, the height of the mandible in the midline should account for approximately two-thirds of the lower face height (sn–gn).

I have found that significant increases in chin height (greater than 3 mm) are best accomplished with horizontal osteotomy and vertical lengthening.

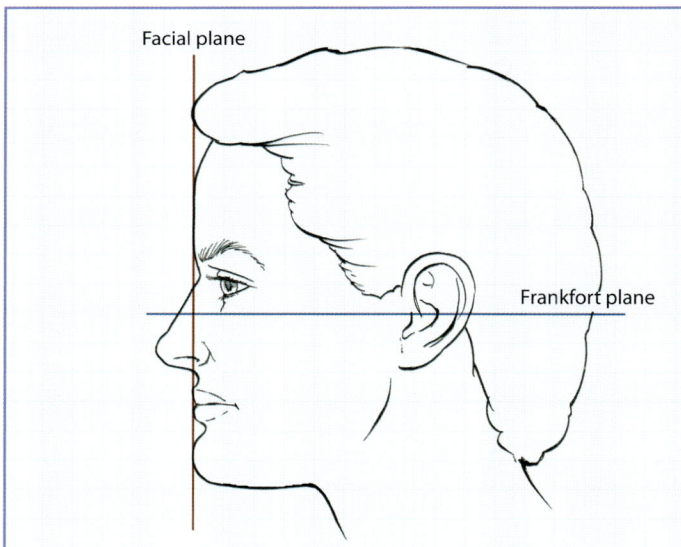

Figure 10.4 Gonzalez-Ulloa's ideal facial plane was a vertical line that extended down from the nasion to meet the Frankfort horizontal. The anteriormost projection of the lips and chin meets this line. This profile is determined by subjective analyses and does not agree with data obtained from normal individuals.

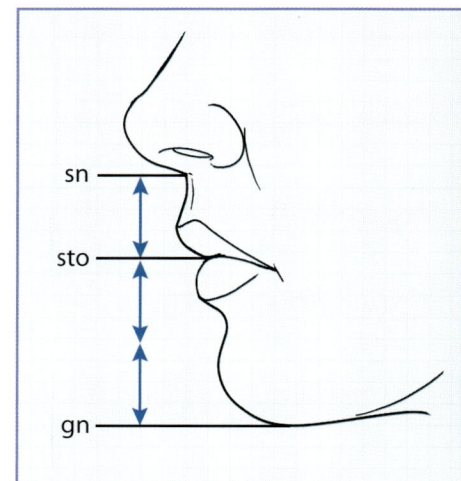

Figure 10.5 Average dimensions of both male and female faces. The distance from the base of the nose (subnasion, sn) to mouth opening (stomion, sto) is half of the distance from sn to gnathion (gn). In other words, the height of the mandible in the midline (sto–gn) should account for two-thirds of the lower face height (sn–gn).

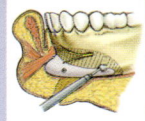

Implants that project maximally at the inferior border of the mandible and have a small wraparound at the border will give a small amount (1–2 mm) of real lengthening. Increasing vertical length by greater amounts with implants can look contrived. An illusion of increased length can be obtained by moving the most projecting part of the chin inferiorly by implant augmentation.

Horizontal projection (chin width)
The width of the chin should be appropriate for the vertical projection. This is the rationale for extended chin implants that allow a transition between the augmented chin point and the anterior mandibular body. Because women's mandibles are disproportionately narrower (relative to overall body size) than men's, care should be taken not to overaugment either the anterior or posterior mandible, so as to avoid masculinization of a woman's face (Fig. 10.6).[7,18]

Predicting the soft tissue response to skeletal augmentation
Objective analyses showed that the soft tissue to hard tissue changes in patients undergoing alloplastic augmentation of the chin averaged between 77.7 and 90%.[19–21] One would anticipate variations in the soft tissue response because of the variability in the thickness of the chin soft tissue envelope. The thicker the overlying soft tissue envelope, the less its surface response to the underlying skeletal augmentation. The thickness in the soft tissue envelope overlying the chin varies within the individual, varies between individuals for any given area, and is usually thicker in males than in females.[22]

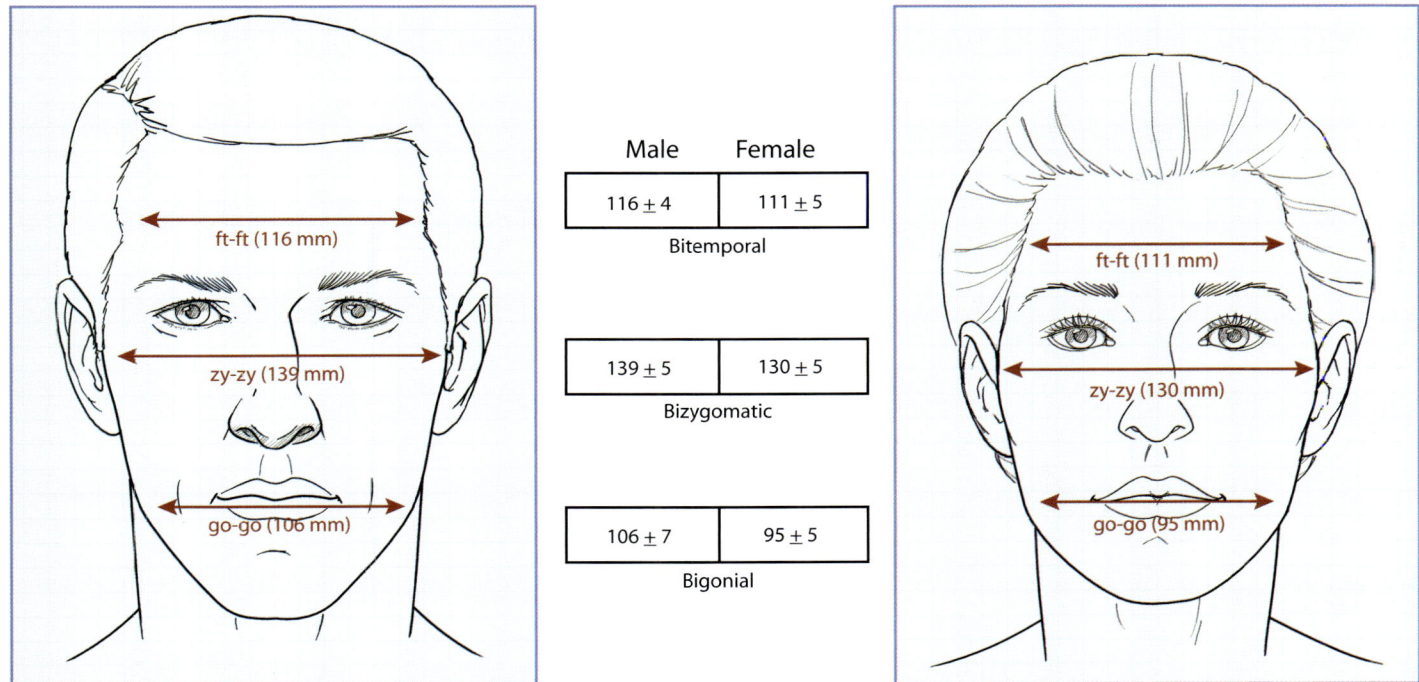

	Male	Female
Bitemporal	116 ± 4	111 ± 5
Bizygomatic	139 ± 5	130 ± 5
Bigonial	106 ± 7	95 ± 5

Figure 10.6 Normal values (mm) for upper, middle, and lower facial width in North American white adult men (ages 19–25) (n = 109) and young adult women (n = 199).[7] Bitemporal (ft–ft) distance is measured from frontotemporal (ft) to frontotemporal, which is the point on each side of the forehead laterally from the elevation of the linea temporalis. Bizygomatic (zy–zy) distance is measured from zygion (zy) to zygion, which is the most lateral point of each zygomatic arch. The bigonial (go–go) distance is measured from gonion (go) to gonion, which is the most lateral point of the mandibular angle close to the bony gonion.

SURGICAL ANATOMY

Structures susceptible to iatrogenic injury during chin augmentation include the mental nerve and the lower lip retractors and elevators. Their anatomy is depicted in Figure 10.7.

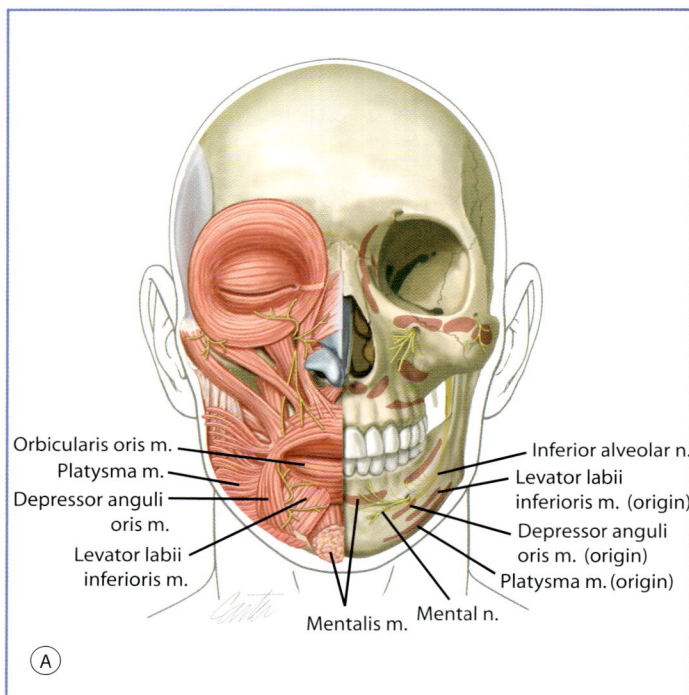

Orbicularis oris m.
Platysma m.
Depressor anguli oris m.
Levator labii inferioris m.
Mentalis m.
Mental n.
Inferior alveolar n.
Levator labii inferioris m. (origin)
Depressor anguli oris m. (origin)
Platysma m. (origin)

(A)

Figure 10.7 Anatomy of the lower lip elevators and retractors, as well as the path of the mental nerve relative to the mandible. These structures are susceptible to injury during chin augmentation. (**A**) Frontal view with facial musculature and position of infraorbital and mental nerves. (**B**) Lateral view with facial musculature origins and path of inferior alveolar nerve.

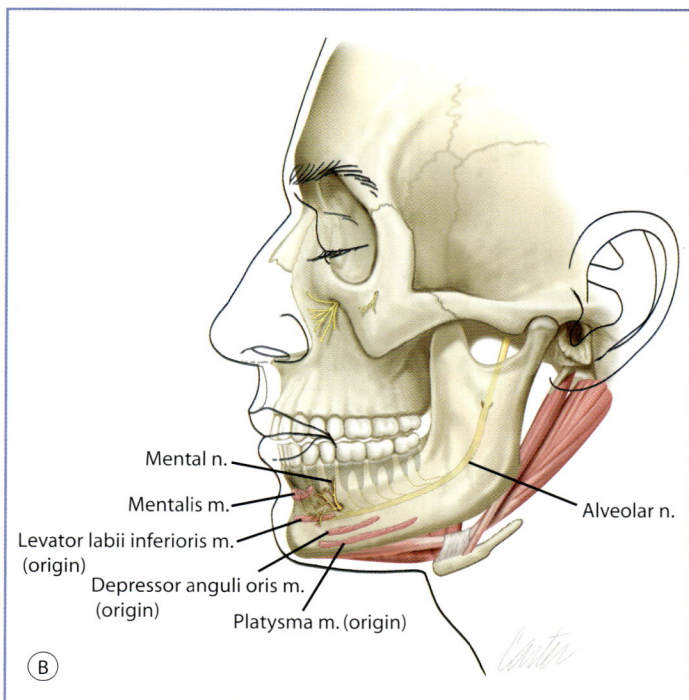

Mental n.
Mentalis m.
Levator labii inferioris m. (origin)
Depressor anguli oris m. (origin)
Platysma m. (origin)
Alveolar n.

(B)

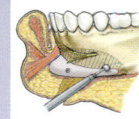

Mental nerve

The inferior alveolar nerve is a branch of the mandibular nerve (V3). It enters the mandibular canal with the inferior alveolar vessels through the mandibular foramen, which is located in the inner aspect of the ramus of the mandible. The nerve and vessels course obliquely from the ramus to the body, where it exits as the mental nerve through the mental foramen, which is located at the level of the first or second premolar.

Hwang et al. documented the course of the inferior alveolar nerve in Korean cadavers. They found that the foramen was located below the second premolar tooth in approximately two-thirds of the cadavers studied. Vertically, the mental foramen was located almost halfway from the tip of the alveolar process to the lower border of the mandible. They also found that the terminal mandibular canal was an average of 4.5 mm under the mental foramen, and that it advances 5 mm anteriorly, loops, and ends at the foramen.

The potential location of this nerve is important to recognize when placing screws or performing horizontal osteotomies of the mandible. Any cuts or holes made in the bone should be placed at least 6 mm beneath the foramen. After exiting the foramen, the mental nerve divides into two or three branches to supply sensation to the mucosa and the skin of the lower lip and chin.

Mentalis muscle

Zide has defined the anatomy of the mentalis and the repercussion of iatrogenic injury to this structure.[23] (See also Zide's discussion of Yaremchuk 2003.[4]) The mentalis muscle is an elevator of the central lower lip. It arises from the mandible at the level of the root of the lower lateral incisor, and therefore defines the inferior limits of the sulcus intraorally. It fans inferiorly as a truncated cone whose base inserts on the skin and therefore dimples the skin when elevating and protruding the lower lip.

This is the most frequently damaged muscle during chin surgery. If it is divided and improperly reapproximated or stripped from its origin and allowed to descend to a more inferior position, the result is inferior malposition of the lower lip, with increased lower incisor show and deepening of the sulcus as well as inferior displacement of the chin pad (Fig. 10.8).[20]

> **PEARL**
>
> The inferior alveolar nerve courses at a level inferior to the mental foramen.

> **PEARL**
>
> The mentalis muscle is the most frequently damaged structure during chin surgery. A submental surgical approach and extended subperiosteal dissection avoid damage to the mentalis muscle.

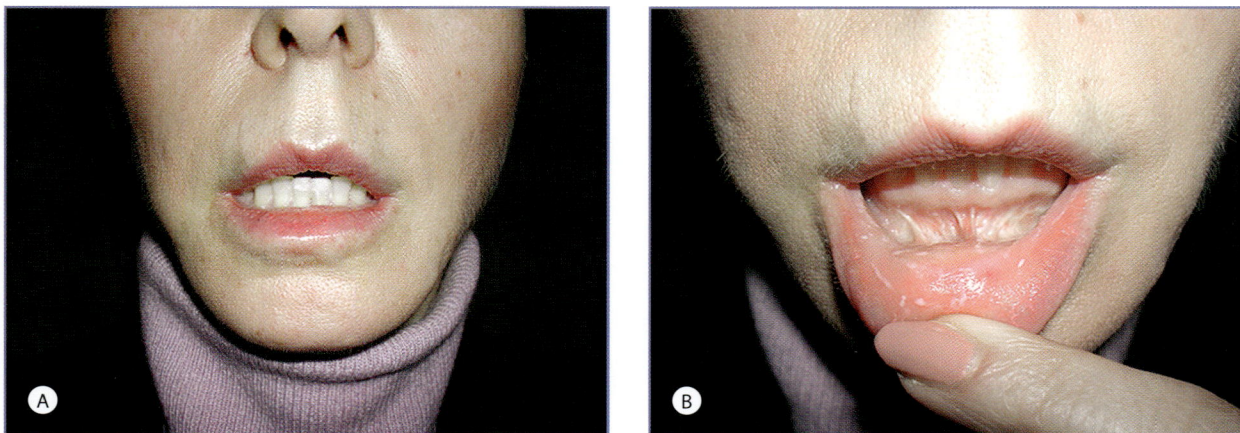

Figure 10.8 Lower lip descent and a deep labiodental sulcus in a patient whose mentalis muscle is divided or stripped and not attached to the mandible during the intraoral approach for chin implant placement. (**A**) Lower lip posture at rest. (**B**) Deep sulcus.

The depressor anguli oris (triangularis), the depressor labii inferioris (quadratus), and the platysma are all depressors of the lower lip. The depressor labii inferioris and depressor anguli oris arise from the oblique line of the mandible to merge with orbicularis oris and skin of the lower lip. The platysma muscle sends fibers that originate from the mandible beneath the oblique line and merge with the lip depressors. Subperiosteal dissection separates these muscles as a continuum from the bone. Failure to stay in the subperiosteal plane may cause damage, usually short-lived, to these muscles. Clinically, this injury mimics that of marginal mandibular branch palsy, because the marginal branch innervates the lower lip depressors. Temporary palsy to this musculature may last 1–2 weeks after primary surgery and 2–3 months after revisional surgeries (Fig. 10.9).

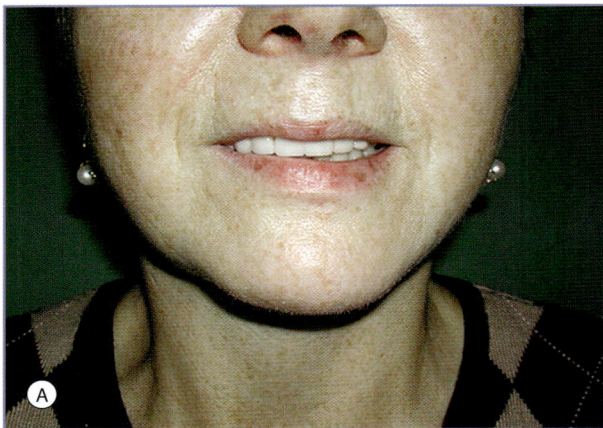

Figure 10.9 Palsy of lower lip depressors. (**A**) Two weeks after tertiary chin implant surgery. (**B**) Resolution of palsy 10 weeks postoperatively.

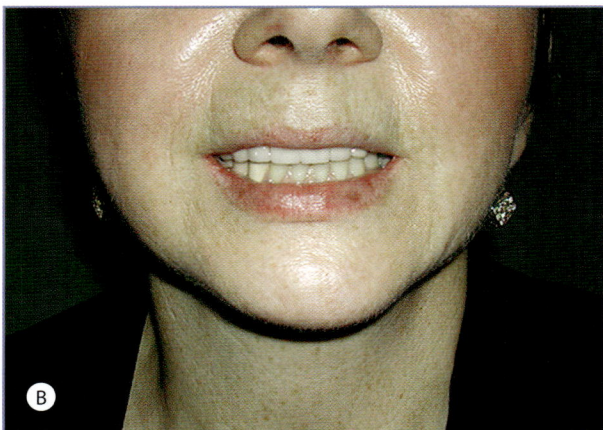

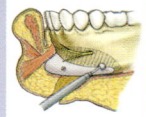

THE IMPLANT

The goal of surgery is to create an anatomically correct and stable mandibular contour. The design and composition of the implant should help accomplish this. Through trial and error with custom-carved chin implants, an easily adaptable implant design has evolved (Fig. 10.10).[4] Its shape and dimensions roughly resemble those of the popular 'extended' silicone chin implant design. It differs in two important aspects. The chin implant comes in two pieces: a right half and a left half. Segmentation facilitates placement of the relatively long and stiff, porous implant. The two-piece design also provides flexibility in positioning the lateral extensions of the implants, ensuring that it mimics the inclination of the patient's mandibular body (Fig. 10.11).

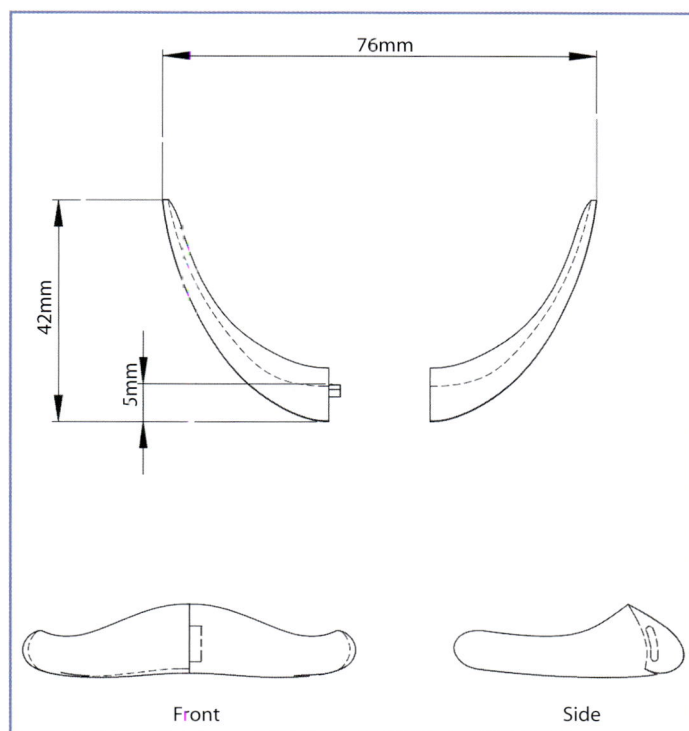

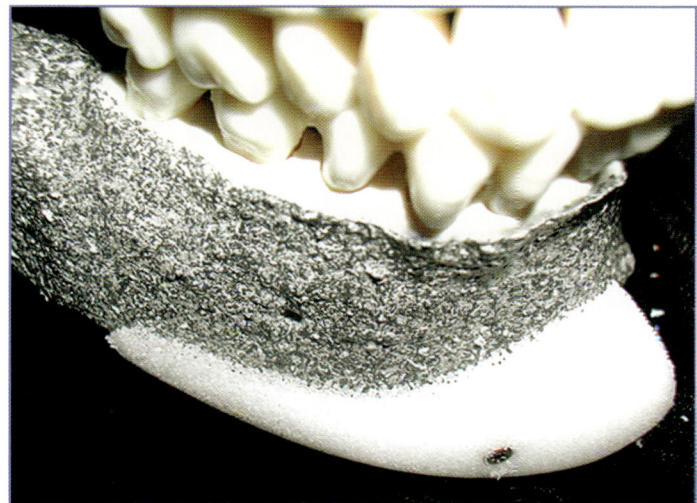

Figure 10.11 Right half of a large, two-piece implant fixed to a skull model. Note how the border of the implant parallels the mandible border.

Front   Side

Figure 10.10 Dimensions of a two-piece implant preferred by the author. The drawing represents an implant that provides 5 mm of anterior projection. The two-piece design allows flexibility and implant positioning. The central connecting tab provided by the manufacturer is rarely used by the author, because it effectively creates a one-piece implant that precludes its adjustment.

The manufacturer (Porex, Fairburn, Georgia) provides a tab insert that is designed to lock the right and left halves of the chin implant. I rarely use this connecting tab, because it dictates the position of the lateral limbs of the implant as well as the width of the central portion of the implant. It effectively makes it a one-piece implant.

A one-piece implant, particularly one with lateral extensions, is unlikely to have an arc, projection, and inclination appropriate for every mandible (Fig. 10.12).

PEARL

The inferior border of an extended one-piece implant rarely mimics the inclination of the mandibular border.

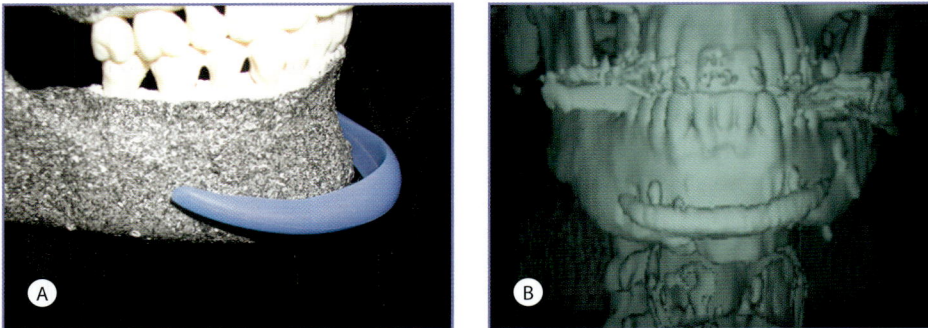

Figure 10.12 The arc, the inclination of its limbs, and the contour of its posterior surface of an extended one-piece implant may all be inappropriate for the shape of a mandible. (**A**) An extended one-piece design implant placed on a skull model. (**B**) Three-dimensional computed tomography scan demonstrating a clinical example.

A two-piece design allows adaptation of each of these parameters for a given mandible. When placed through the submental approach, the two-piece implant limits asymmetry in the horizontal plane. With one-piece implants, asymmetry in horizontal positioning increases as one proceeds laterally. It is not uncommon to find one end of an extended silicone implant impinging on the mental nerve, while the other end extends beyond the edge of the mandibular border (Fig. 10.13).

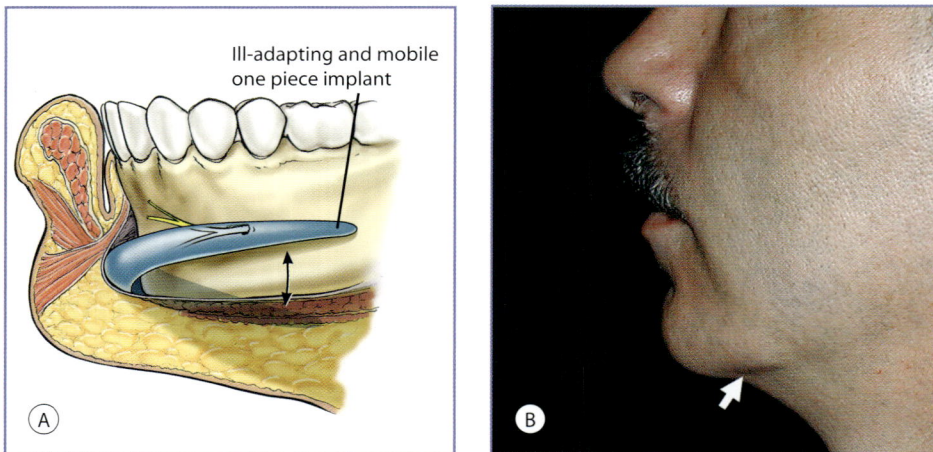

Figure 10.13 Ill-positioned one-piece extended implant. (**A**) When placed through an intraoral approach, it is common for one end to extend beyond the mandibular border while the other end impinges on the mental nerve. (**B**) Clinical example of an extended one-piece implant protruding beyond the mandibular border. Arrow points to protruding implant.

Ill-adapting and mobile one piece implant

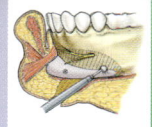

The lateral extensions differ from 'extended implants' in that they have a greater vertical height and more gradual taper. This shape provides a better transition between the implant and the mandible. These features allow the implant to be placed along the mandibular border, thereby creating a new, 'anatomically correct' shape.

Alloplastic augmentation with certain shaped implants can create unnatural chin contours. Implants that augment only the chin point produce an abrupt, protruding chin rather than a jaw–chin continuum (Fig. 10.14).[13,24]

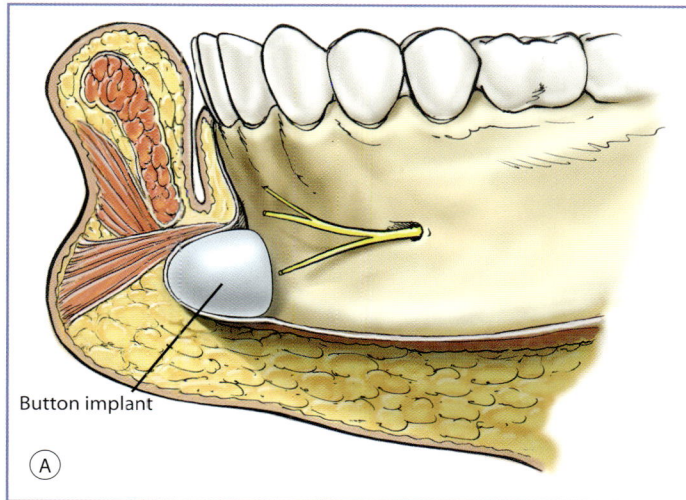

Button implant

(A)

(B)

Figure 10.14 (A) Illustration and (B) clinical example of a large button chin implant resulting in a poor implant–mandible transition with a stuck-on appearance.

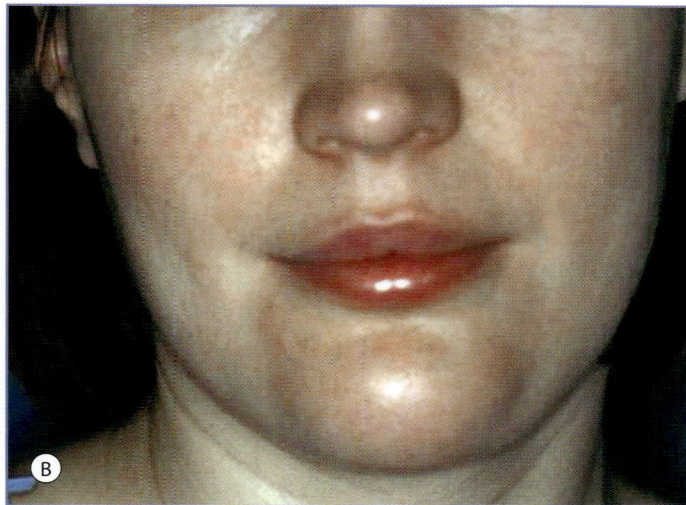

OPERATIVE TECHNIQUE

Anesthesia

It is my preference to perform chin and mandibular augmentation under general nasotracheal anesthesia. This provides a panoramic view of the operative field. If intraoral incisions are necessary, the airway is protected while the oral cavity can be optimally prepared (Fig. 10.15).

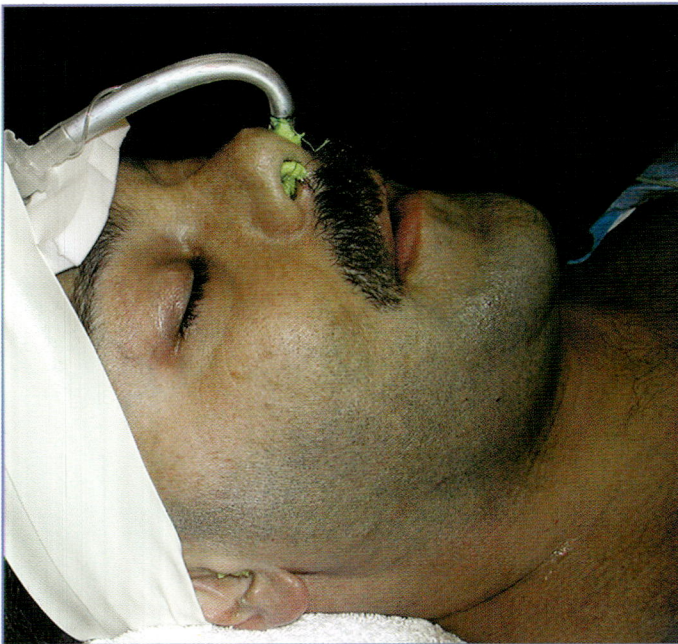

Figure 10.15 General anesthesia using nasotracheal intubation is ideal for chin and mandible augmentation. The airway is protected and controlled. A panoramic view of the operative area is provided.

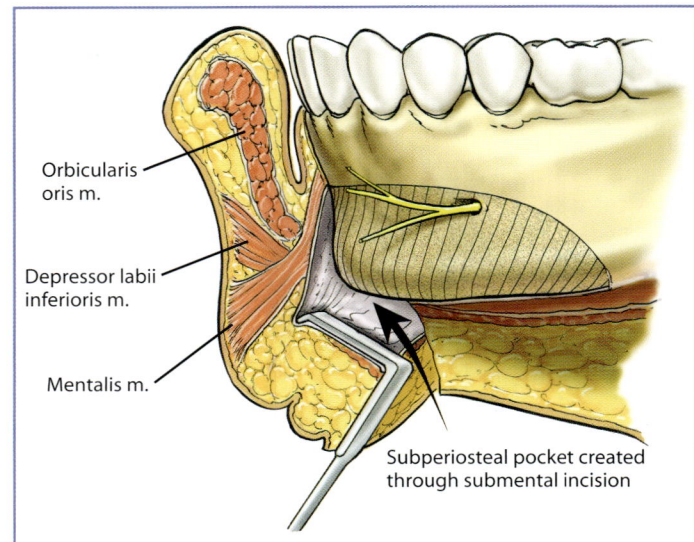

Figure 10.16 Surgical access to the chin and anterior mandibular border. A submental skin and subcutaneous incision is telescoped over the chin where the periosteum is incised with electrocautery. The striped area denotes the area of subperiosteal dissection. Note that a pocket larger than the implant is dissected to allow ease of implant insertion and to provide a panoramic view of the area to be augmented. (From Yaremchuk 2003,[4] with permission.)

Submental incision (Fig. 10.16)

The chin and the lower anterior mandible are accessed through a submental skin and subcutaneous incision. The soft tissues are then telescoped over the inferior border of the mandible, where the periosteum is incised with needle tip electrocautery. The midline of the chin is marked on the pogonion as a reference point. Wide subperiosteal dissection is performed. The upper limits of the dissection are the origin of the mentalis muscle. Laterally, the mental foramen with its exiting nerve and the inferior border of the mandible body are exposed. Lateral dissection extends approximately 1 cm beyond the area of augmentation.

PEARL

Mark the midline of the chin for orientation.

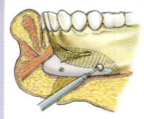

The submental approach and extended dissection avoid damage to the mentalis muscle, allow visualization of the mental nerve, and provide a panoramic view of the complex and varying contours of the mandible to allow precise implant placement. The technique of intraoral placement of chin implants avoids a cutaneous scar but provides limited exposure to the menton without compromising the mentalis muscle. As a result, the intraoral approach is associated with superior malposition of implants (Fig. 10.17)[23] and lower lip dysfunction resulting from mentalis muscle division or detachment (Fig. 10.8).[23] After reviewing his series of more than 100 cases of postoperative chin problems, Zide noted that almost all chin implant problems that he has seen were caused by implants that were placed transorally.[3]

Implant positioning

On the basis of the preoperative assessment and intraoperative findings, an appropriate size implant is placed on the area to be augmented, which usually includes the pogonion, gnathion, and menton centrally and the mandibular border laterally. One or two titanium screws (Synthes Corp., Paoli, Pennsylvania), 6–8 mm in length, are used to fix the implant to the mandible. Screw fixation is performed for several reasons. It allows precise, stable positioning of the implant. It adapts the posterior surface of the implant to the anterior surface of the mandible, thereby obliterating gaps between the implant and the mandible (gaps between the implant and the mandible will result in an undesirable increase in augmentation in the gap area). Immobilizing the implant with screws allows final in-place contouring of the implant to ensure proper implant projection and an imperceptible transition between the implant and the mandible (Figs 10.18 and 10.19).

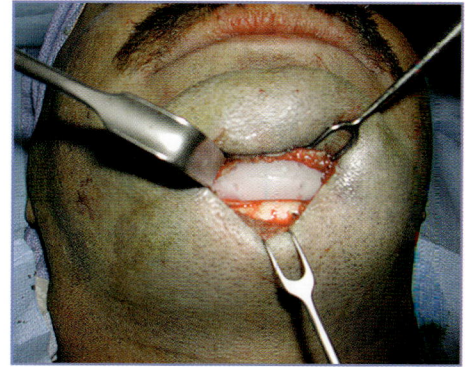

Figure 10.17 Submental exposure during revisional surgery of silicone implant previously placed through an intraoral incision. Note that the implant has been positioned too high, well above the gnathion.

> **PEARL**
>
> Many chin implant problems are caused by transoral placement.

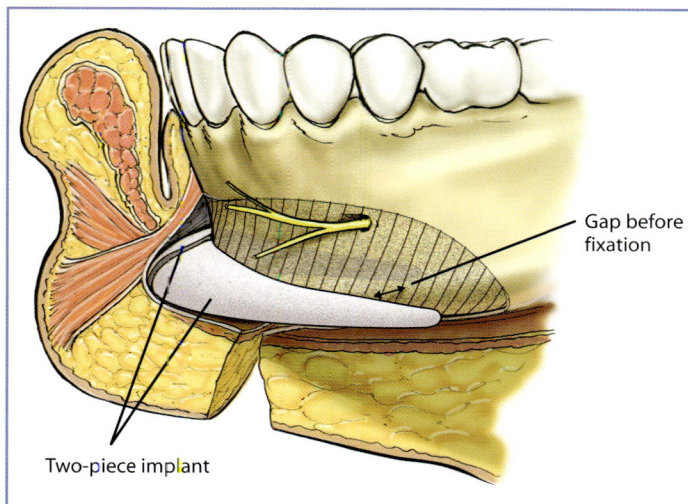

Figure 10.18 A two-piece porous polyethylene implant placed in a subperiosteal pocket. Note the two-piece design, which allows the lateral extension of the implant to follow the inclination of the mandibular border. Note that because the contour of the posterior surface of the implant does not mimic the contour of the anterior surface of the mandible, there is a gap between the mandible and the implant. (From Yaremchuk 2003,[4] with permission.)

Screw fixation

Contouring distal transition

(A)

(B)

(C)

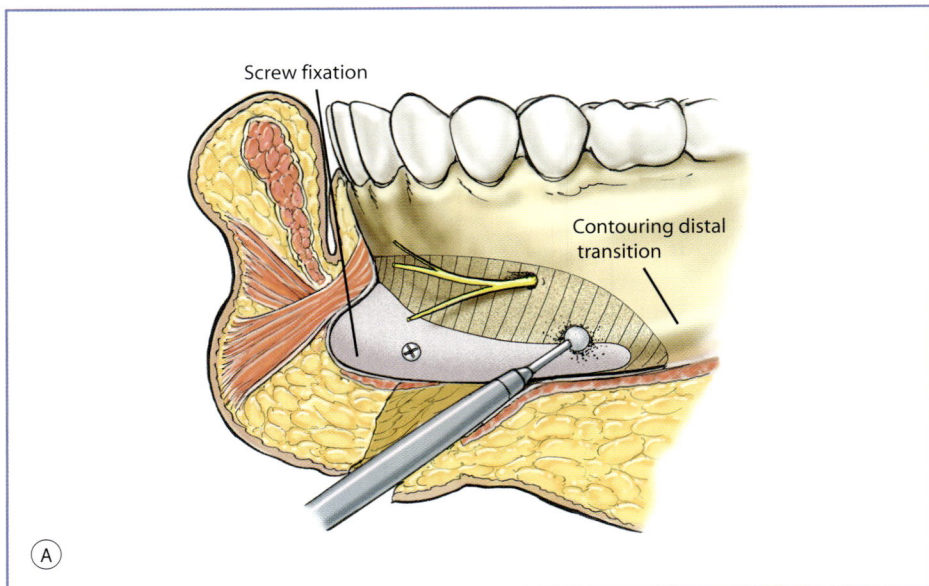

Figure 10.19 Screw fixation of the implant to the mandible prevents implant movement and obliterates gaps between the implant and the anterior surface of the mandible. Screw fixation also allows 'in-place' contouring of the implant to ensure desired contour and an imperceptible implant–skeleton transition. (**A**) In-place contouring of the implant fixed to the mandible with titanium screws. (From Yaremchuk 2003,[4] with permission.) (**B**) Clinical example of screw-fixed two-piece porous polyethylene chin implant exposed through a submental incision. (**C**) Clinical photograph of screw-immobilized chin implant being contoured with high-speed burr. The inferior border is being reduced to ensure proper vertical height of the chin.

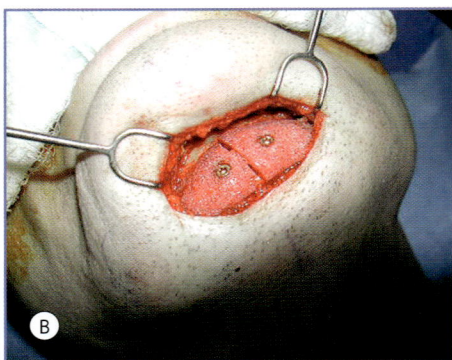

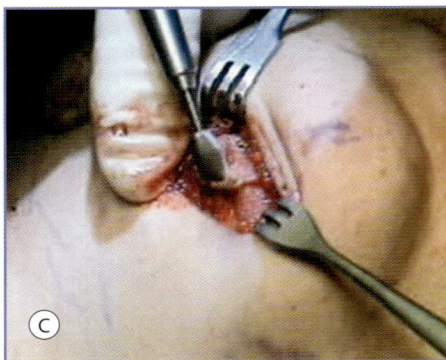

The wound is closed in layers. A mild compressive dressing is placed and then removed in 48–72 h.

Submental lipectomy

Many patients benefit from defatting the submental area. Precise defatting improves neck contour and improves mandibular border definition. My preference is to use the submental incision to create a full-thickness skin and subcutaneous flap by dissecting directly on the platysma. The fat is trimmed from the full-thickness flap with scissors. The wound is closed in layers and a mildly compressive dressing applied.

Defatting could also be done with liposuction. I prefer excision under direct observation, because it avoids irregularities and possible overresection that, in my hands, is more possible with liposuction.

Unless the patient is obese, I rarely remove fat from beneath the platysma or strap muscles. Overdefatting can create a submental depression that is disfiguring.

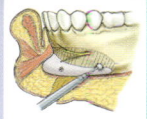

Clinical examples

Patients who have undergone primary chin augmentation using the above-described techniques are shown in Figures 10.20–10.24.

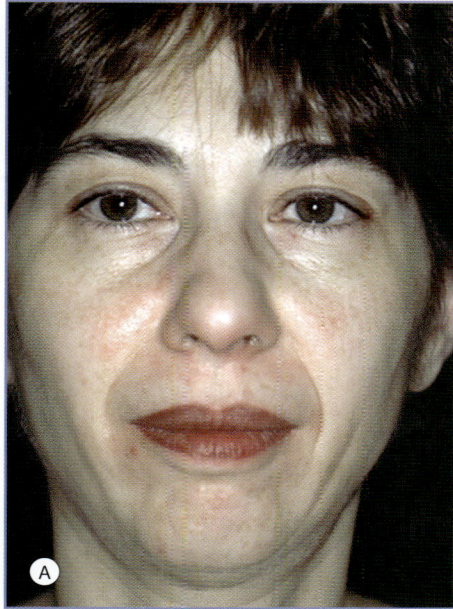

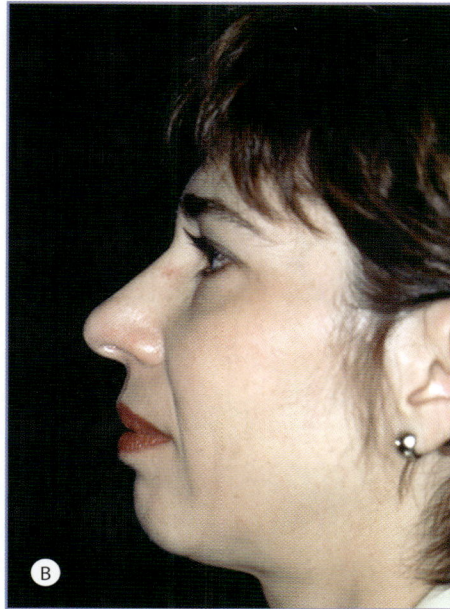

A

B

Figure 10.20 A 50-year-old woman underwent chin augmentation with a 3-mm, two-piece, porous polyethylene implant at the time of rhytidectomy. It was placed to lower the most projecting point of the chin. (**A** and **B**) Preoperative frontal and lateral views. (**C–E**) Postoperative frontal, lateral, and oblique views. (From Yaremchuk 2003,[4] with permission.)

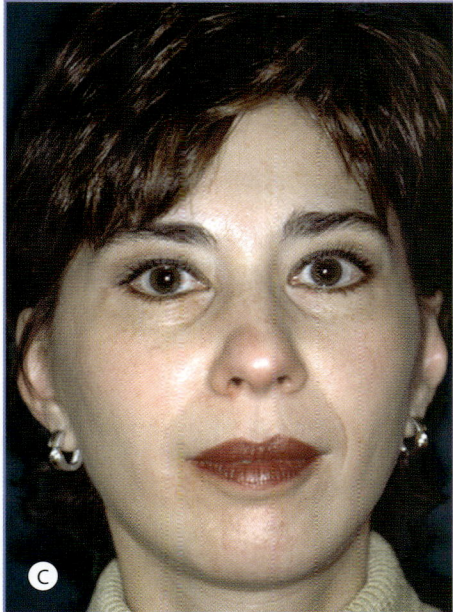

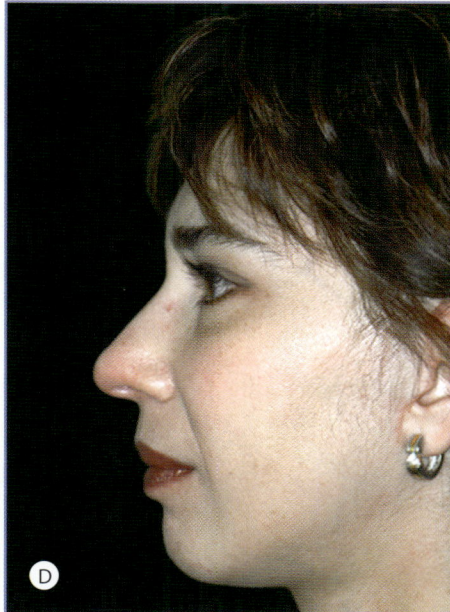

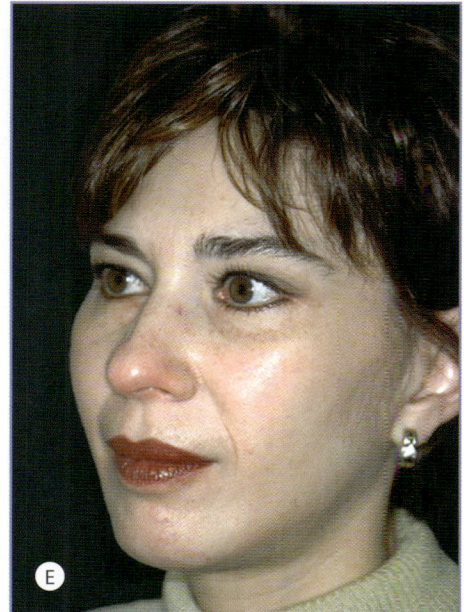

C

D

E

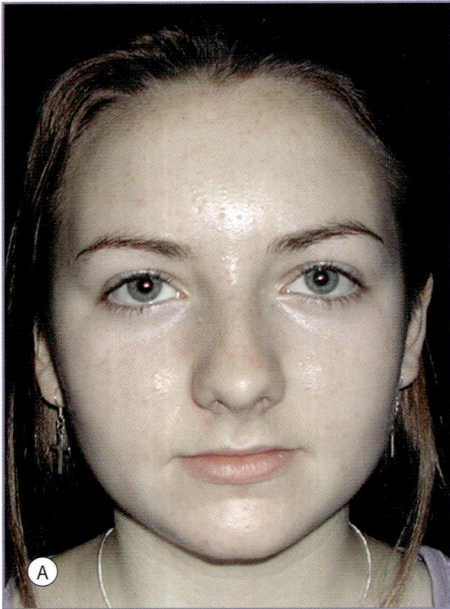

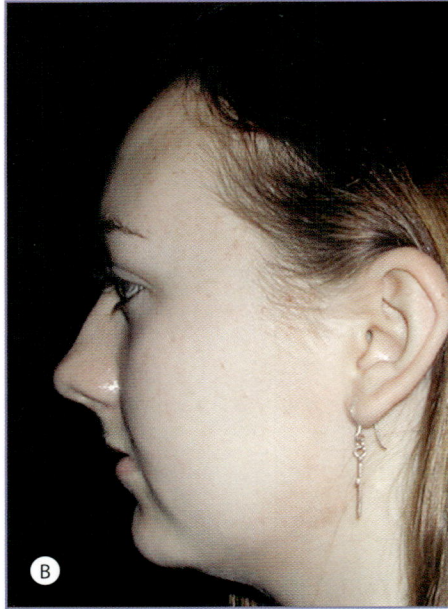

Figure 10.21 An 18-year-old woman desired more strength and definition to her lower face. A two-piece, 5-mm projection, porous polyethylene implant was placed. A submental lipectomy and a buccal lipectomy were also performed. The nasal spine was rongeured. (**A** and **B**) Preoperative frontal and lateral views. (**C–E**) Postoperative frontal, lateral, and oblique views. Note also how increasing the chin projection almost to that of the lower lip further exaggerates the depth of the labiomental fold. (From Yaremchuk 2003,[4] with permission.)

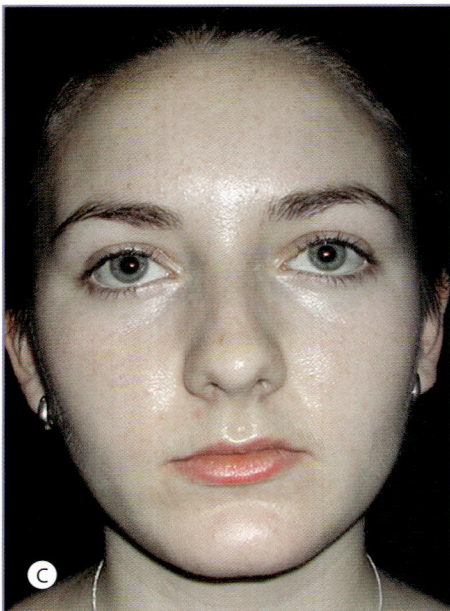

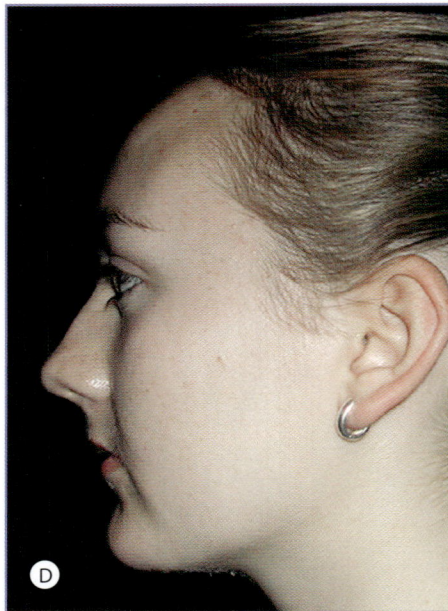

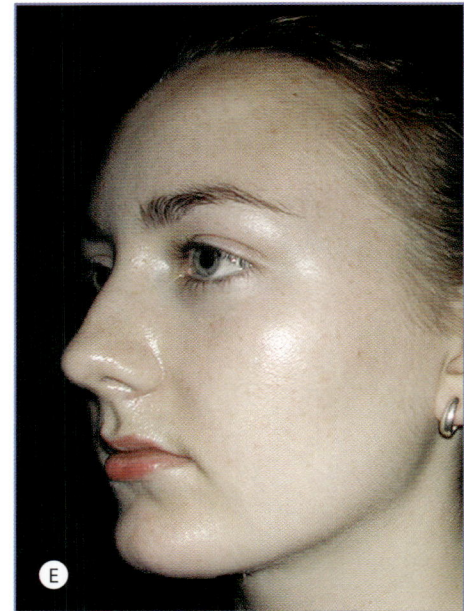

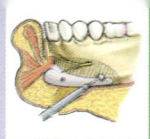

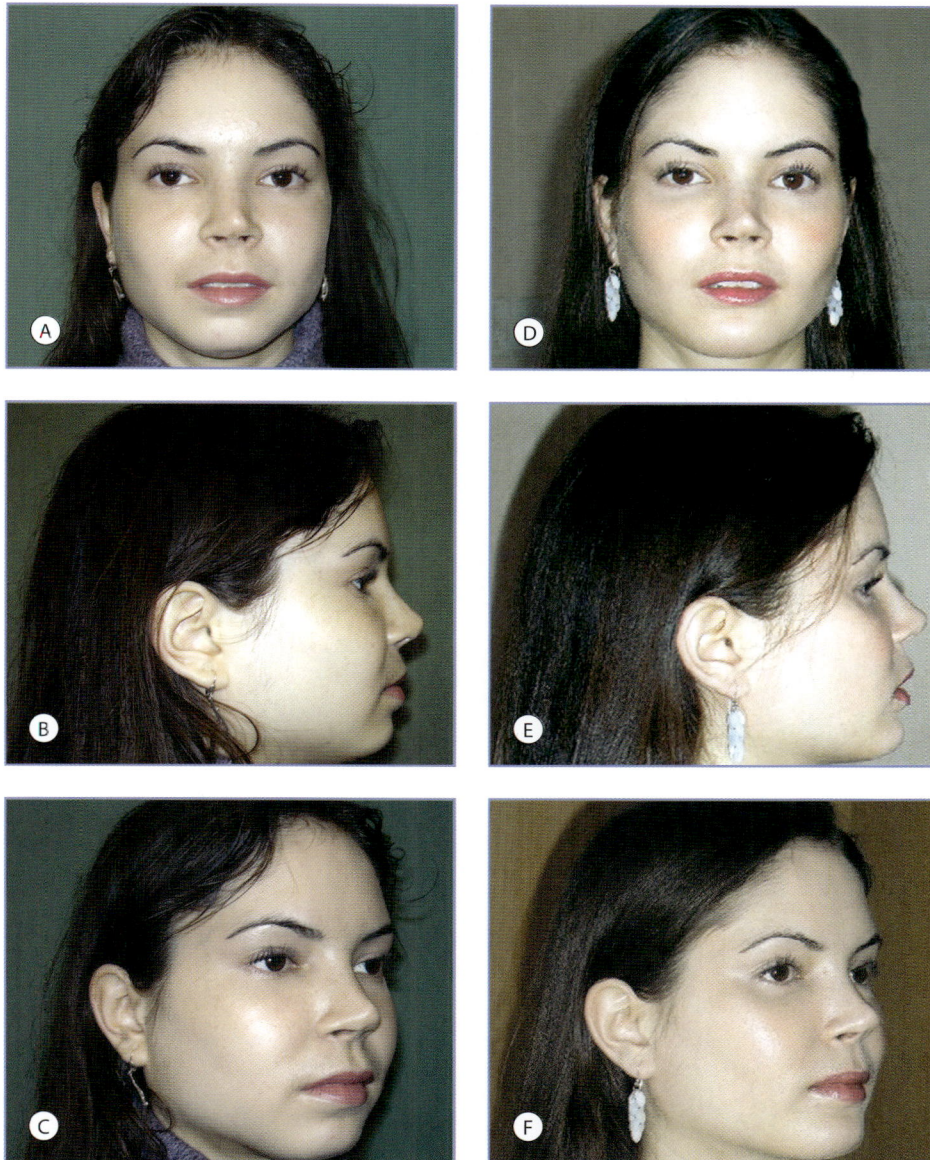

Figure 10.22 A 24-year-old woman underwent malar augmentation, chin augmentation with a 5-mm implant, and submental lipectomy. (**A–C**) Preoperative frontal, lateral, and oblique views. (**D–F**) Postoperative frontal, lateral, and oblique views.

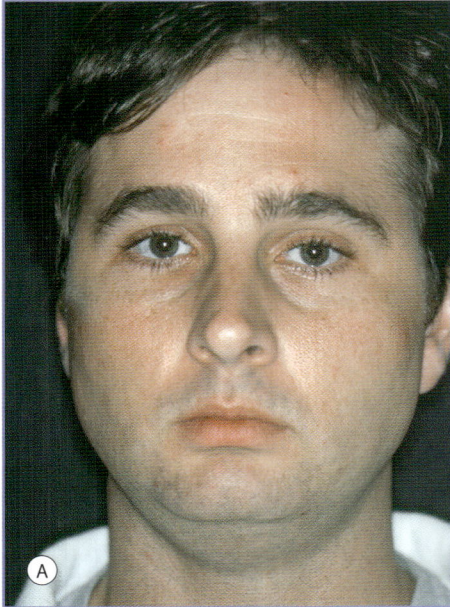

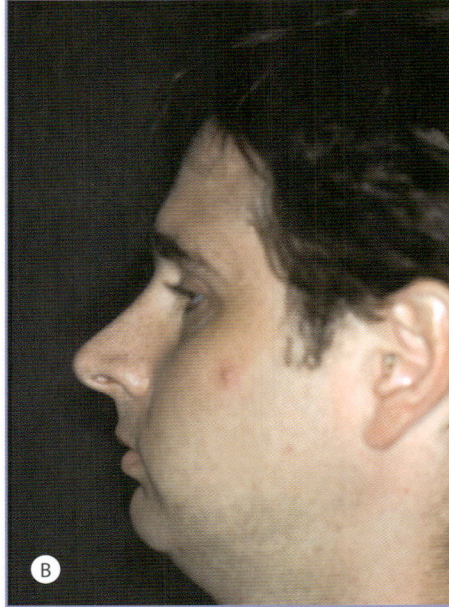

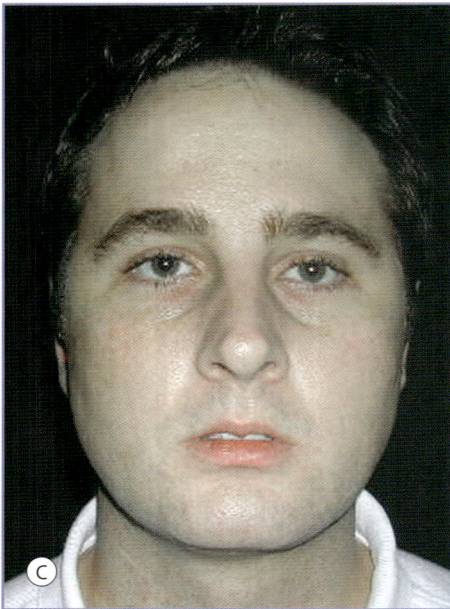

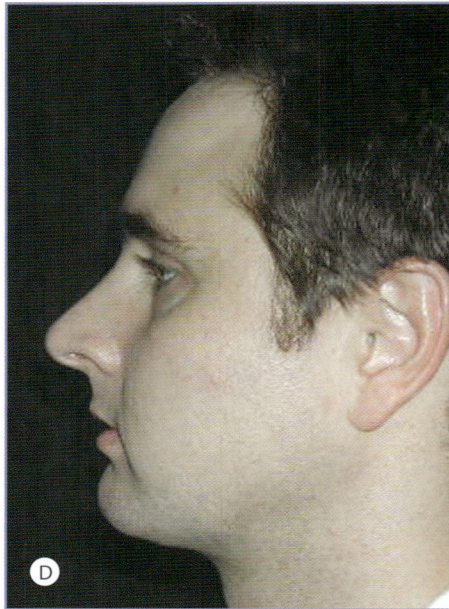

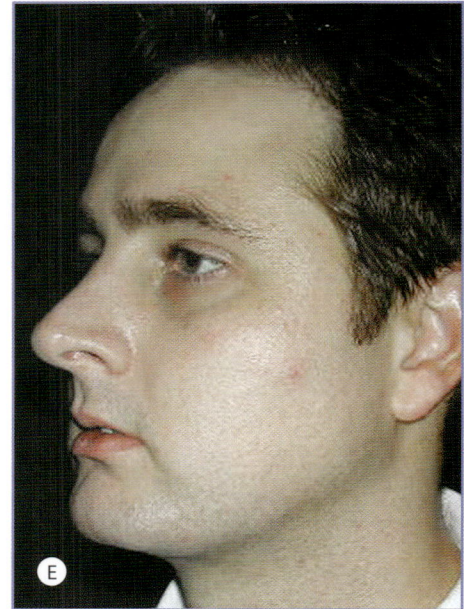

Figure 10.23 A 31-year-old man underwent chin augmentation with a 7-mm projection, two-piece, porous polyethylene implant. A submental lipectomy was performed. (**A** and **B**) Preoperative frontal and lateral views. (**C–E**) Postoperative frontal, lateral, and oblique views. (From Yaremchuk 2003,[4] with permission.)

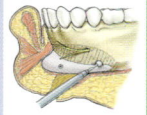

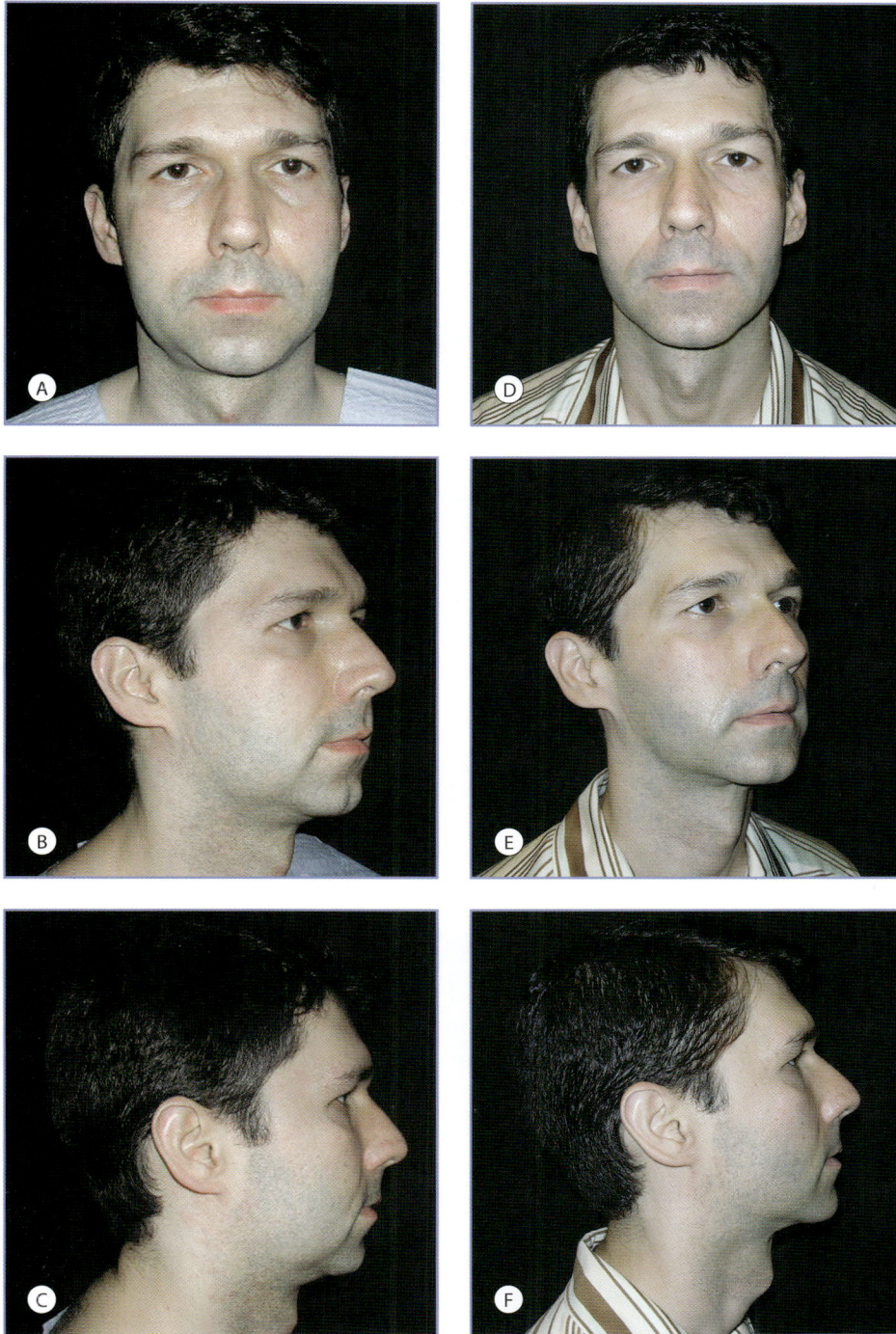

Figure 10.24 A 43-year-old man underwent chin augmentation with a 5-mm projection porous polyethylene implant. A submental lipectomy was performed. (**A–C**) Preoperative frontal, lateral, and oblique views. (**D–F**) Postoperative frontal, lateral, and oblique views.

SKELETAL ASYMMETRIES

Congenital asymmetries of the facial skeleton are usually more complex than localized areas of volume excess or deficiency. Rather, they resemble a warping or twisting of the facial skeleton. This is difficult to discern on physical examination or plain x-rays, but becomes obvious with three-dimensional CT imaging. CT data also allow fabrication of models. These models are useful for planning (Fig. 10.25) or fabrication of custom implants.

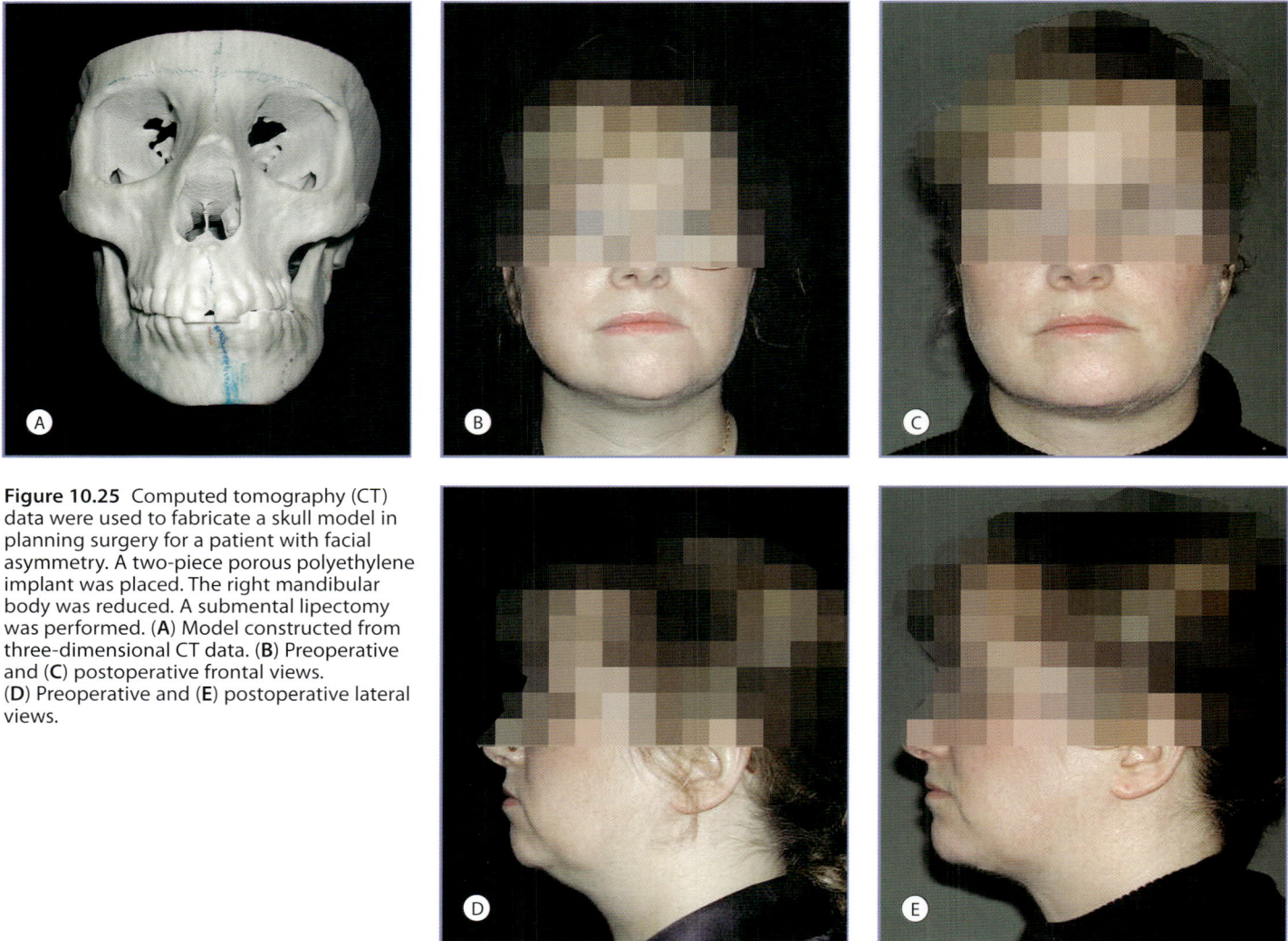

Figure 10.25 Computed tomography (CT) data were used to fabricate a skull model in planning surgery for a patient with facial asymmetry. A two-piece porous polyethylene implant was placed. The right mandibular body was reduced. A submental lipectomy was performed. (**A**) Model constructed from three-dimensional CT data. (**B**) Preoperative and (**C**) postoperative frontal views. (**D**) Preoperative and (**E**) postoperative lateral views.

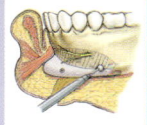

SECONDARY SURGERY

In my experience, and similar to Zide's,[23] most patients presenting for additional surgery had implants placed through an intraoral approach. Some of these patients have problems related to mentalis dysfunction, which includes lower lip descent with increased lower incisor show, a deep sulcus, and often chin pad ptosis. Correction of these deformities requires resuspension of the mentalis—a technically demanding procedure (Fig. 10.26).

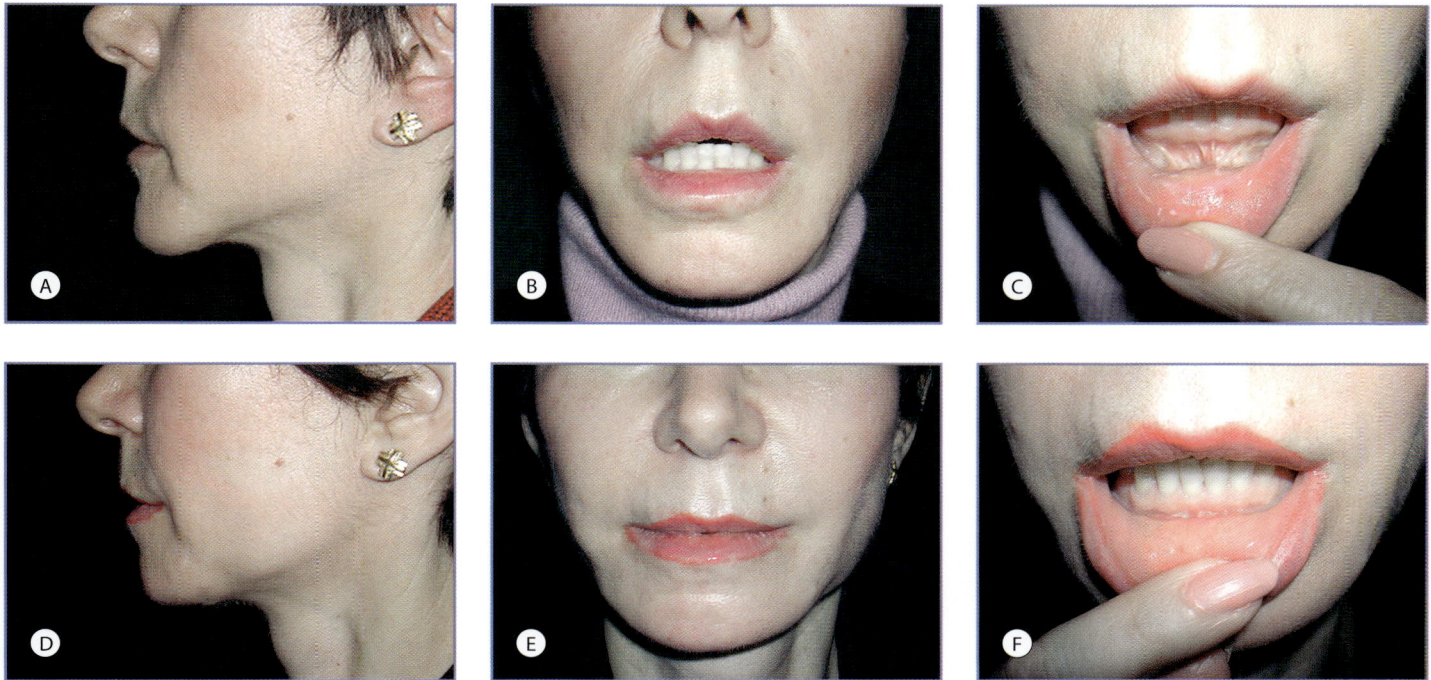

Figure 10.26 A patient exhibiting deformity due to mentalis muscle damage. (**A**) Chin pad ptosis. (**B**) Lower lip descent. (**C**) Deep sulcus due to loss of mentalis continuity or detachment. (**D**) Corrected chin ptosis. (**E**) Restored lip posture. (**F**) Restored sulcus.

My preference is to totally free the chin in a subperiosteal plane to a point above the lowered sulcus. A Mitek (Mitek Worldwide, Norwood, Massachusetts) anchor is then placed between the tooth roots and is used as a post to attach the elevated chin pad, which is purchased on its posterior surface with figure-of-eight sutures. This requires a submental approach for exposure, and often a small intraoral approach to allow suture tying. The chin must have enough projection to support the elevated chin pad. If projection is inadequate, chin augmentation is required.

Most often, patients complain of implant asymmetry—particularly with extended implants, implant malposition, and poor implant to native mandible transition—usually due to large button implant (Fig. 10.14). These deformities may be exaggerated over time in patients with thin skin as the soft tissues contract over smooth-surfaced implants. The bone erosion that is inevitable beneath smooth implants is usually not clinically apparent but may complicate revisional surgery.

Revisional surgery requires implant removal and replacement with an appropriately sized, shaped, and positioned implant. Removal of a smooth-surfaced implant often reveals a distorted soft tissue envelope. The distortion will worsen with time due to ongoing soft tissue contraction forces. This distortion can be lessened if the soft tissue envelope is redraped over another implant. If a smooth implant is removed, soft tissue contraction deformity may arise from progression of the soft tissue contraction process initiated by this smooth implant. For this reason, placing a smaller implant to limit this process is advocated (Figs 10.27 and 10.28).

<table>
<tr><td>**PEARL**</td></tr>
<tr><td>If a smooth implant is removed, place a smaller implant to limit the soft tissue contraction deformity.</td></tr>
</table>

<table>
<tr><td>**PEARL**</td></tr>
<tr><td>Skeletal contour is much easier to control than soft tissue contour.</td></tr>
</table>

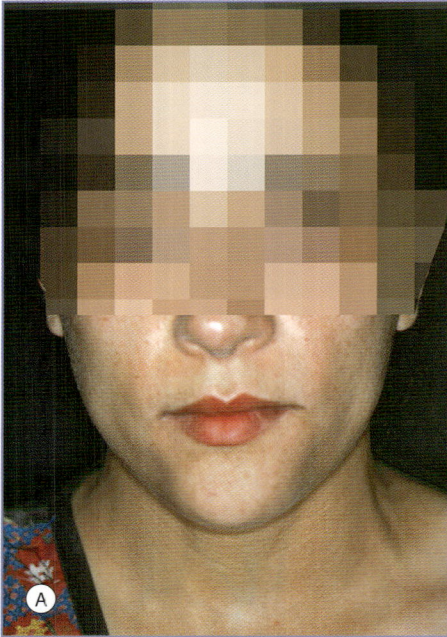

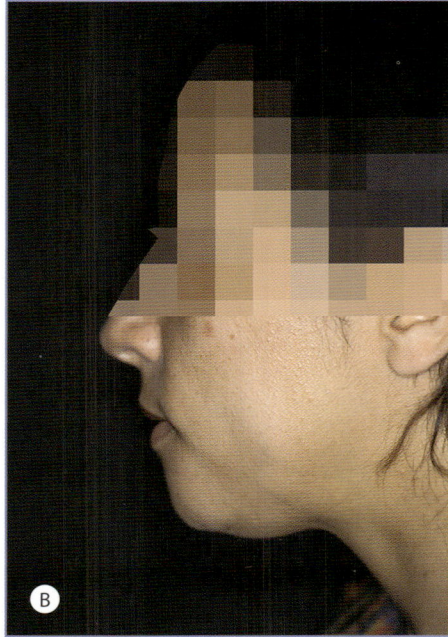

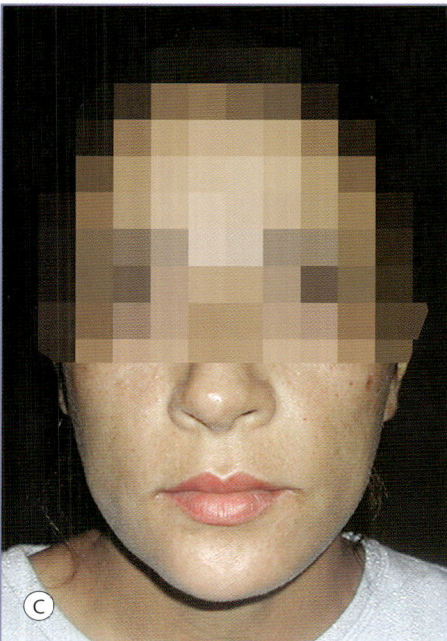

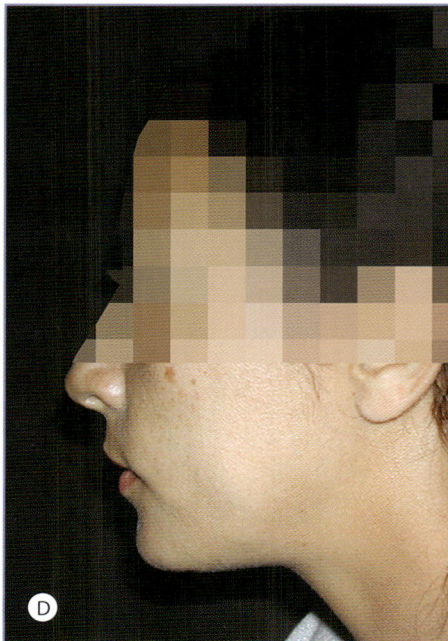

Figure 10.27 A 36-year-old woman presented 17 years after previous smooth silicone chin implant placement. She was displeased with the asymmetry and unnatural appearance of her chin. Through a submental approach, the silicone implant was removed. It was replaced with a two-piece porous polyethylene implant fixed with screws. A submental lipectomy was performed. (**A** and **B**) Preoperative frontal and lateral views. (**C–E**) Postoperative frontal, lateral, and oblique views. Note that despite the replacement with a symmetrically positioned and immobilized implant, asymmetry, although less, persists. This is due to the soft tissue distortion caused by the contraction process encapsulating the malpositioned original implant.

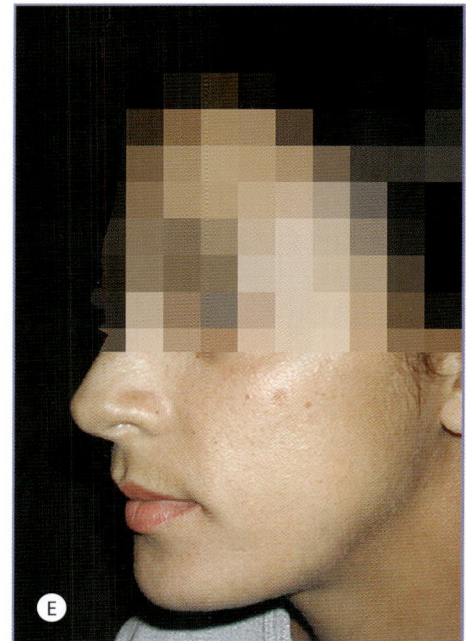

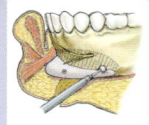

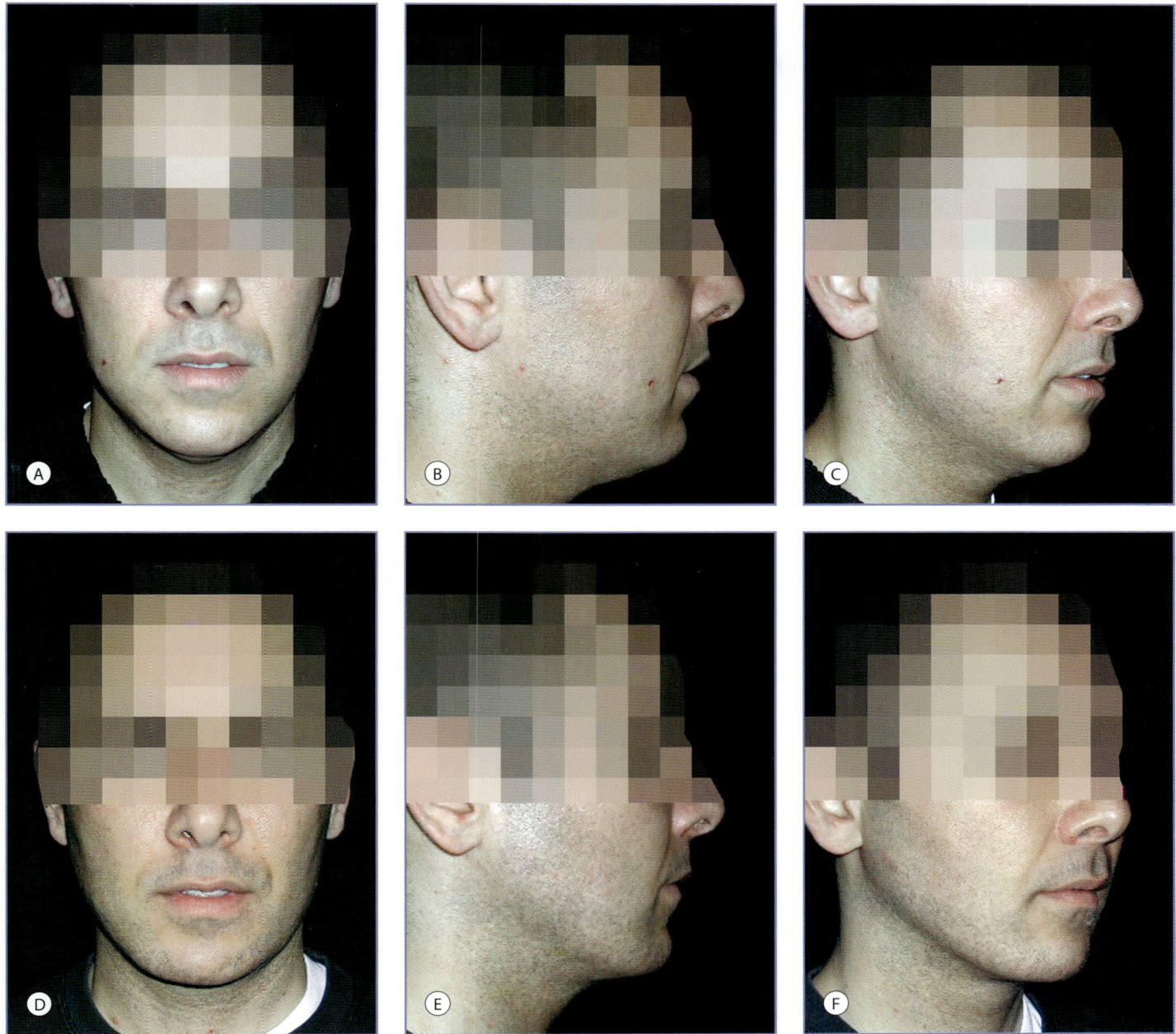

Figure 10.28 A 32-year-old man had chin augmentation performed 10 years earlier. He was displeased with the unnatural contour. The silicone chin implant was removed, and a 7-mm porous polyethylene implant was placed and a submental lipectomy performed. (**A–C**) Preoperative frontal, lateral, and oblique views. (**D–F**) Postoperative frontal, lateral, and oblique views.

SLIDING GENIOPLASTY

Sliding genioplasty involves a horizontal osteotomy of the mandible just beneath the mental foramen. A now freed chin point is positioned as desired, usually anteriorly to increase chin projection but theoretically it can be moved in any direction. Sliding genioplasty is usually performed through an intraoral incision, although I prefer the submental approach. Strap muscles are left attached to the distal bone segment to preserve the vascularity of the free segment. Most often, the distal segment is immobilized in its new position with plates and screws.

The procedure's main advantage over implant augmentation of the chin is its ability to increase the vertical height of the chin. The space between the mandible and the repositioned segment is maintained by filling it with a bone graft or an alloplastic implant. Another advantage of horizontal osteotomy is that when the chin point is advanced, the suprahyoid muscles are put on a stretch, therefore decreasing submental fullness and improving submental contour (Fig. 10.29).

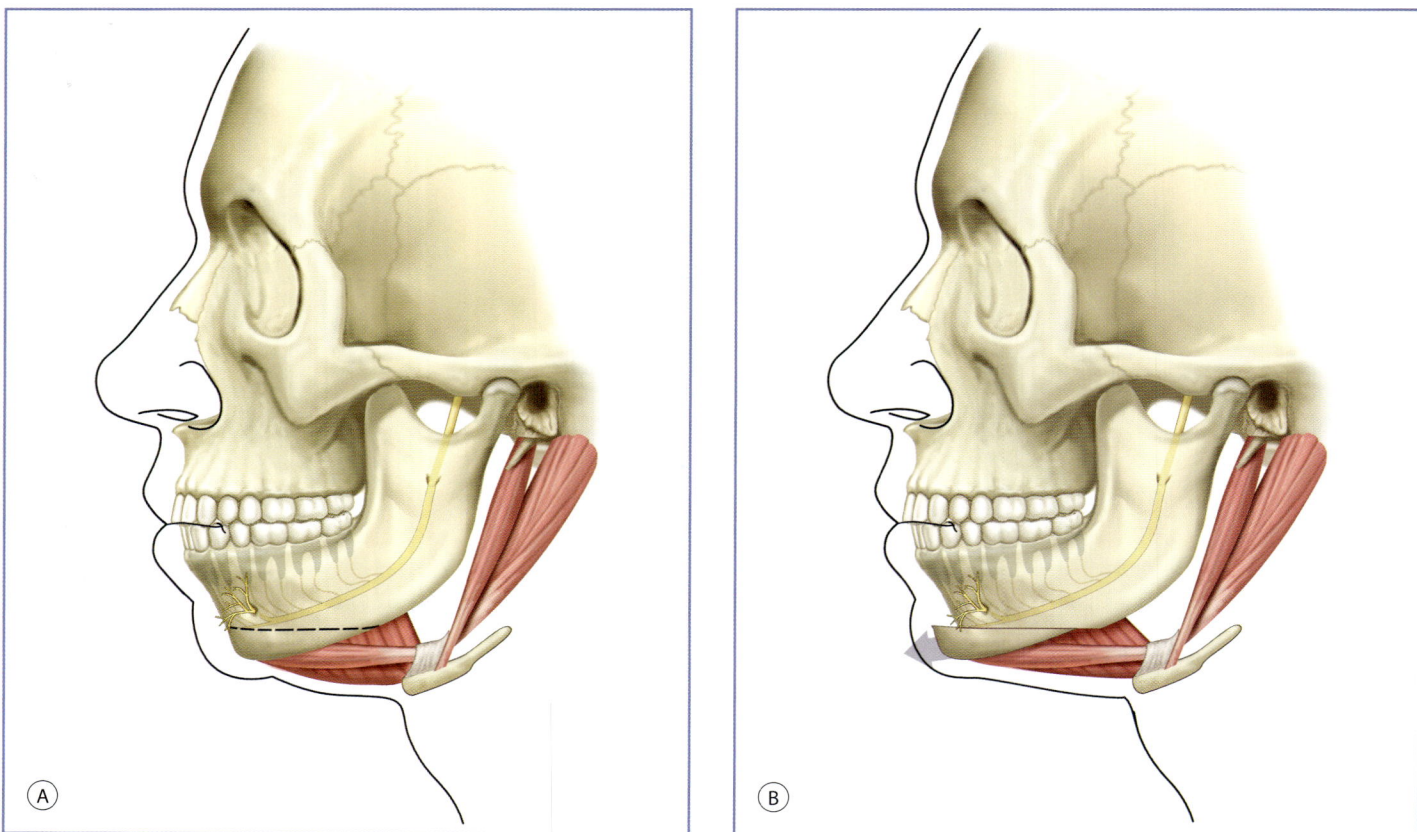

Figure 10.29 Advancement osteotomy of chin results in tightening of the suprahyoid muscles and may decrease submental fullness. (**A**) Before osteotomy. (**B**) After osteotomy and advancement. Note indentation at the osteotomy site along the mandible border.

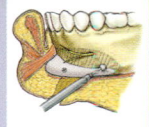

Disadvantages of sliding genioplasty include risk of mentalis muscle damage when performed through an intraoral incision, and possible trauma to and even division of the mental nerve during osteotomy. These problems are avoidable with proper technique. The inevitable disadvantage that is intrinsic to sliding genioplasty is the unnatural body and border contours that accompany the selective movement of the chin point. The contour that results is one that has a poor transition, resulting in a stuck-on appearance of the chin much like a large button implant, as well as the step-off at the site of osteotomy along the mandibular body (Figs 10.29 and 10.30). The notching or indentation is especially detrimental to those who have a preexisting prejowl sulcus. Furthermore, sliding genioplasty requires considerable facility in bone carpentry. Obliquity in the horizontal osteotomy can either lengthen or shorten the vertical height of the chin post advancement. Free segment malposition or improper fixation can lead to obvious asymmetries.

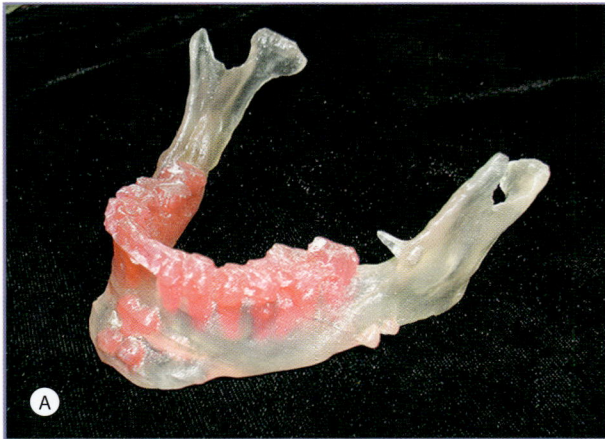

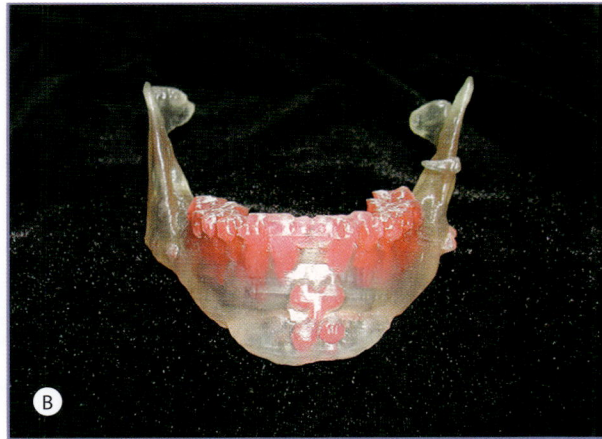

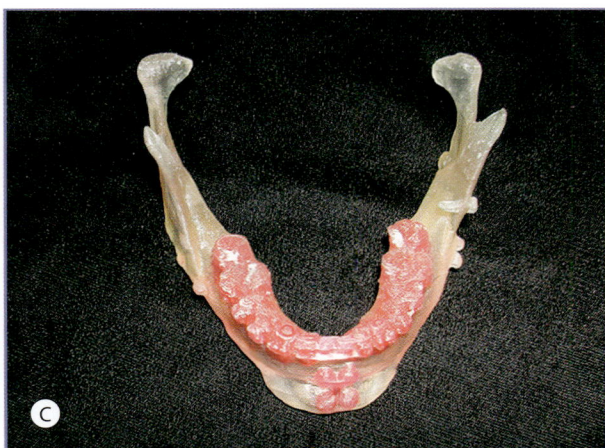

Figure 10.30 Acrylic model made from computed tomography data of a patient who had undergone sliding genioplasty and sagittal split osteotomy. It demonstrates a poor transition between the advanced chin segment and mandible, as well as indentation along the mandible border at osteotomy sites.

After sliding genioplasty

The mandibular border step-off deformity (notch), and to some extent the lack of transition with the repositioned chin, can be corrected with implants. Custom-carved implants can be placed through submental and lateral sulcus incisions to fill these depressions. Implants are fixed with screws. It is critical to feather all transitions between the implant and native mandible. A patient who had this surgery is presented in Figure 10.31.

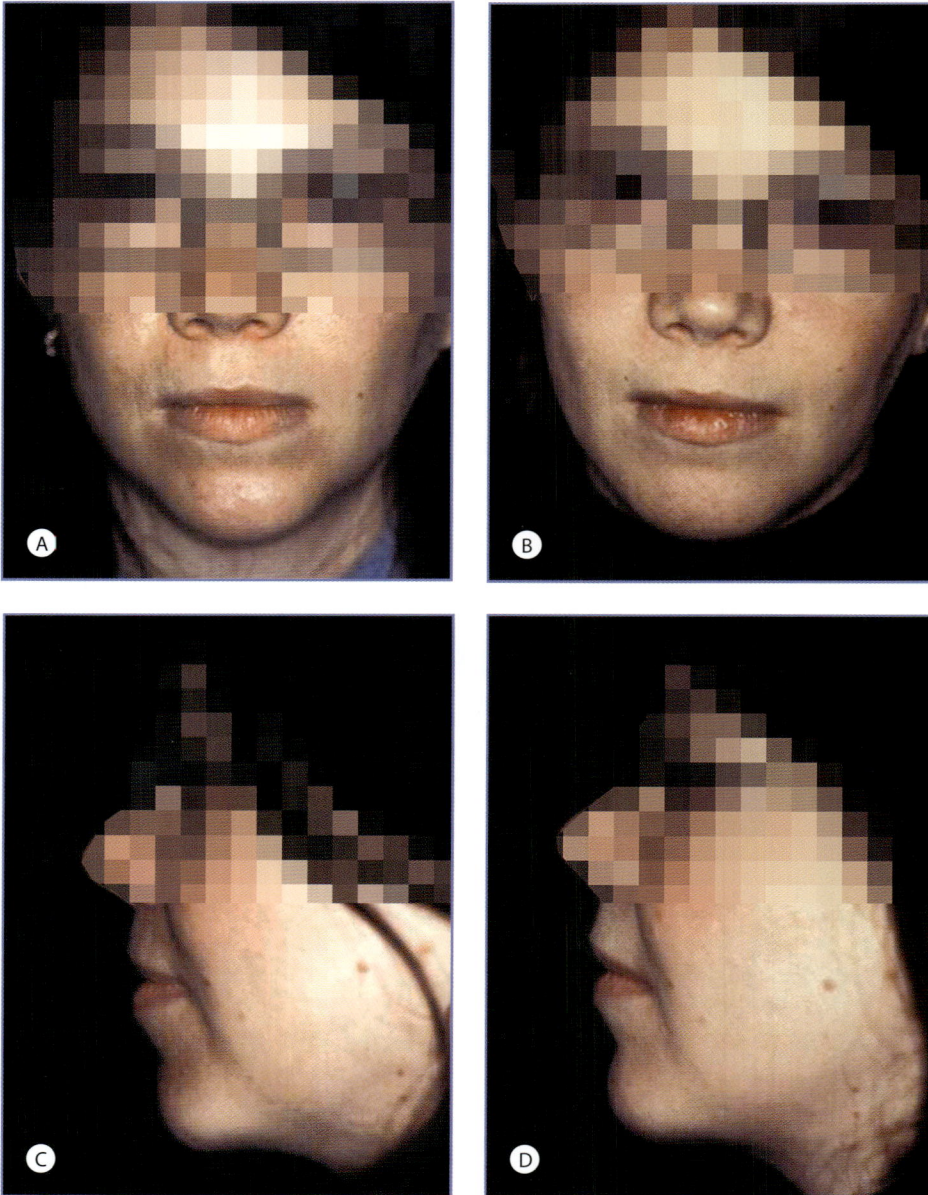

Figure 10.31 A 32-year-old woman was displeased with the notch deformities after sliding genioplasty. The indentation was filled with a custom-contoured porous polyethylene implant placed through intraoral and submental incisions. (**A**) Preoperative and (**B**) postoperative frontal views. (**C**) Preoperative and (**D**) postoperative lateral views.

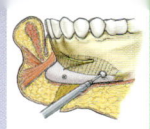

REFERENCES

1. Millard DR. Adjuncts in augmentation mentoplasty and corrective rhinoplasty. Plast Reconstr Surg 1965; 36:48–61.
2. Spear SL, Kassan M. Genioplasty. Clin Plast Surg 1989; 16(4):695–706.
3. Zide BM, Pfeifer TM, Longaker MT. Chin surgery: I. Augmentation—the allures and the alerts. Plast Reconstr Surg 1999; 104(6):1843–1853.
4. Yaremchuk MJ. Improving aesthetic outcomes after alloplastic chin augmentation. Plast Reconstr Surg 2003; 112(5):1422–1432; discussion 1433–1434.
5. Newman J, Dolsky RL, Mai ST. Submental liposuction extraction with hard chin augmentation. Arch Otolaryngol 1984; 11:454.
6. Courtiss EH. Suction lipectomy of the neck. Plast Reconstr Surg 1985; 76(6):882–889.
7. Farkas LG, Hreczko TA, Katic MJ. Appendix A. Craniofacial norms in North American Caucasians from birth (one year) to adulthood. In: Farkas LG, ed. Anthropometry of the head and face. 2nd edn. New York: Raven Press; 1994.
8. Steiner CC. Cephalometrics in clinical practice. Angle Orthod 1959; 29:8.
9. Hambleton RS. Tissue covering of the skeletal face as related to orthodontic problems. Am J Orthod 1964; 50:405.
10. Burstone CJ. Lip posture and its significance in treatment planning. Am J Orthod 1967; 53(4):262–284.
11. Ricketts RM. Esthetics, environment and the law of lip relation. Am J Orthod 1968; 54(4):272–289.
12. Legan HL, Burstone CJ. Soft tissue cephalometric analysis for orthognathic surgery. J Oral Surg 1980; 38(1):744–751.
13. Flowers RS. Alloplastic augmentation of the anterior mandible. Clin Plast Surg 1991; 18:107–137.
14. McCarthy JG, Ruff GL. The chin. Clin Plast Surg 1988; 15(1):125–137.
15. Farkas LG, Sohm P, Kolar JC, et al. Inclinations of the facial profile: art versus reality. Plast Reconstr Surg 1985; 75(4):509–519.
16. Gonzalez-Ulloa M. Quantitative principles in cosmetic surgery of the face (profileplasty). Plast Reconstr Surg 1962; 29:186–198.
17. Gonzalez-Ulloa M, Stevens E. The role of chin correction in profileplasty. Plast Reconstr Surg 1968; 41(5):477–486.
18. Yaremchuk MJ. Mandibular augmentation. Plast Reconstr Surg 2000; 106:697–706.
19. Dann JJ, Epker BM. Proplast genioplasty: a retrospective study with treatment recommendations. Angle Orthod 1977; 47(3):173–185.
20. Moenning JE, Wolford LM. Chin augmentation with various alloplastic materials: a comparative study. Int J Adult Orthodon Orthognath Surg 1989; 4(3):175–187.
21. Karas SC, Wolford LM. Augmentation genioplasty with hard tissues replacement implants. J Oral Maxillofac Surg 1981; 11:912.
22. Michelow BJ, Guyuron B. The chin: skeletal and soft tissue components. Plast Reconstr Surg 1993; 95:473–478.
23. Zide BM. The mentalis muscle: an essential component of chin and lower lip position. Plast Reconstr Surg 1989; 83(3):413–420.
24. Terino EO. Alloplastic contouring in the malar–mid-face–middle third facial aesthetic unit. In: Terino EO, Flowers RS, eds. The art of alloplastic facial contouring. St. Louis: Mosby; 2000.

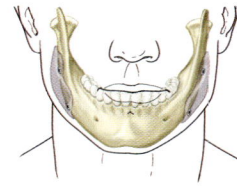

Chapter 11

Mandible

INDICATIONS

Three groups of patients benefit from implant augmentation of the mandibular body, angle, and ramus. These include patients with normal, deficient, or surgically altered anatomy.

Normal dimensions

Most patients who desire mandible augmentation have lower face horizontal dimensions that relate to the upper and middle thirds of the face within a normal range (Figs 11.1 and 11.2).[1]

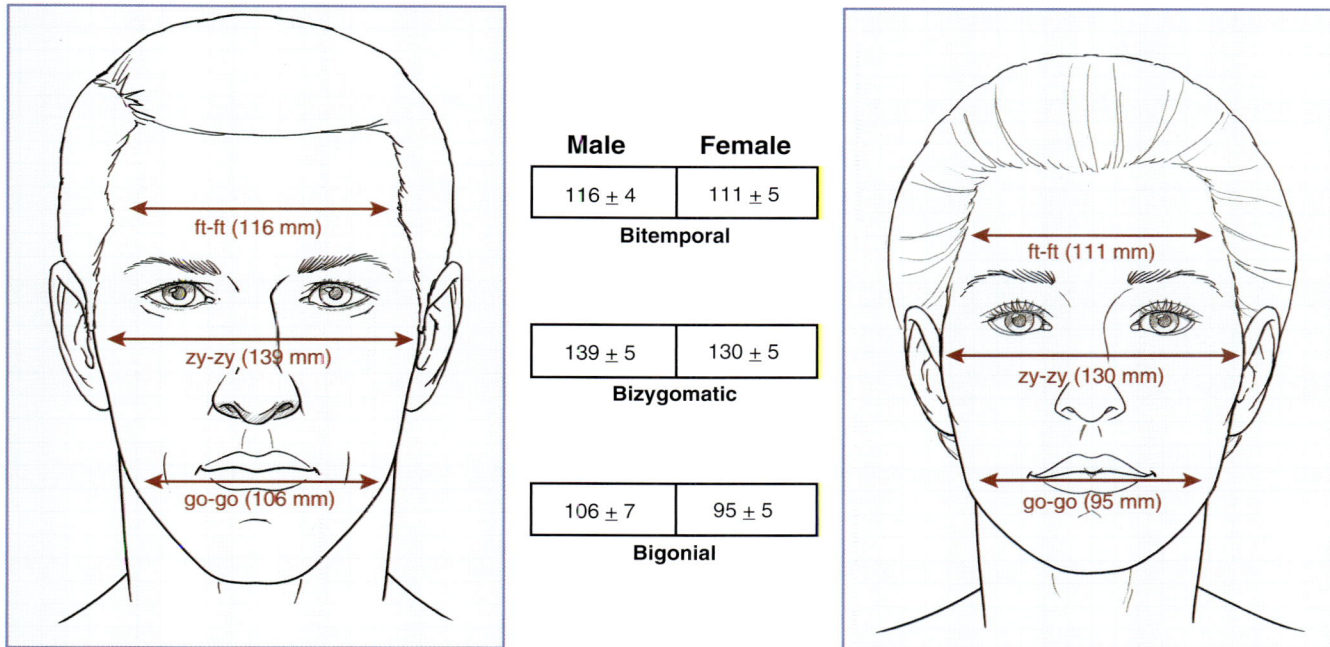

	Male	Female
Bitemporal	116 ± 4	111 ± 5
Bizygomatic	139 ± 5	130 ± 5
Bigonial	106 ± 7	95 ± 5

Figure 11.1 Normal values (mm) for upper, middle, and lower facial width in North American white adult men (ages 19–25) ($n = 109$) and young adult women ($n = 200$).[1] Bitemporal distance (ft–ft) is measured from frontotemporal (ft) to frontotemporal, which is the point on each side of the forehead laterally from the elevation of the linea temporalis. Bizygomatic distance (zy–zy) is measured from zygion (zy) to zygion, which is the most lateral point of each zygomatic arch. The bigonial distance (go–go) is measured from gonion (go) to gonion, which is the most lateral point of the mandibular angle close to the bony gonion. Note that the male lower face is both relatively and absolutely wider than that of the female.

197

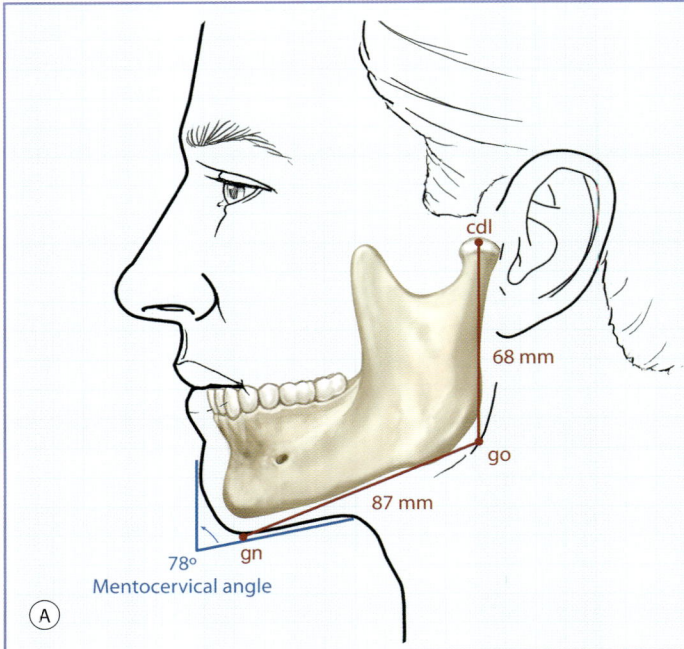

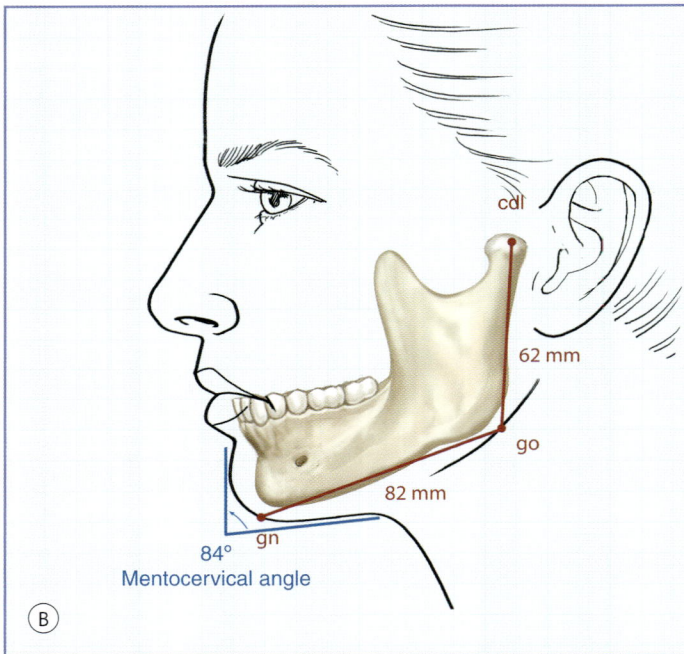

Figure 11.2 Normal values for mentocervical angle, height of the mandible ramus (go–cdl), and depth of the lower face (go–gn) in North American white adult men (ages 19–25) (**A**) and young adult women (**B**).[1] Menton (or gnathion) (gn) is the lowest median landmark on the lower border of the mandible. It is identified by palpation and is identical to the bony gnathion. Condylion laterale (cdl) is the most lateral point on the surface of the condyle of the mandible. It is identified by palpation at each temporomandibular joint when the jaw is open. The gonion (go) is the most lateral point of the mandibular angle close to the bony gonion. The mentocervical angle is formed by the upper contour of the chin and the surface beneath the mandible.

These patients, usually men, perceive a wider lower face as desirable. This group benefits from implants designed to augment the ramus and posterior body of the mandible, and in so doing increase the bigonial distance. Other patients desire more definition and angularity to the mandibular border. Implants that augment the anterior mandible back to the ramus can achieve this.

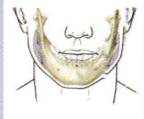

Skeletal deficiency

Another group of patients who benefit from mandible augmentation are those with skeletal mandibular deficiency (Fig. 11.3).[2] It has been estimated that approximately 5% of the total US population has skeletal mandibular deficiency resulting in a class II occlusal problem. The majority of these patients (approximately 80%) can have their dental relationships normalized through orthodontic tooth movement. The remaining 20%, or 1% of the total population, have mandibular deficiency that is so severe that surgical mandibular advancement would be needed to correct it.[2]

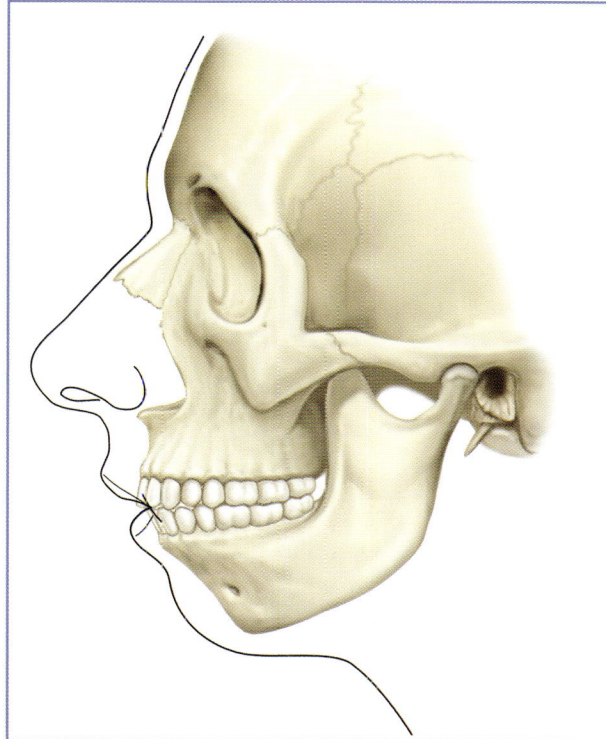

Figure 11.3 Soft tissue contour and skeletal configuration of a patient with mandibular deficiency and corrected occlusion. Note the obtuse mandibular and mentocervical angles, with steep mandibular plane.

The classic method of correcting class II dental malocclusion in patients with significant mandibular deficiency, in addition to preoperative and postoperative orthodontic treatment, includes sagittal split ramus osteotomy and sliding advancement genioplasty, with possible LeFort I maxillary impaction. This combination of procedures can provide a class I dental relationship while normalizing the skeletal contour. In patients with mandibular deficiency who have had their malocclusion corrected through orthodontics alone, mandibular osteotomy would disturb these dental relationships, requiring extensive perioperative orthodontic treatment. This type of treatment is both costly and time-consuming. Alloplastic augmentation of the mandible can provide a visual effect similar, and in my opinion superior, to that of sagittal osteotomy with advancement, employing an outpatient surgical procedure that avoids any further dental manipulation.

The anatomy associated with mandibular deficiency, which can be camouflaged with implants, includes the obtuse mandible angle with steep mentocervical angle, as well as the decreased vertical (gonion–condylion laterale) and transverse ramus (gonion–gnathion) dimensions. The addition of an extended chin implant will camouflage the poorly projecting chin.

Surgically altered anatomy

A third group of patients who may benefit from alloplastic augmentation of the mandible are patients who have had their class II dental malocclusion due to mandibular deficiency corrected by sagittal split osteotomy with advancement of the distal segment. This procedure splits or separates the tooth-bearing symphysis and adjacent bodies from the non-tooth-bearing but articulating rami. Requisites for positioning the resultant anterior and posterior segments to improve occlusion, allow bone healing, and continue joint function may result in displeasing postoperative contour. The advancement of the distal, or tooth-bearing, segment is dictated by occlusal relations. It inevitably creates a contour irregularity at the site of the body osteotomy and distal segment advancement. This area of narrowing may be visible, and even disfiguring, in certain individuals. Positioning of the posterior segment requires that the condyle be seated in the glenoid fossa, and that there be sufficient segment contact to allow bone healing. Fulfillment of these requisites dictates the position of the ramus and its angle. This may result in an aesthetically displeasing position of the ramus angle, with insufficient height, insufficient width, or asymmetry (Fig. 11.4). Mandible implants can be used to improve contour in these patients.[3]

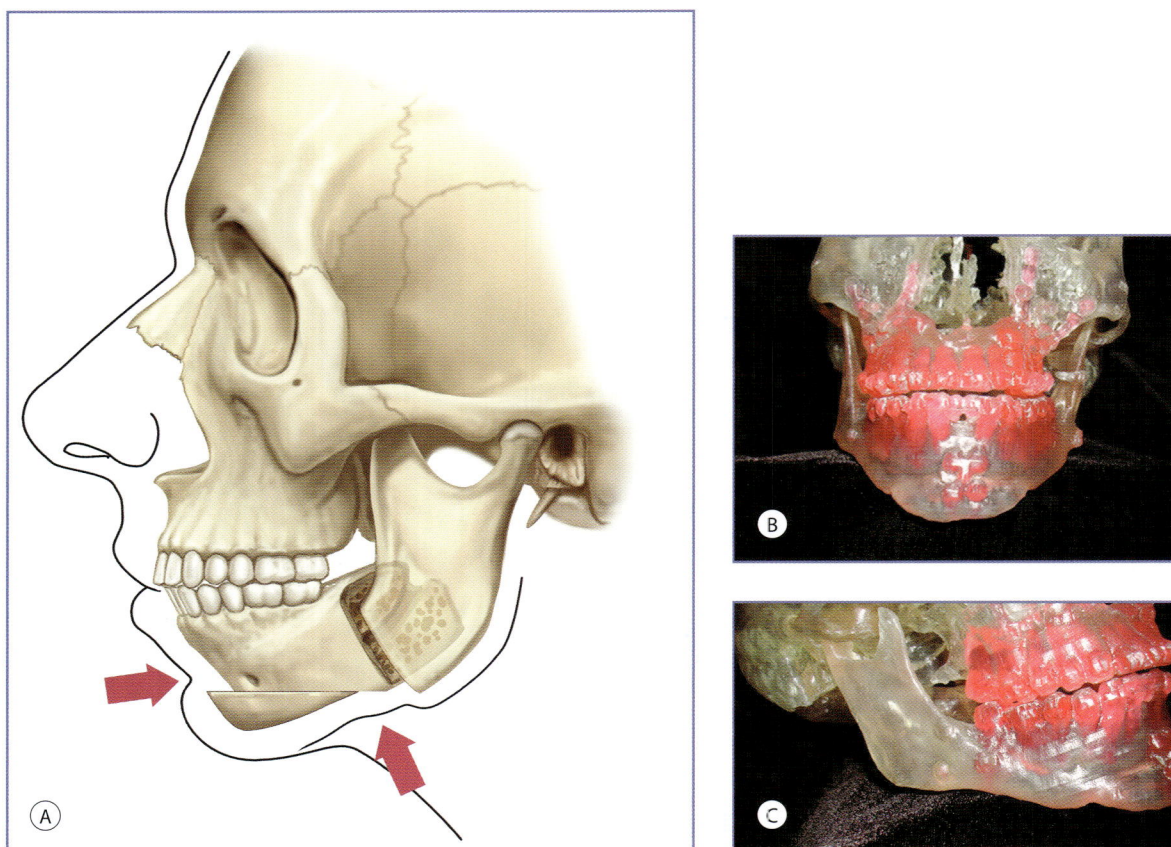

Figure 11.4 Skeletal contour after sagittal split osteotomy and advancement of distal segment, as well as sliding advancement genioplasty of deficient mandible. Note that there is an indentation along the mandibular border at the sites of osteotomy and advancement. (**A**) Artist's depiction. Arrows point to the contour irregularity along the mandibular border at the site of osteotomy. (**B**) Acrylic model obtained from computed tomographic scan data of a patient who had undergone sagittal split and horizontal maxillary osteotomies. Note contour irregularities along the mandibular border. Note also the asymmetries in posterior segment position. These will lead to discrepancies in lower face width and height.

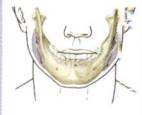

Beware of overaugmenting the normal-shaped but aging mandible to reinflate the aging soft tissue envelope. Unless the patient is edentulous, the amount of bone loss is not great, and implant augmentation risks the result of distorted dimensions with undesirable looks. The result is an oversized mandible, especially in women. One should also be aware that the external appearance obtained with augmenting the skeleton is different from that obtained by augmenting the soft tissues. Skeletal augmentation increases bony projection and provides angularity. Soft tissue augmentation lessens the transmission of the underlying skeleton by increasing the thickness of its overlying envelope. Soft tissue augmentation may increase prominence but decreases angularity.

Mandibular body and ramus augmentation in women with normal-dimensioned mandibles risks masculinization of the patient's appearance. The anthropometric measurements provided by Farkas (Fig. 11.1) help in understanding our visual interpretation of male and female patients with normal mandibular morphology and dimensions who undergo mandibular augmentation.[1] These data show that all transverse facial dimensions are greater in men than in women, and that the bigonial distance is the transverse facial dimension that has the greatest difference between sexes. In other words, the lower one-third of women's faces tends to be absolutely and relatively narrower than that of men. Hence, when normal male mandibles undergo augmentation, they may be perceived as stronger. However, when normal female mandibles undergo augmentation, they may be perceived as masculinized.

EVALUATION AND PLANNING

Physical examination

Physical examination is the most important element in preoperative assessment and planning. Reviewing life-sized posteroanterior and lateral photographs with the patient can be helpful when discussing aesthetic concerns and goals. To allow the patient to understand the scale and scope of augmentation, it is useful to have sample implants available to demonstrate on a model skull and to apply these implants to the relevant area of the patient's face.

X-rays

Posteroanterior and lateral cephalograms provide data that help the surgeon determine how the dimension of the implant might be altered to best suit the patient. Three-dimensional computed tomographic scans and the models obtained from their data can be invaluable when attempting to correct asymmetries associated with congenital, posttraumatic, or postsurgical deformities.

In general, however, the size and position of the implant are largely aesthetic judgments. An approximately 1:1 ratio of augmentation to resultant projection is anticipated.

PEARL

Skeletal augmentation provides a different visual effect to that of soft tissue augmentation.

PEARL

Aggressive augmentation of the female mandible risks its masculinization.

201

SURGICAL ANATOMY

Skeleton

The mandible consists of the tooth-bearing body and the ramus that extends upward from the angle. The ramus, including the angle, is covered on its external surface by the masseter muscle. The gonion is the tip of the outer surface of the angle. The outer surface of the angle may be embellished by a masseteric tuberosity denoting the insertion of the masseter muscle. (Its inner surface may be raised by a pterygoid tuberosity where the medial pterygoid muscle inserts.) The upper aspect of the ramus ends posteriorly in a condylar process, and anteriorly in a coronoid process separated by the mandibular notch.

The oblique line runs forward and downward from the anterior border of the ramus. It affords attachment for the depressor labii inferioris and depressor anguli oris. The platysma is attached near the inferior border of the mandible. The buccinator muscle is attached to the outer lip of the superior border of the mandible as far forward as the first molar tooth. The mental foramen lies approximately at the interspace between the two premolars, and about midway in the height of the dentulous adult mandible. As the body proceeds anteriorly toward the midline, it swells out to form the mental protuberance (Fig. 11.5A).

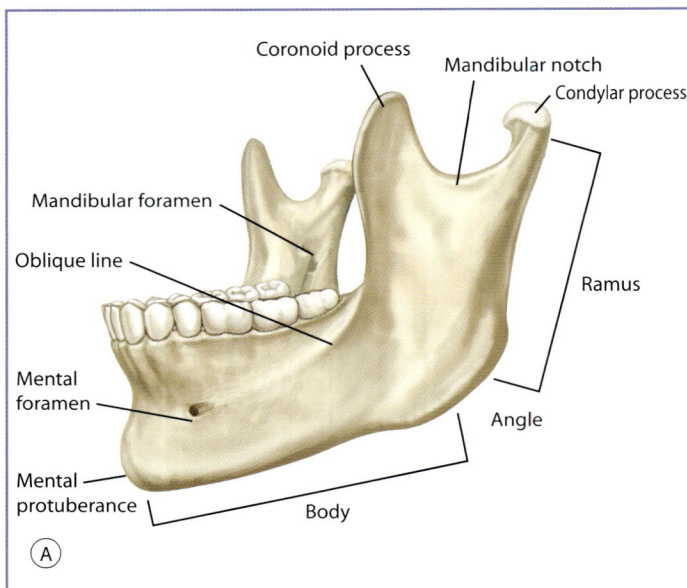

Figure 11.5 (**A**) Mandible anatomy. Surface topography.

Musculature

There are four muscles predominantly responsible for the movement of the mandible: the masseter, the temporal, the medial pterygoid, and the lateral pterygoid. Only the masseter and indirectly the medial pterygoid, as part of the mandibular sling, are encountered during mandibular augmentation. The masseter muscle consists of superficial and deep portions. The larger superficial portion arises from the zygomatic process of the maxilla and from the anterior two-thirds of the inferior border of the zygomatic arch. Its fibers pass inferiorly and posteriorly to insert into the angle and inferior half of the lateral surface of the ramus of the mandible. The masseter and the medial pterygoid muscle are so positioned that they form a sling around the inferior border of the mandible, and therefore suspend the angle of the mandible.

When placing a mandibular angle implant, it is necessary to separate the superficial portion of the masseter and its sling component from the mandible in a subperiosteal plane. Tearing the periosteum at the inferior border may disrupt the sling mechanism and allow the freed masseter to ride up, causing a depression in the soft tissues overlying the angle. This depression is exaggerated when the muscle is contracted. The smaller, deep portion of the masseter arises from the posterior third of the inferior border and from the whole of the medial surface of the zygomatic arch. This portion of the muscle passes anteriorly and inferiorly to insert into the superior half of the ramus and the lateral surface of the coronoid process (Fig. 11.5B).

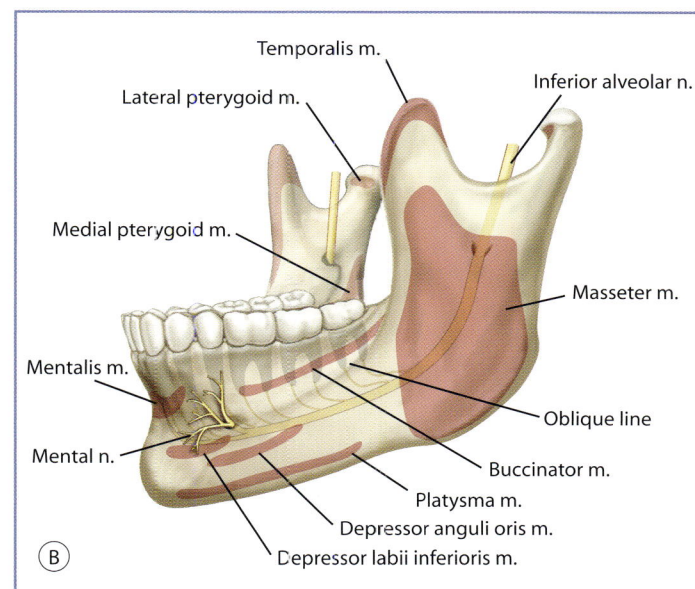

Figure 11.5 (*Cont'd*) (**B**) Muscle origins and insertions.

The buccinator is another muscle that is encountered during exposure of the mandible during mandibular augmentation. The buccinator is the principal muscle of the cheek. It forms the lateral wall of the oral cavity. It occupies the area between the mandible and the maxilla, and originates in part from both structures. It originates from the outer surface of the alveolar processes of the maxilla above and the mandible below, adjacent to their three molar teeth. The other origin of this quadrilateral muscle is the pterygomandibular raphe, which stretches from the medial pterygoid process to the inner surface of the mandible. Its fibers pass forward to become continuous with the orbicularis oris.

Inferior alveolar nerve

The inferior alveolar nerve is a branch of the mandibular nerve (V3). It enters the mandibular canal with the inferior alveolar vessels through the mandibular foramen, which is located in the inner aspect of the ramus of the mandible approximately halfway between its anterior and posterior borders. It is important to visualize the path of the inferior alveolar nerve when placing screws to immobilize mandibular implants.

IMPLANT DESIGNS

Ramus and body implants are capable of changing the shape of the mandible in three dimensions—bigonial width (gonion–gonion), ramus height (gonion–condylion laterale), and body length (gonion–gnathion)—as well as the inclination of the mandibular border. Figure 11.6 depicts an implant design often used for men who want a wider lower face. These patients benefit from dimension D (the added thickness provided over the ramus and posterior body, which increases bigonial distance or the width of the lower face). Dimensions A and B are sufficient in size to provide a transition with the rest of the mandible appropriate for the amount of dimension D (lower facial width) increase. Note that dimension E remains constant so that the inclination of the mandible does not change, and increases ramus height only slightly. The flange allows the implant to adapt to the mandibular border.

> **PEARL**
>
> Mandibular implants can change the width (transverse dimension), height (vertical dimension), and depth (posterior dimension) of the mandible, as well as the inclination of the mandibular plane.

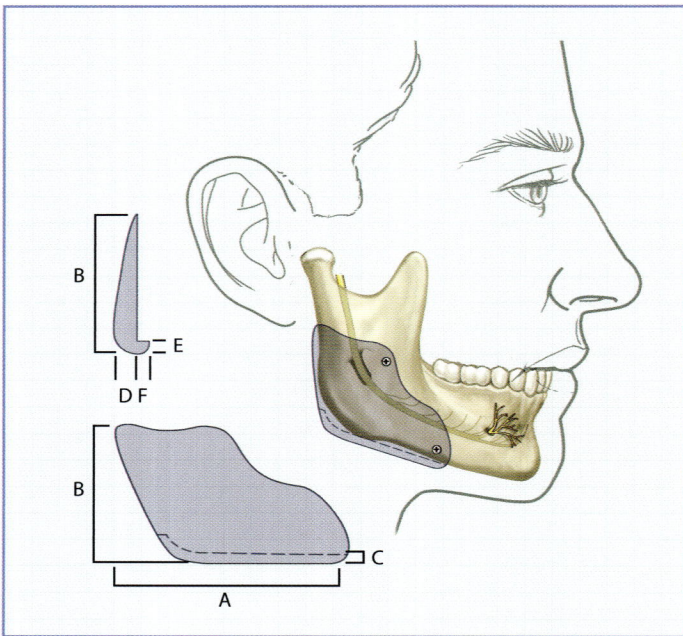

Figure 11.6 Configuration and dimensions of mandibular ramus and posterior body implant used to increase lower facial width. Screw fixation guarantees position and ensures application of implant to skeleton. A = 47 mm, B = 37 mm, C = 3 mm, D = 6.5 mm, and E = 3 mm.

The other implant is used to augment the congenitally deficient mandible. Its dimensions are presented in Figure 11.7. It differs from the other implant in several ways. In addition to augmentation of the ramus and posterior body, its greater length (A) allows it to augment the anterior body of the mandible. It therefore increases not only posterior but also anterior mandibular width. Its tapering projection beyond the inferior edge of the mandible (C and E) allows it to change the inclination of the plane of the mandibular border. Because it also projects beyond the posterior border, in addition to extending beyond the inferior edge of the ramus, it can lessen the obliquity of the mandibular angle. The implant is often used with a chin implant for deficient mandibles.

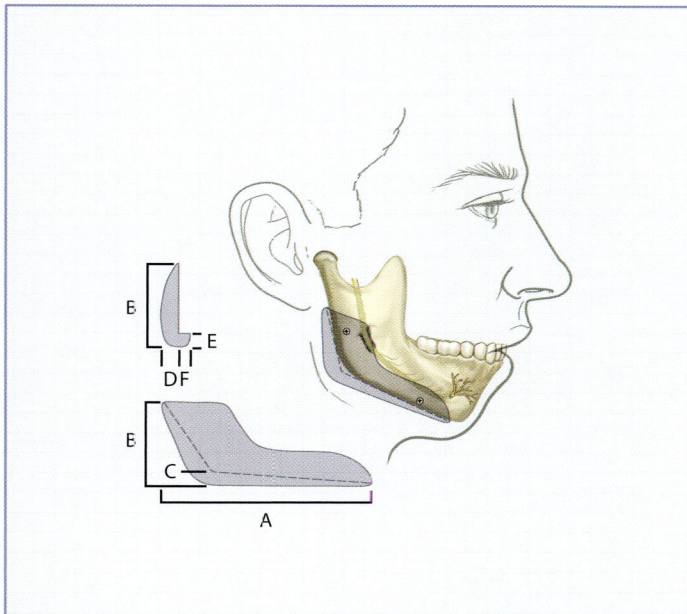

Figure 11.7 Configuration and dimension of mandibular ramus and mandibular body implant used to augment the deficient mandible. Because it extends beyond the posterior border of the ramus and inferior edge of the ramus and body, it closes the mandibular angle and levels the plane of the mandibular border. Screw fixation guarantees position and ensures application of implant to skeleton. A = 79 mm, B = 32 mm, C = 5 or 10 mm, D = 7 mm, and E = 10 mm.

Figure 11.8 shows how a mandibular body and angle implant can be used with the chin implant to augment all dimensions of the congenitally deficient mandible. These implant designs and concepts are developed from the work of Terino,[4,5] Whitaker,[6] Aiche,[7] Taylor and Teenier,[8] and Ramirez,[9] as well as this author.[10]

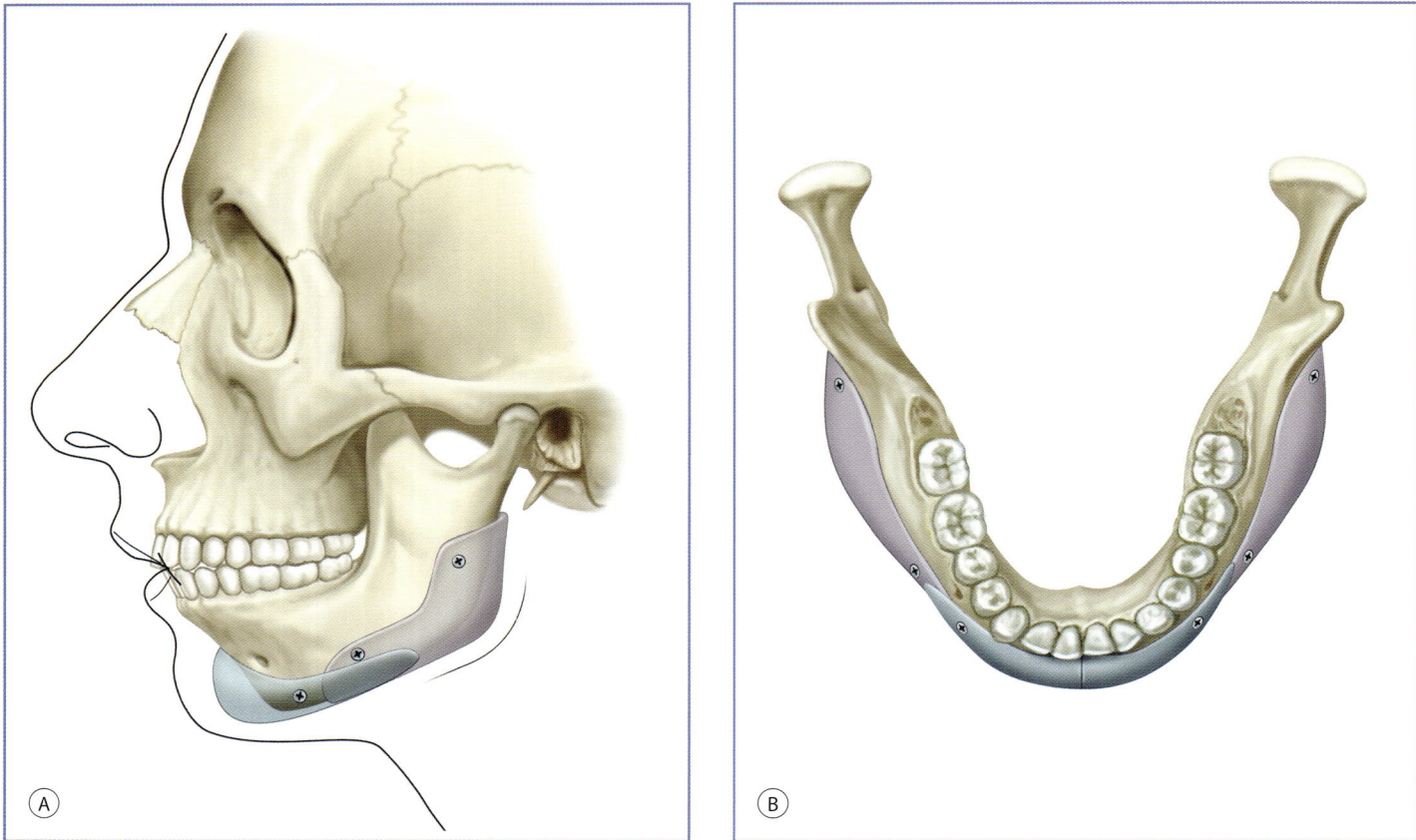

Figure 11.8 Mandibular body and angle implant used in combination with a chin implant. This combination is often used for patients with class 2 mandibular deficiency. (**A**) Lateral and (**B**) axial views.

OPERATIVE TECHNIQUE

Anesthesia

It is my preference to perform chin and mandibular augmentation under general nasotracheal anesthesia. This provides a panoramic view of the operative field. The airway is protected while the oral cavity can be optimally prepared. The face and oral cavity are prepared with an iodine solution after placement of a throat pack. The operative site is infiltrated with 1:200 000 adrenaline (epinephrine) solution to provide hemostasis.

Incisions

A generous intraoral mucosal incision is made to expose the ramus and body of the mandible. It is made at least 1 cm above the sulcus on its labial side (Fig. 11.9). The anterior ramus and body of the mandible are freed from their soft tissues. If the mental area is also being augmented, a submental incision is made for access and exposure of the anterior mandible. The mental nerve is visualized as it exits its foramen, to avoid its injury. It is important to free both the inferior and the posterior borders of the mandible of soft tissue attachments to allow implant placement (Fig. 11.10).

As determined by preoperative assessment, the implant is trimmed with a scalpel or mechanical burr before its placement on the mandible.

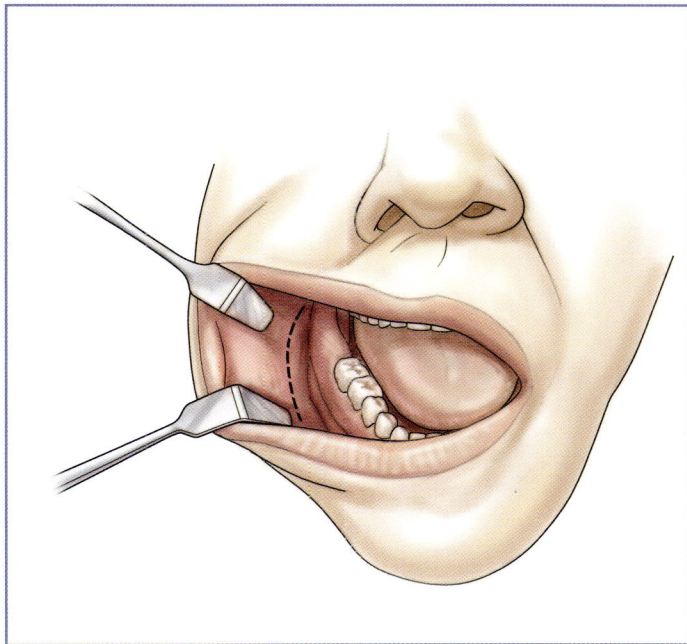

Figure 11.9 An intraoral mucosal incision is made along the ramus and posterior body of the mandible. It is made approximately 1 cm above the sulcus on its labial side.

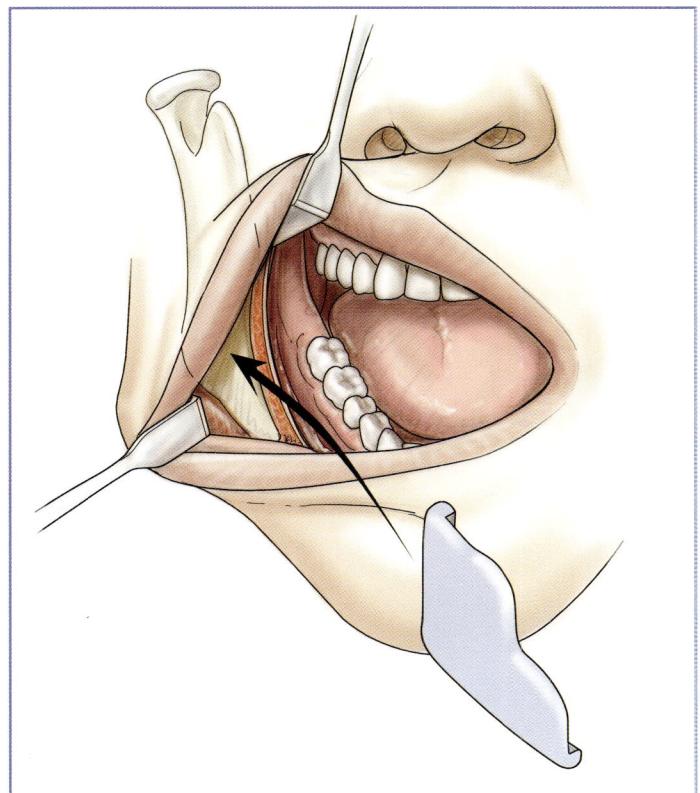

Figure 11.10 Subperiosteal pocket created for placement of a mandibular implant.

Implant positioning

To ensure the desired placement of the implant and its application to the surface of the mandible, the implant is fixed to the mandible with titanium screws. A long guarded drill facilitates screw hole drilling. (As originally described, self-drilling screws were used.[9] However, I abandoned the use of self-drilling screws when I found that the thick cortex of the mandible often made screw penetration difficult). With vigorous retraction, implant fixation can be done through the intraoral incision (Fig. 11.11).

An implant used to augment only the mandibular border may have insufficient vertical height to allow screw placement from the intraoral approach. In this case, when screw fixation is deemed critical, stab wound incisions (2–3 mm in length) are made in the neck skin beneath the inferior border of the mandible. A trocar and sheath can be used to protect the skin from the drill and screw placement. This allows strategic unicortical screw fixation of the implant to the mandible (Fig. 11.12).

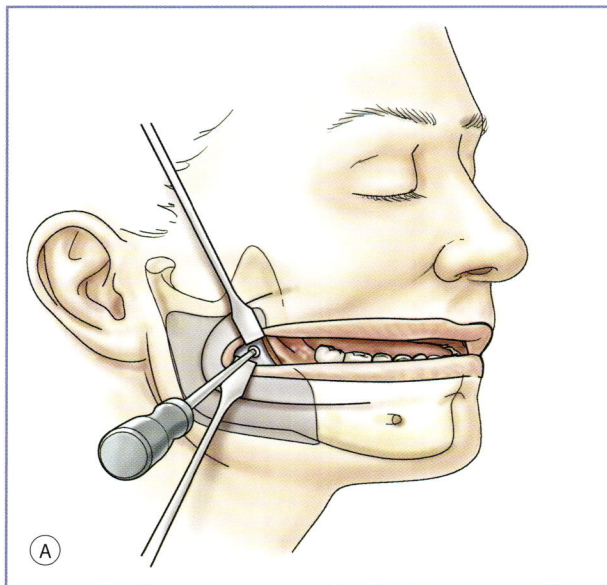

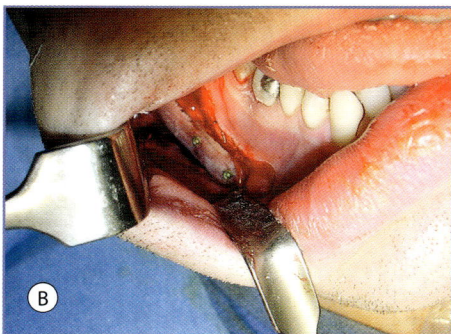

(A)

(B)

Figure 11.11 Screw fixation of the implant to the mandible through an intraoral approach. (**A**) Artist's depiction. (**B**) Clinical photograph during mandibular augmentation. The lower lip is being retracted. The portion of the implant augmenting the mandibular body is being exposed. Note screw fixation.

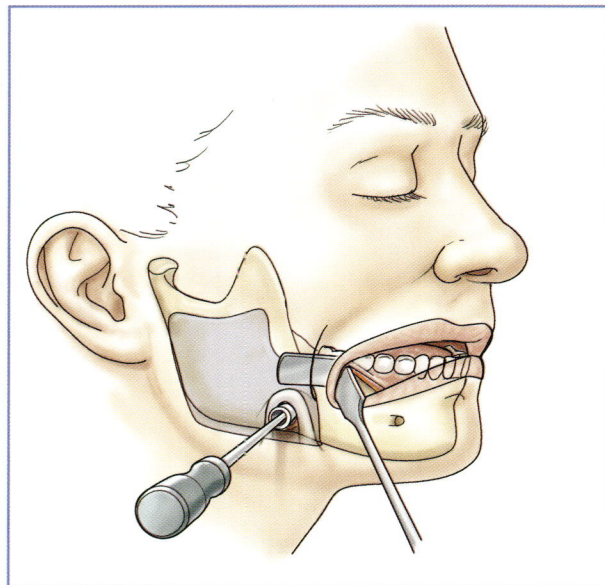

Figure 11.12 Screw fixation of the implant to the mandible through an extraoral approach. A stab wound incision is made in the neck skin and telescoped superiorly to allow axial drilling of the screw hole and screw fixation of the implant.

Usually, two or three screws are used to obliterate any gaps between the mandible and the implant (Fig. 11.13). Screws are placed to avoid the anticipated path of the inferior alveolar nerve before its exit from the mental foramen. Gaps may also arise when there are significant prominences on the surface of the mandible. This is often the case at the oblique line of the mandible body. Reduction of these prominences allows the posterior surface of the implant to be congruent with the anterior surface of the implant, thereby avoiding gaps.

It is crucial to soften any transitions between the implant and the mandible, particularly where the implant extends beyond the anterior mandibular border's inferior edge. Any step-offs between the implant and the mandible in this area may be visible in thin patients. Screw fixation of the implants allows scalpel or mechanical burr final contouring with the implants in place.

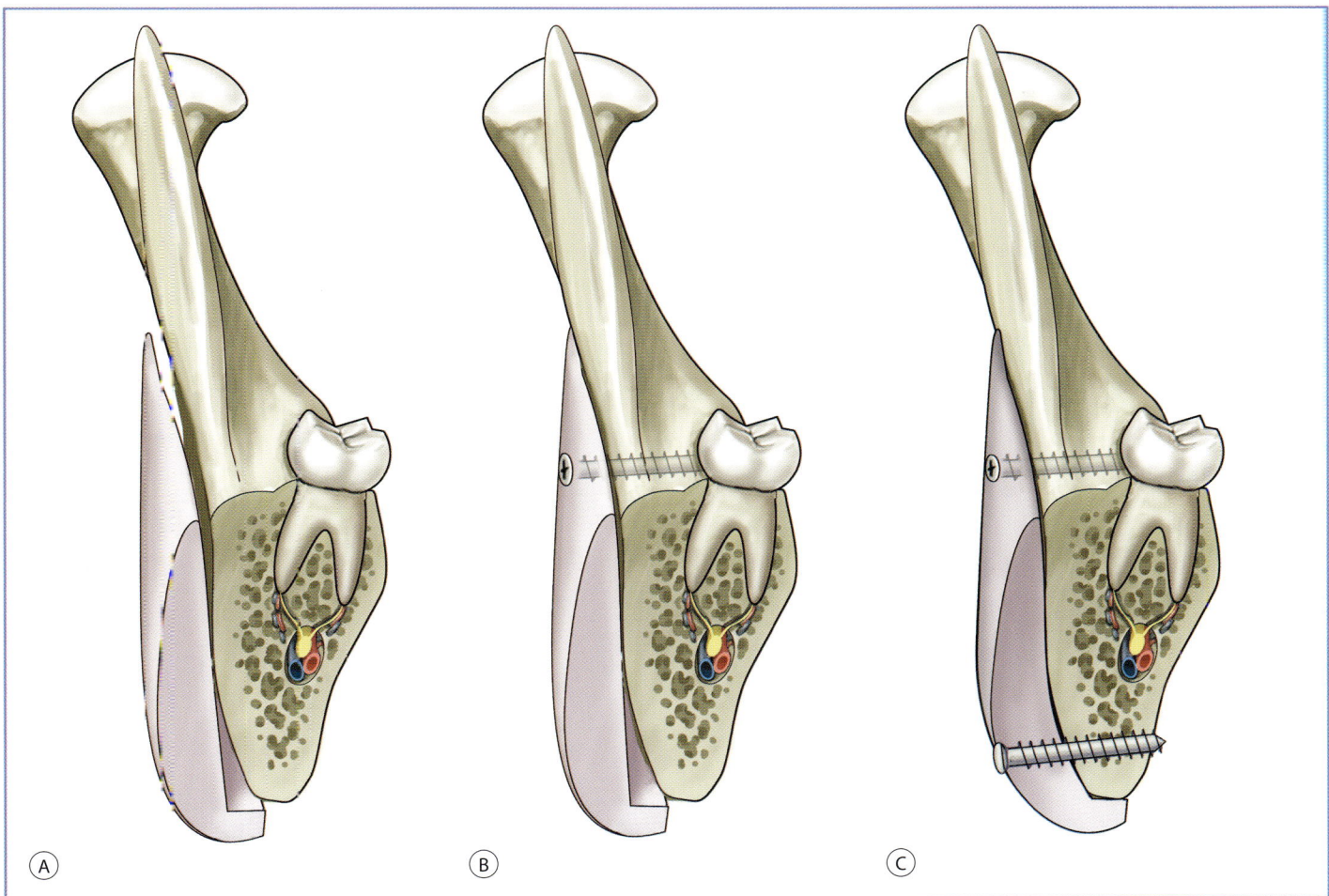

Figure 11.13 Screw fixation applies the implant to the skeleton and obliterates the gaps. (Gaps are equivalent to an increase in augmentation.) (**A**) Coronal view shows discrepancy in contour between anterior surface of mandible and posterior surface of implant, resulting in gaps. (**B**) The upper screw is in place and has fixed and immobilized the implant to the skeleton. (**C**) The lower screw has been placed. The posterior surface of the implant is now congruent with the anterior surface of the mandible.

The incision is closed in two layers with absorbable sutures. Care is taken to evert the mucosal edges. Neither the operative field nor the implants have been treated with antibiotic solutions. A small suction drain is left in until the next morning. I prefer one with a trocar that allows the skin exit site to be located behind the ear lobule. An elastic tape external dressing is used to help apply the soft tissues to the implant and avoid hematoma formation.

Patients are administered broad-spectrum antibiotics (cephalosporins) intravenously immediately before the procedure. Oral antibiotics are administered for 5 days postoperatively.

A liquid diet is prescribed for the first 3 days postoperatively and a soft diet for the next 5 days. Frequent mouth washes are advised, as well as very careful tooth brushing.

PEARL

Meticulous two-layer incision closure is part of the strategy to avoid mandible implant contamination with saliva postoperatively.

CLINICAL EXAMPLES

Clinical examples are shown in Figures 11.14–11.22.

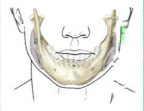

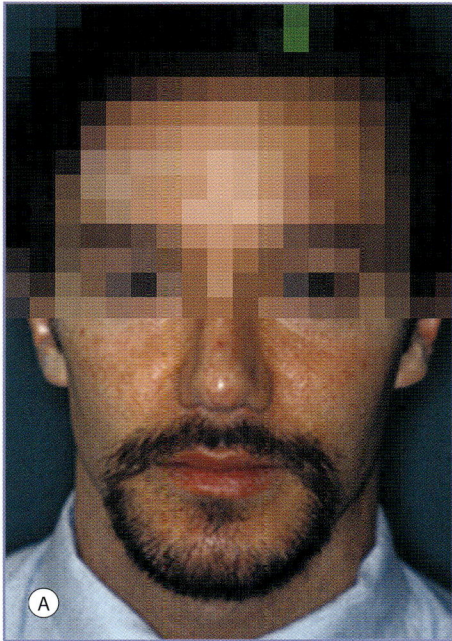

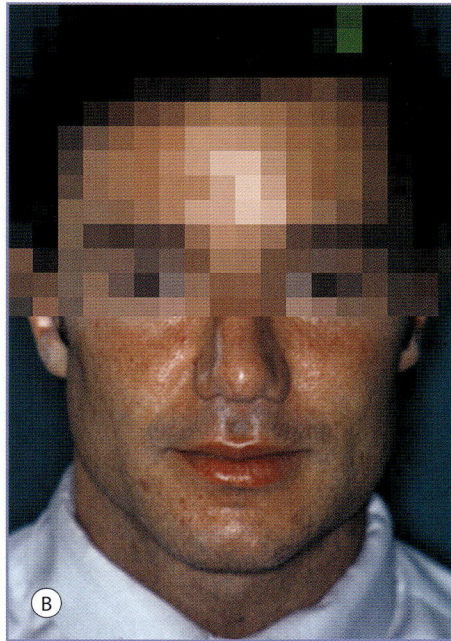

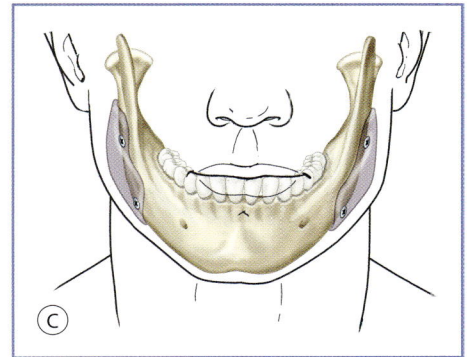

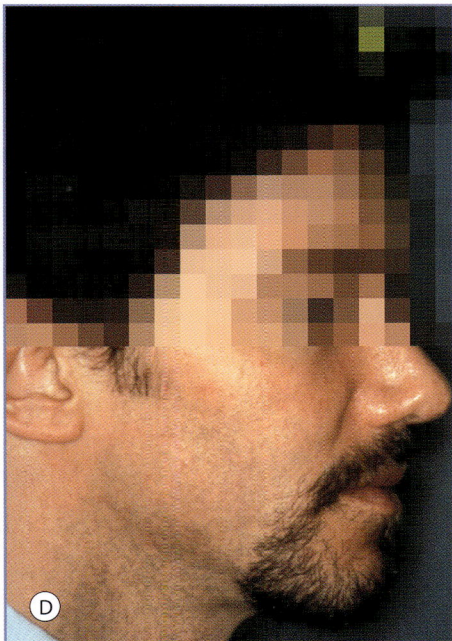

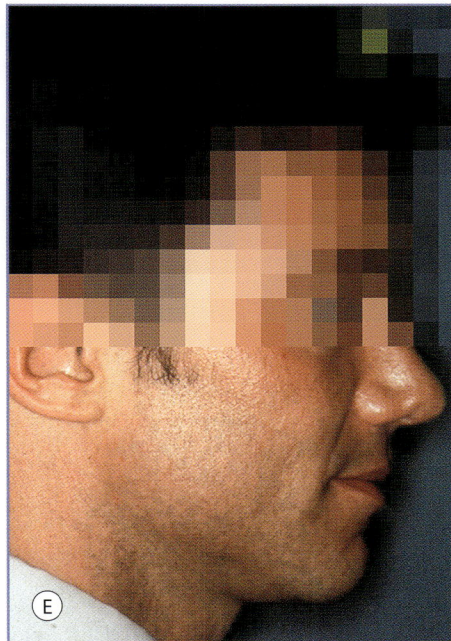

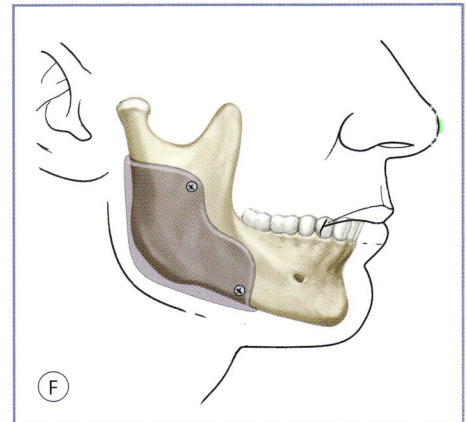

Figure 11.14 A 30-year-old actor with normal facial dimensions and class I dental occlusion desired more 'strength' to his jaw and requested chin augmentation. After evaluation, a mandible ramus and posterior body augmentation with the implants described in Figure 11.6 was performed, as well as a tertiary rhinoplasty. (**A**) Preoperative frontal and (**B**) postoperative frontal views. (**C**) Artist's simulation of implant surgery, frontal view. (**D**) Preoperative and (**E**) postoperative lateral views. (**F**) Artist's simulation of implant surgery, lateral view. (From Yaremchuk 2000,[10] with permission.)

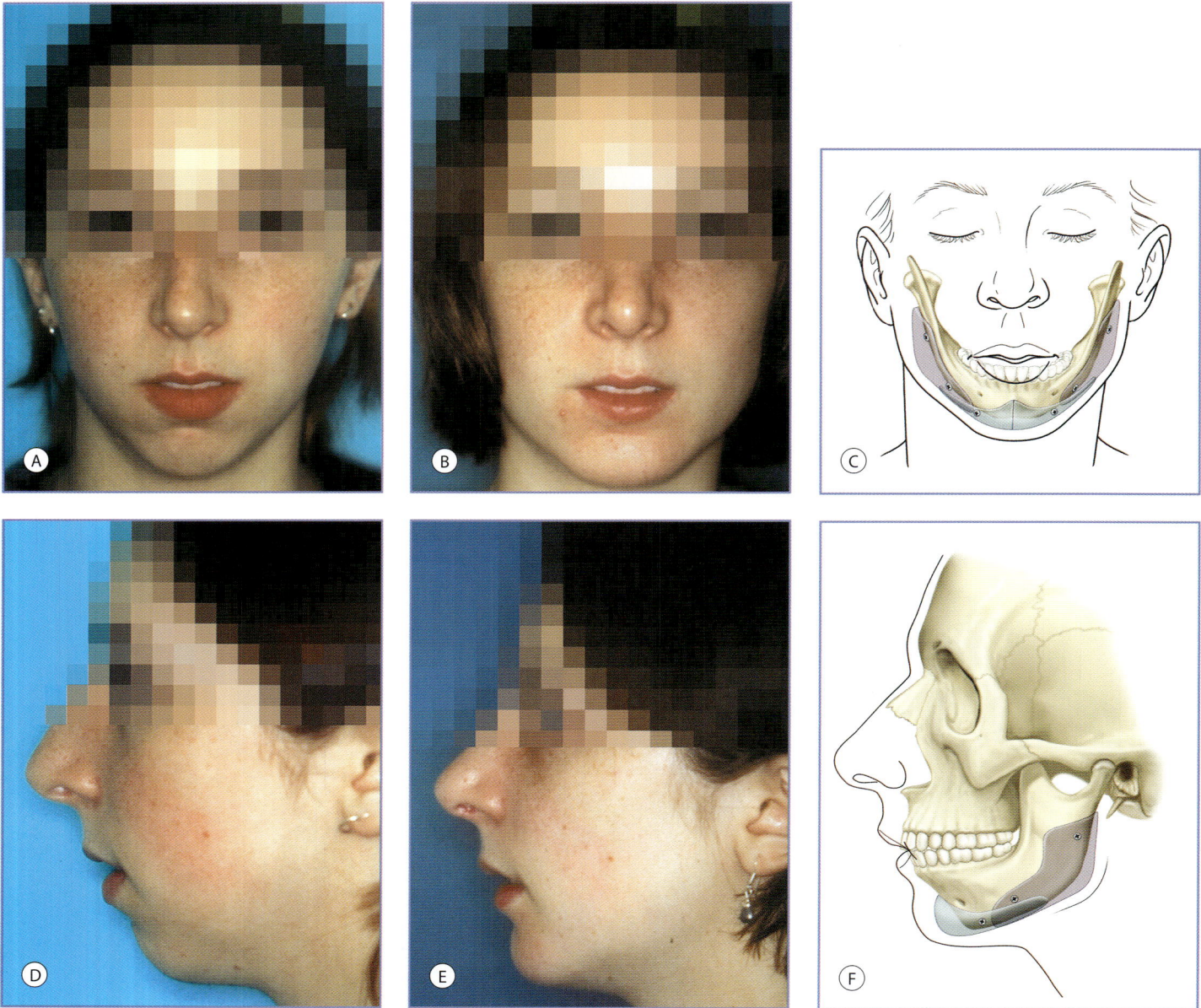

Figure 11.15 A 21-year-old woman who had undergone orthodontic correction of her class II malocclusion desired improved nasal and mandibular contour. Rhinoplasty and mandibular augmentation with mandibular ramus and body implants (Fig. 11.7), as well as extended chin implant, were placed. The configuration employed in Figure 11.8 is similar to that employed in this patient. (**A**) Preoperative and (**B**) postoperative frontal views. (**C**) Artist's simulation of implant surgery, frontal view. (**D**) Preoperative and (**E**) postoperative lateral views. (**F**) Artist's simulation of implant surgery, lateral view. (From Yaremchuk 2000,[10] with permission.)

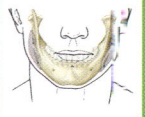

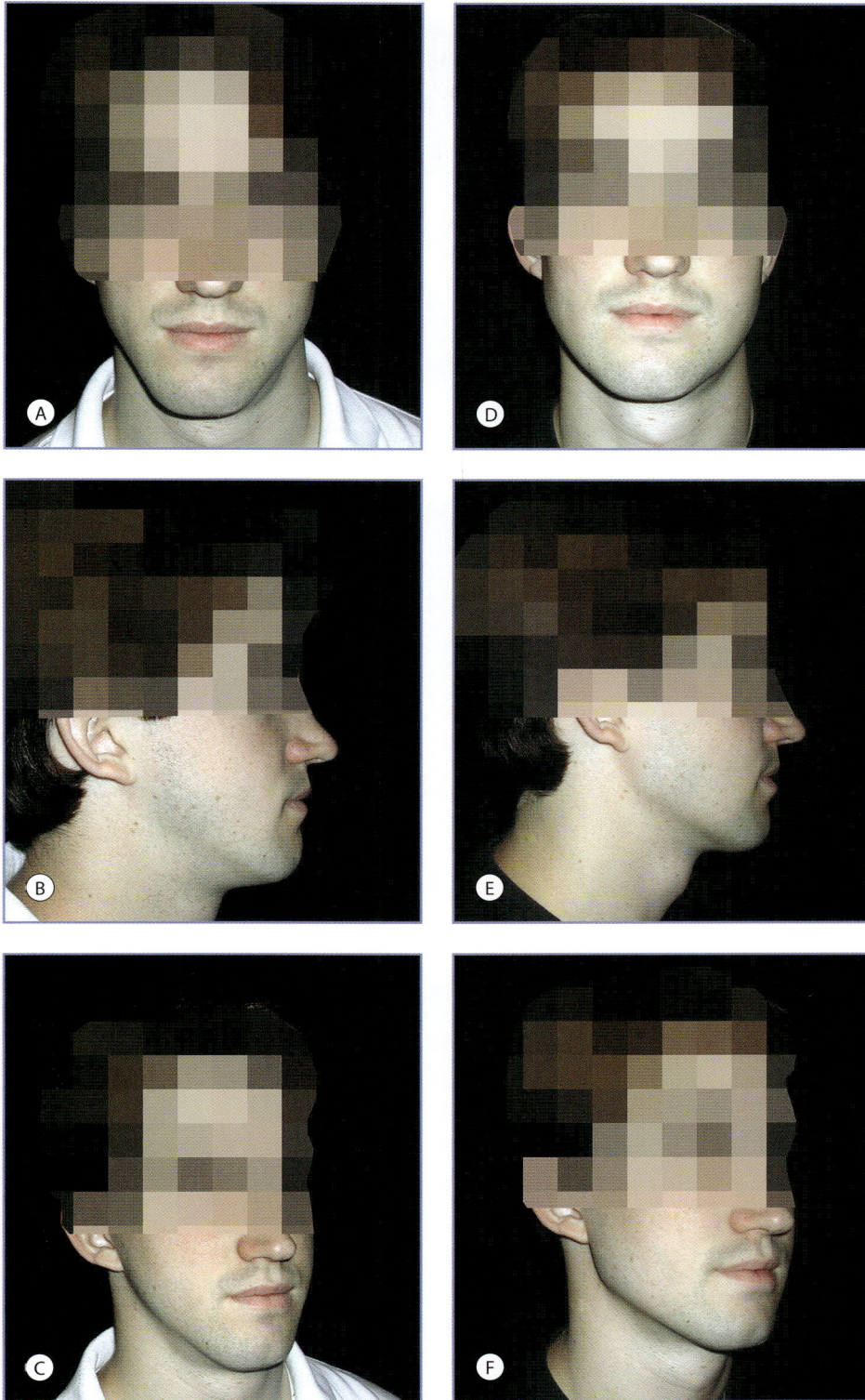

Figure 11.16 A 24-year-old man desired better balance to his face. Malar and mandible implants were placed. (**A–C**) Preoperative frontal, lateral, and oblique views. (**D–F**) Postoperative frontal, lateral, and oblique views.

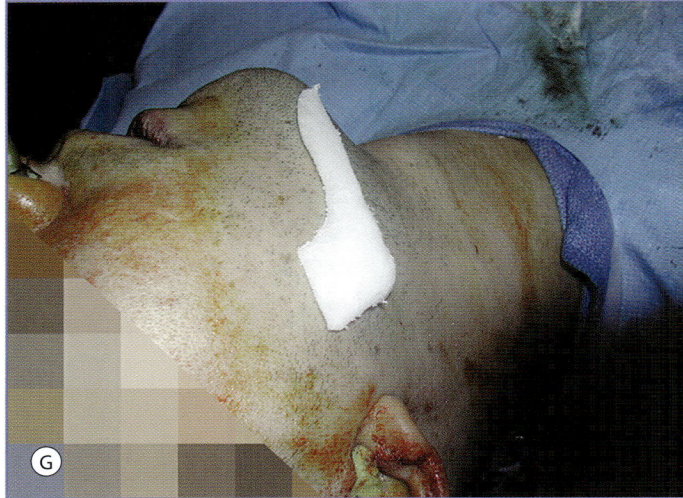

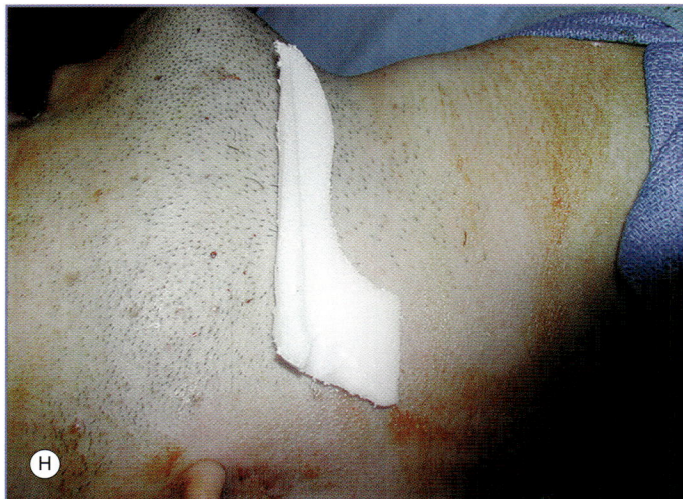

Figure 11.16 (*Cont'd*) A 24-year-old man desired better balance to his face. Malar and mandible implants were placed. (G) Intraoperative view shows the anterior surface of the implant used. (**H**) The posterior surface shows that the implant was trimmed so that the mandibular border inclination (mentocervical angle) was decreased, but the depth of the lower jaw was not changed (gonion–gnathion). The ramus height was increased (gonion–condylion laterale).

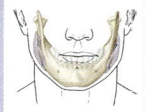

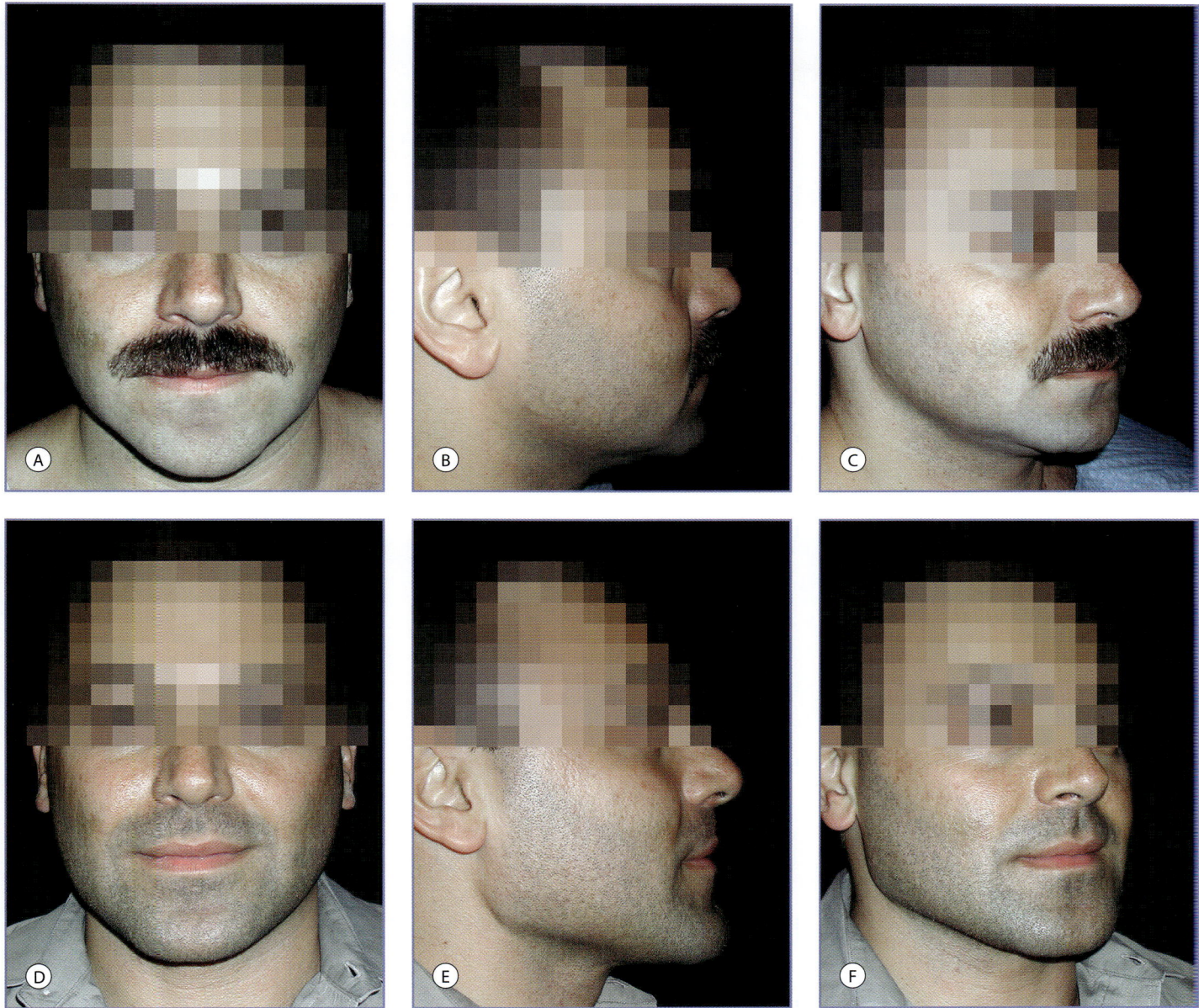

Figure 11.17 A 35-year-old man had five previous chin operations. He desired a very strong mandible. A silicone chin implant was removed. A 9-mm porous polyethylene chin implant and a mandibular angle implant were placed. The chin pad was resuspended. (**A–C**) Preoperative frontal, lateral, and oblique views. (**D–F**) Postoperative frontal, lateral, and oblique views.

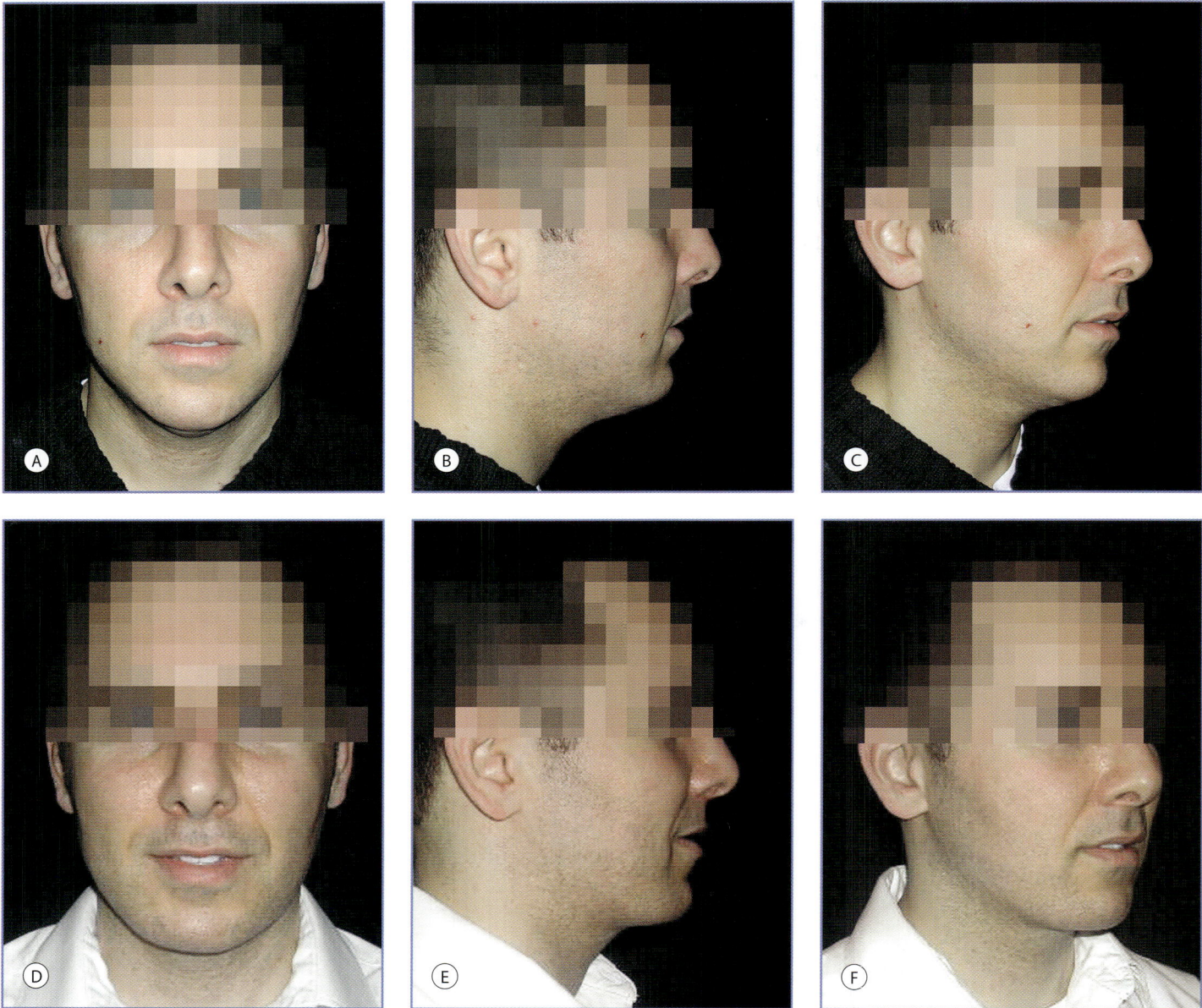

Figure 11.18 A 32-year-old man was displeased with the mandibular contour. He disliked the artificial appearance of the silicone chin implant placed 10 years before and subsequently revised. At the first operation, the silicone chin implant was removed and replaced with a 7-mm porous polyethylene implant. A submental lipectomy was also performed. One year later, a mandible angle implant was placed to increase mandibular definition. (**A–C**) Preoperative frontal, lateral, and oblique views. (**D**) Postoperative frontal view after removal of silicone chin implant and replacement with the two-piece porous polyethylene implant. Despite symmetric implant placement, chin asymmetry persists due to the soft tissue contraction deformity that formed around the malpositioned original smooth implant. (**E**) Postoperative lateral and (**F**) oblique views.

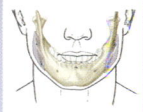

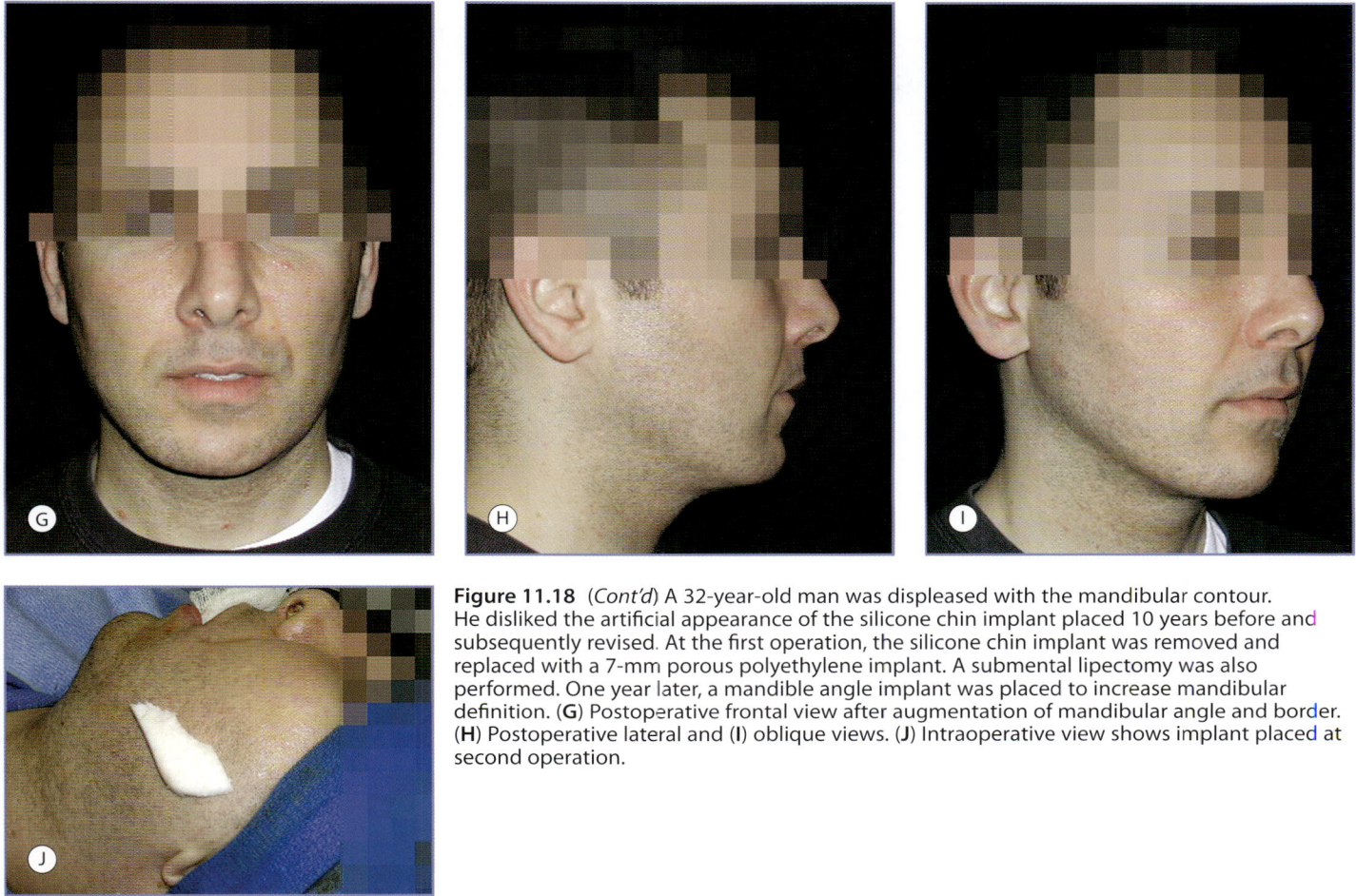

Figure 11.18 (*Cont'd*) A 32-year-old man was displeased with the mandibular contour. He disliked the artificial appearance of the silicone chin implant placed 10 years before and subsequently revised. At the first operation, the silicone chin implant was removed and replaced with a 7-mm porous polyethylene implant. A submental lipectomy was also performed. One year later, a mandible angle implant was placed to increase mandibular definition. (**G**) Postoperative frontal view after augmentation of mandibular angle and border. (**H**) Postoperative lateral and (**I**) oblique views. (**J**) Intraoperative view shows implant placed at second operation.

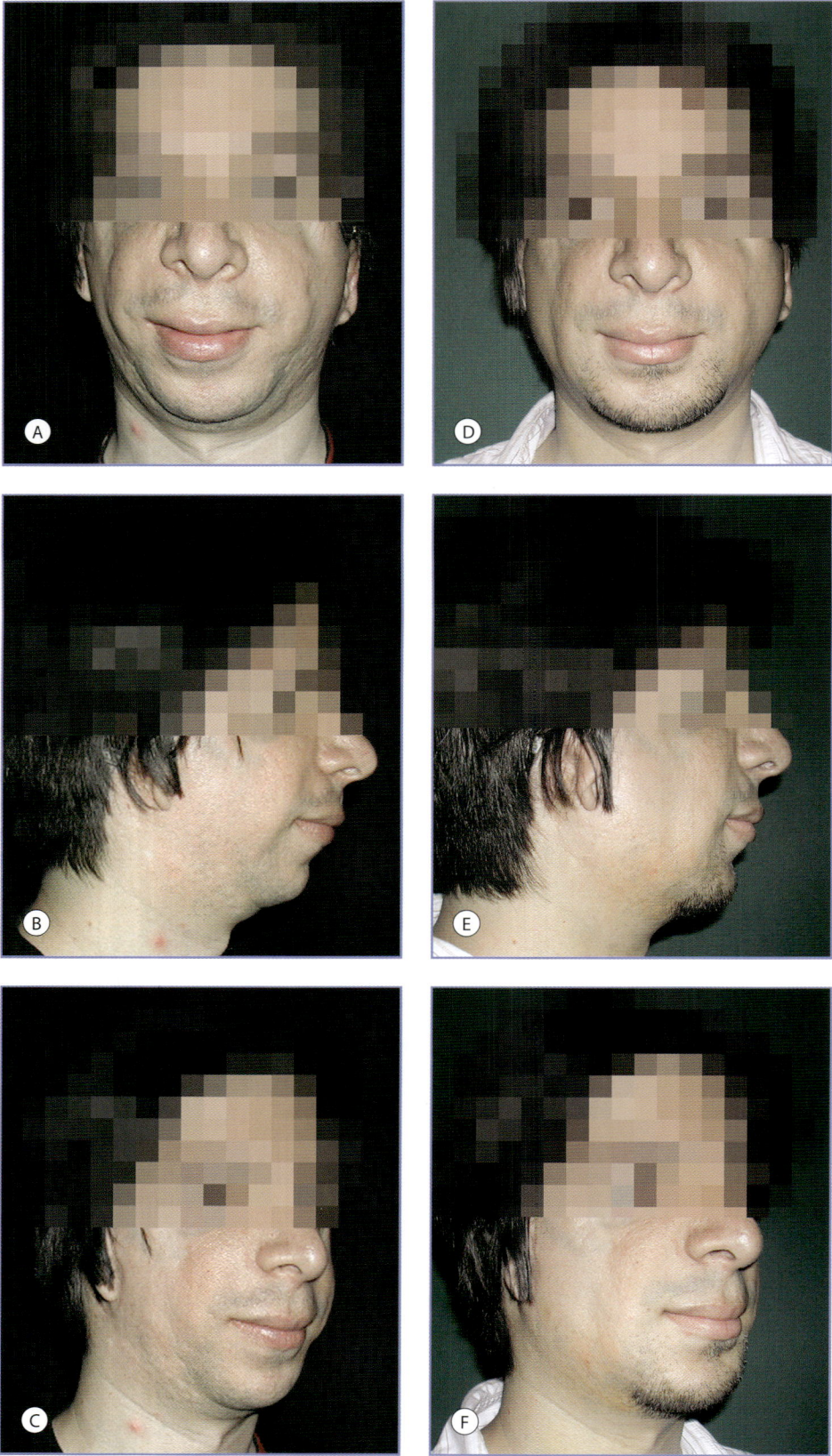

Figure 11.19 A 30-year-old man with Treacher Collins syndrome had had a sliding genioplasty as an adolescent. A 9-mm porous polyethylene chin implant and mandibular implants were placed. (**A–C**) Preoperative frontal, lateral, and oblique views. (**D–F**) Postoperative frontal, lateral, and oblique views.

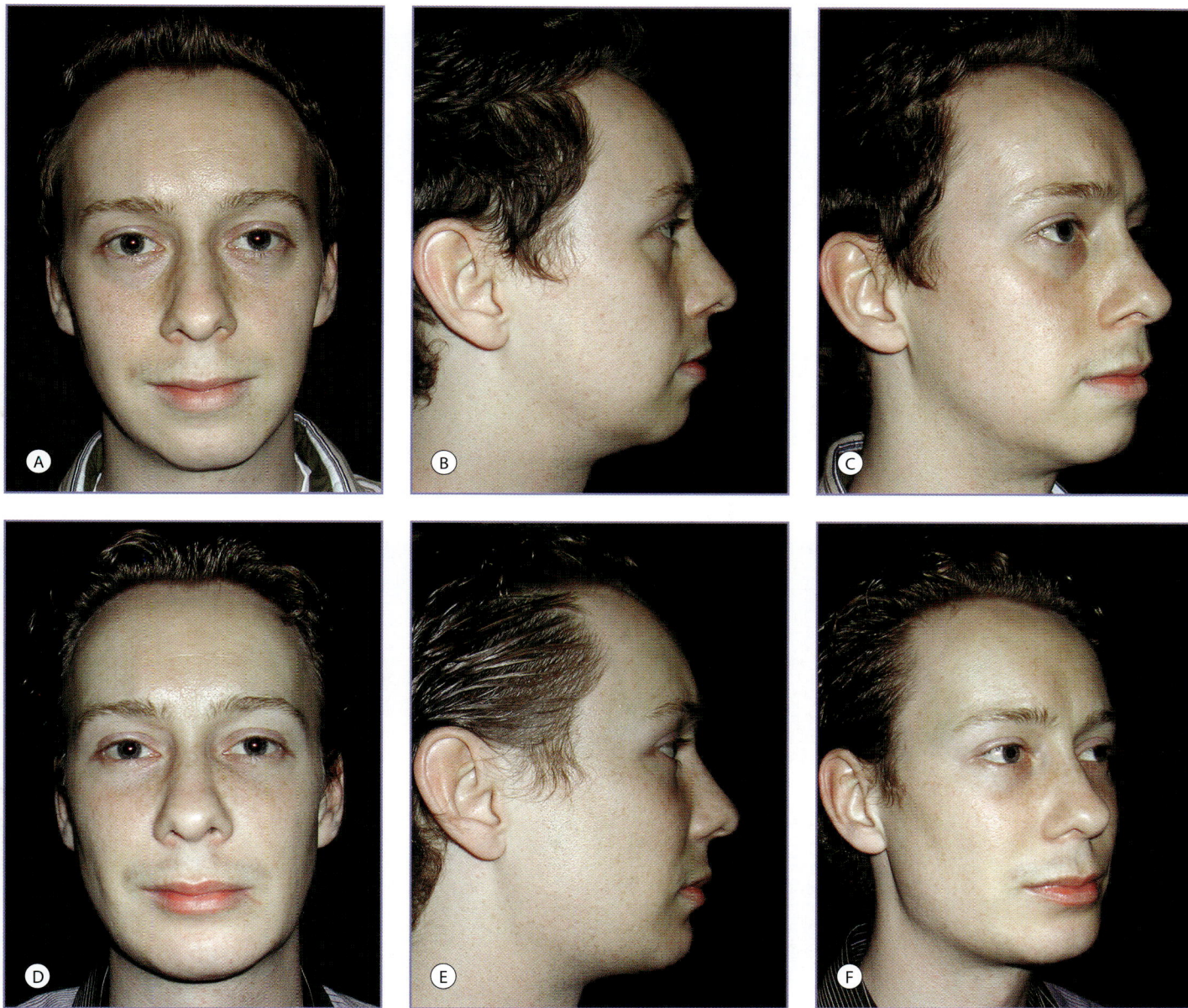

Figure 11.20 A 24-year-old man underwent infraorbital rim, paranasal, and medial malar augmentation as well as a subperiosteal midface lift. He also underwent mandibular and chin augmentation with a 7-mm implant. The vertical height of the chin was shortened by 3 mm. These manipulations (increasing ramus height and decreasing chin height, while increasing chin projection) gave the visual appearance of derotating the mandible. Placement of a chin implant without chin shortening would have resulted in an excessively long chin without sufficient chin projection. (**A–C**) Preoperative frontal, lateral, and oblique views. (**D–F**) Postoperative frontal, lateral, and oblique views.

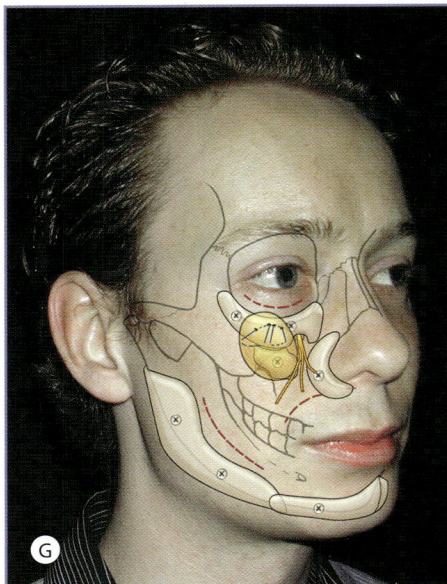

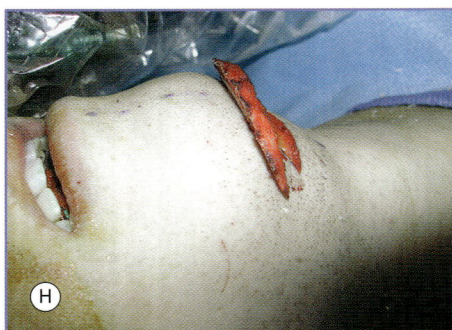

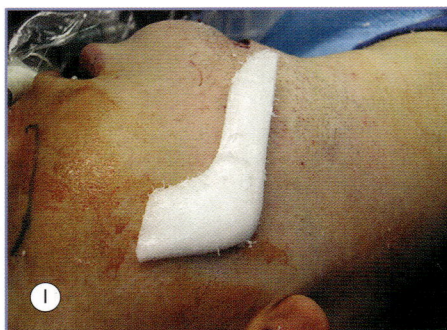

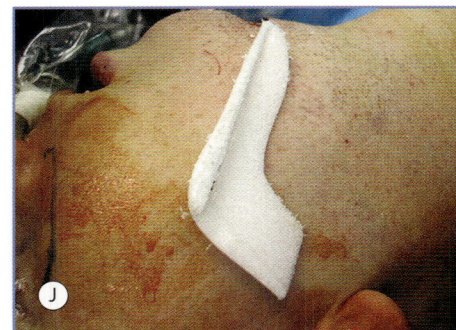

Figure 11.20 (*Cont'd*) A 24-year-old man underwent infraorbital rim, paranasal, and medial malar augmentation as well as a subperiosteal midface lift. He also underwent mandibular and chin augmentation with a 7-mm implant. The vertical height of the chin was shortened by 3 mm. These manipulations (increasing ramus height and decreasing chin height, while increasing chin projection) gave the visual appearance of derotating the mandible. Placement of a chin implant without chin shortening would have resulted in an excessively long chin without sufficient chin projection. (**G**) Diagrammatical representation of the operation. (**H**) Intraoperative view shows the bone removed from the chin. (**I**) Anterior surface of implant used to augment the mandibular body and ramus. (**J**) Posterior surface of implant.

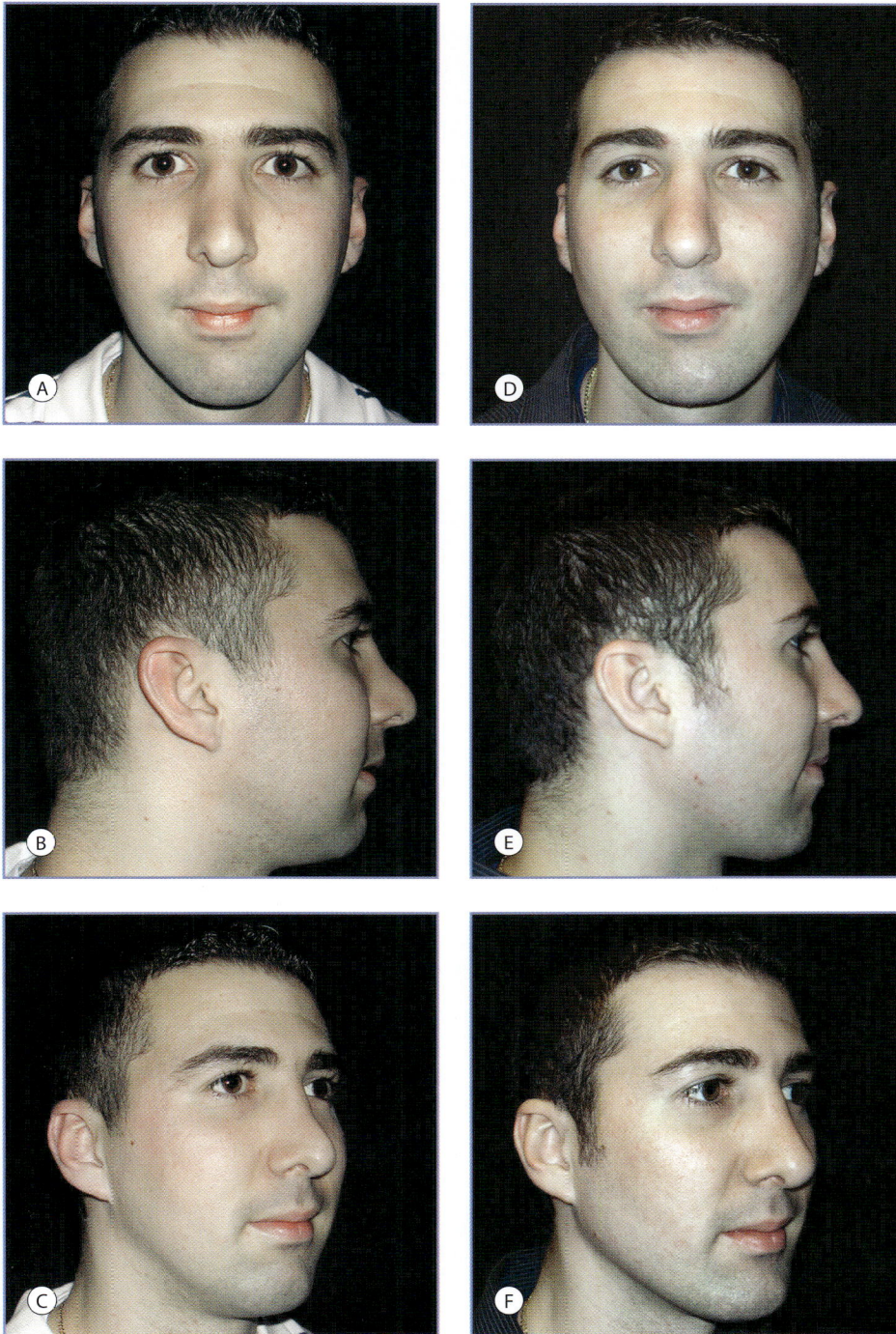

Figure 11.21 A 26-year-old man had undergone previous chin augmentation and two rhinoplasties. The silicone chin implant was removed and replaced with a 7-mm porous polyethylene implant. Mandibular angle implants shown in Figure 11.7 were placed. A tertiary rhinoplasty was performed. (**A–C**) Preoperative frontal, lateral, and oblique views. (**D–F**) Postoperative frontal, lateral, and oblique views.

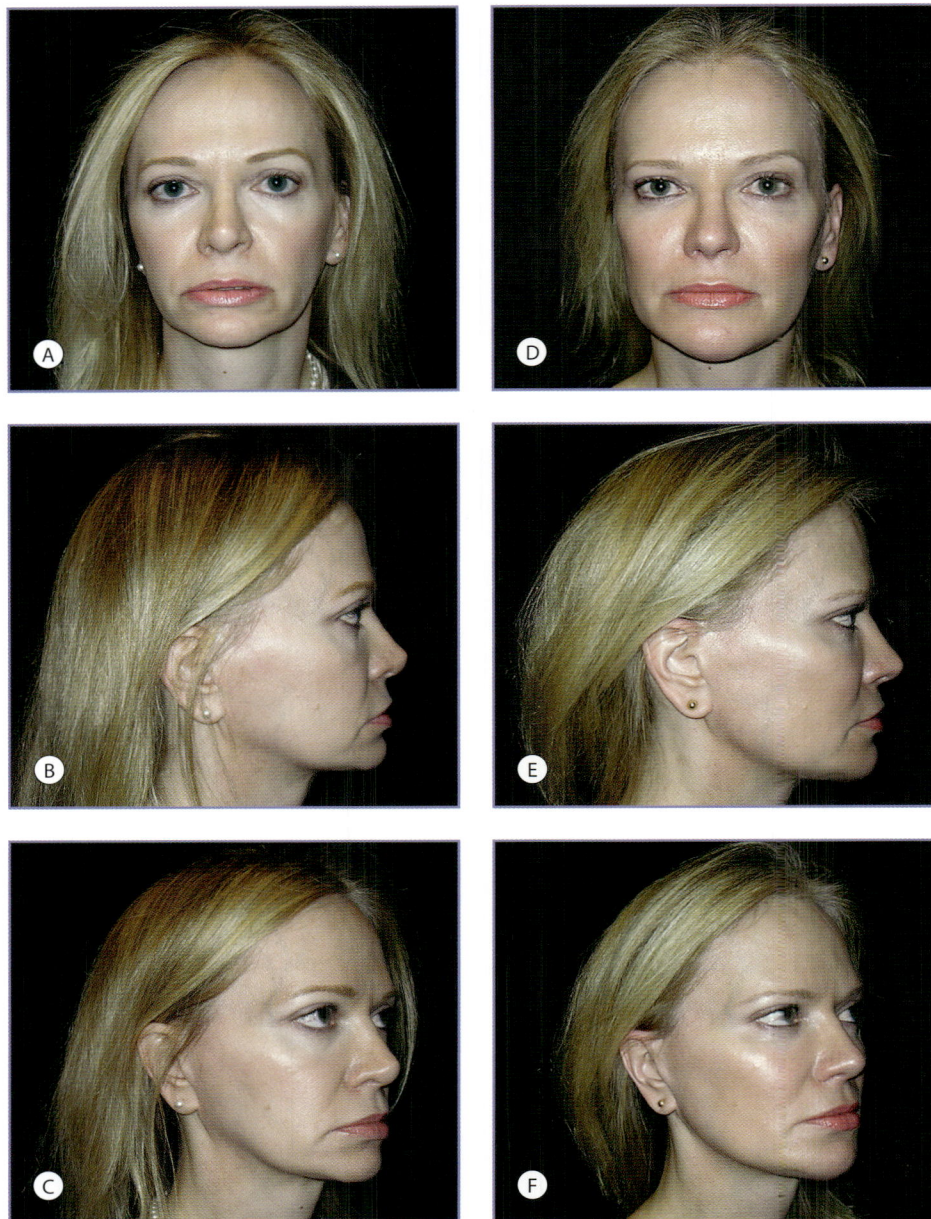

Figure 11.22 This woman had undergone brow lift, face-lift, and lower lid blepharoplasty in the past. In two procedures, the patient underwent hairline and brow lowering, infraorbital rim and malar implant augmentation, midface lift, horizontal osteotomy of the chin with 8-mm vertical elongation, 5-mm chin implant augmentation, and mandibular body and angle implant augmentation. (Another surgeon performed a secondary rhinoplasty.) **(A–C)** Preoperative frontal, lateral, and oblique views. **(D–F)** Postoperative frontal, lateral, and oblique views.

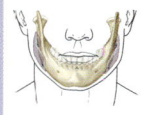

REFERENCES

1. Farkas LG, Hreczko TA, Katic MJ. Appendix A. Craniofacial norms in North American Caucasians from birth (one year) to young adulthood. In: Farkas LG, ed. Anthropometry of the head and face. 2nd edn. New York: Raven Press; 1994.
2. Bell WH, Proffit WR, Chase DL, et al. Mandibular deficiency. In: Bell WH, Proffit WR, White RP, eds. Surgical correction of dentofacial deformities, vol 1. Philadelphia: Saunders; 1980.
3. Semergidis TG, Migliore SA, Sotereanos GC. Alloplastic augmentation of the mandibular angle. J Oral Maxillofac Surg 1996; 54(12):1417–1423.
4. Terino EO. Alloplastic facial contouring: surgery of the fourth plane. Aesthetic Plast Surg 1992; 16(3):195–212.
5. Terino EO. Unique mandibular implants, including lateral and posterior angle implants. Facial Plast Surg Clin North Am 1994; 2:311.
6. Whitaker LA. Aesthetic augmentation of the posterior mandible. Plast Reconstr Surg 1991; 87(2):268–275.
7. Aiche AE. Mandibular angle implants. Aesthetic Plast Surg 1992; 16:3490.
8. Taylor CO, Teenier TJ. Evaluation and augmentation of the mandibular angle region. Facial Plast Surg Clin North Am 1994; 3:329.
9. Ramirez OM. Mandibular matrix implant system: a method to restore skeletal support to the lower face. Plast Reconstr Surg 2000; 106(1):176–189.
10. Yaremchuk MJ. Mandibular augmentation. Plast Reconstr Surg 2000; 106:697.

Index